ECG WORKOUT

EXERCISES IN ARRHYTHMIA INTERPRETATION

SIXTH EDITION

Jane Huff, RN, CCRN

Education Coordinator, Critical Care Unit
Arrhythmia Instructor
Advanced Cardiac Life Support (ACLS) Instructor
White County Medical Center
Searcy, Arkansas

Guest Faculty, Physician Assistant Program
Harding University
Searcy, Arkansas

Wolters Kluwer | Lippincott Williams & Wilkins
Health

Philadelphia • Baltimore • New York • London
Buenos Aires • Hong Kong • Sydney • Tokyo

STAFF

Publisher
J. Christopher Burghardt

Acquisitions Editor
Bill Lamsback

Product Director
David Moreau

Senior Product Manager
Diane Labus

Editors
Karen Comerford, Heather Ditch,
Erika Kors

Editorial Assistants
Karen J. Kirk, Jeri O'Shea, Linda
K. Ruhf

Creative Director
Doug Smock

Art Director
Elaine Kasmer

Illustrator
Joseph Clark

Vendor Manager
Beth Martz

Senior Manufacturing Coordinator
Beth J. Welsh

Production Services
SPi Global

Printed in China.
ECGWO06010810-040215

Library of Congress Cataloging-in-Publication Data
Huff, Jane, RN.
ECG workout : exercises in arrhythmia interpretation / Jane Huff.—6th ed.
    p. ; cm.
  Includes index.
  ISBN 978-1-4511-1553-6
 1. Arrhythmia—Diagnosis—Problems, exercises, etc. 2. Electrocardiography—Interpretation—Problems, exercises, etc. I. Title.
  [DNLM: 1. Arrhythmias, Cardiac—diagnosis—Problems and Exercises.
2. Electrocardiography—Problems and Exercises. WG 18.2]
  RC685.A65H84 2012
  616.1'2807547076—dc23
                          2011014268

Contents

Preface

ECG Workout: Exercises in Arrhythmia Interpretation, Sixth Edition, was written to assist physicians, nurses, medical and nursing students, paramedics, emergency medical technicians, telemetry technicians, and other allied health personnel in acquiring the knowledge and skills essential for identifying basic arrhythmias. It may also be used as a reference for electrocardiogram (ECG) review for those already knowledgeable in ECG interpretation.

The text is written in a simple manner and illustrated with figures, tables, boxes, and ECG tracings. Each chapter is designed to build on the knowledge base from the previous chapters so that the beginning student can quickly understand and grasp the basic concepts of electrocardiography. An effort has been made not only to provide *good quality ECG tracings,* but also to provide a sufficient number and variety of ECG practice strips so the learner feels confident in arrhythmia interpretation. There are *over 600 practice strips — more than any book on the market.*

Chapter 1 provides a discussion of basic anatomy and physiology of the heart. The electrical basis of electrocardiology is discussed in Chapter 2. The components of the ECG tracing (waveforms, intervals, segments, and complexes) are described in Chapter 3. This chapter also includes practice tracings on waveform identification. Cardiac monitors, lead systems, lead placement, ECG artifacts, and troubleshooting monitor problems are discussed in Chapter 4. A step-by-step guide to rhythm strip analysis is provided in Chapter 5, in addition to practice tracings on rhythm strip analysis. The individual rhythm chapters (Chapters 6 through 9) include a description of each arrhythmia, arrhythmia examples, causes, and management protocols. Current advanced cardiac life support (ACLS) guidelines are incorporated into each arrhythmia chapter as applicable to the rhythm discussion. Each arrhythmia chapter also includes approximately 100 strips for self-evaluation. Chapter 10 presents a general discussion of cardiac pacemakers (types, indications, function, pacemaker terminology, malfunctions, and pacemaker analysis), along with practice tracings. Chapter 11 is a posttest consisting of a mix of rhythm strips that can be used as a self-evaluation tool or for testing purposes.

The text has been thoughtfully revised and expanded to include new figures, updated boxes and tables, additional glossary terms, and even more practice rhythm strips. *Skillbuilder rhythm strips,* which are new to this edition, appear immediately following the practice rhythm strips in Chapters 7, 8, and 9. Each Skillbuilder section provides a mix of strips that test not only your understanding of information learned in that arrhythmia chapter but also the concepts and skills learned in the chapter(s) immediately preceding it. For example, the Skillbuilder strips in Chapter 7 (Atrial arrhythmias) include atrial rhythm strips as well as strips on sinus arrhythmias (covered in Chapter 6); Chapter 8 (Junctional arrhythmias and AV blocks) includes junctional arrhythmias and AV blocks, as well as atrial and sinus arrhythmias; and Chapter 9 (Ventricular arrhythmias and bundle-branch block), a mix of all of the arrhythmias covered in Chapters 6 through 9. Such practice with mixed strips will enhance your ability to differentiate between rhythm groups as you progress through the book — a definite advantage when you get to the Posttest. A handy pull-out section consisting of 48 individual flashcards further challenges your ability to identify different types of arrhythmias.

The ECG tracings included in this book are actual strips from patients. Above each rhythm strip are 3-second indicators for rapid-rate calculation. For precise rate calculation, an *ECG conversion table for heart rate* is printed on the inside back cover. For convenience, a removable plastic version is also attached to the inside back cover. The heart rates for regular rhythms listed in the answer keys were determined by the precise rate calculation method and will not always coincide with the rapid-rate calculation method. Rate calculation methods are discussed in Chapter 5.

The author and publisher have made every attempt to check the content, especially drug dosages and management protocols, for accuracy. Medicine is continually changing, and the reader has the responsibility to keep informed of local care protocols and changes in emergency care procedures.

*This book is dedicated to
Novell Grace, a "**busy**" little girl.*

1 Anatomy and physiology of the heart

Description and location of the heart

The heart is a hollow, four-chambered muscular organ that lies in the middle of the thoracic cavity between the lungs, behind the sternum, in front of the spinal column, and just above the diaphragm (Figure 1-1). The top of the heart (the *base*) is at approximately the level of the second intercostal space. The bottom of the heart (the *apex*) is formed by the tip of the left ventricle and is positioned just above the diaphragm to the left of the sternum at the fifth intercostal space, midclavicular line. There, the apex can be palpated during ventricular contraction. This physical examination landmark is referred to as the *point of maximal impulse* (PMI) and is an indicator of the heart's position within the thorax.

The heart is tilted forward and to the left so that the right side of the heart lies toward the front. About two-thirds of the heart lies to the left of the body's midline and one-third extends to the right. The average adult heart is approximately 5″ (12 cm) long, 3½″ (8 to 9 cm) wide, and 2½″ (6 cm thick) — a little larger than a normal-sized fist. The heart weighs between 7 and 15 oz (200 and 425 grams). Heart size and weight are influenced by age, weight, body build, frequency of exercise, and heart disease.

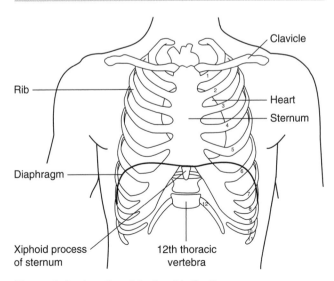

Figure 1-1. Location of the heart in the thorax.

Function of the heart

The heart is the hardest working organ in the body. The heart functions primarily as a pump to circulate blood and supply the body with oxygen and nutrients. Each day the average heart beats over 100,000 times. During an average lifetime, the human heart will beat more than 3 billion times.

The heart is capable of adjusting its pump performance to meet the needs of the body. As needs increase, as with exercise, the heart responds by accelerating the heart rate to propel more blood to the body. As needs decrease, as with sleep, the heart responds by decreasing the heart rate, resulting in less blood flow to the body.

The heart consists of:
- four chambers
  - two atria that receive incoming blood
  - two ventricles that pump blood out of the heart
- four valves that control the flow of blood through the heart
- an electrical conduction system that conducts electrical impulses to the heart, resulting in muscle contraction.

Heart surfaces

There are four main heart surfaces to consider when discussing the heart: *anterior*, *posterior*, *inferior*, and *lateral* (Figure 1-2). The heart surfaces are explained below:
- anterior — the front
- posterior — the back
- inferior — the bottom
- lateral — the side.

Structure of the heart wall

The heart wall is arranged in three layers (Figure 1-3):
- the *pericardium* — the outermost layer
- the *myocardium* — the middle muscular layer
- the *endocardium* — the inner layer.

Enclosing and protecting the heart is the pericardium, which consists of an outer fibrous sac (the *fibrous pericardium*) and an inner two-layered, fluid-secreting membrane (the *serous pericardium*). The outer fibrous pericardium comes in direct contact with the covering of the lung (the pleura) and is attached to the center of the diaphragm inferiorly, to the sternum anteriorly, and to the esophagus, trachea, and main bronchi posteriorly. This position

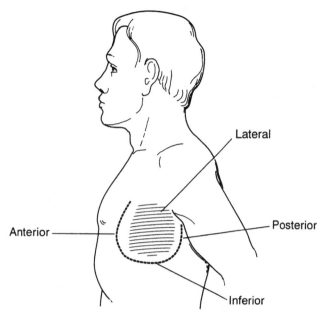

Figure 1-2.   Heart surfaces.

anchors the heart to the chest and prevents it from shifting about in the thorax. The serous pericardium is a continuous membrane that forms two layers: the parietal layer lines the inner surface of the fibrous sac and the visceral layer (also called *epicardium*) lines the outer surface of the heart muscle. Between the two layers of the serous pericardium is the pericardial space, or cavity, which is usually filled with 10 to 30 mL of thin, clear fluid (the pericardial fluid) secreted by the serous layers. The primary function of the pericardial fluid is to provide lubrication, preventing

friction as the heart beats. In certain conditions, large accumulations of fluid, blood, or exudates can enter the pericardial space and may interfere with ventricular filling and the heart's ability to contract.

The *myocardium* is the thick, middle, muscular layer that makes up the bulk of the heart wall. This layer is composed primarily of cardiac muscle cells and is responsible for the heart's ability to contract. The thickness of the myocardium varies from one heart chamber to another. Chamber thickness is related to the amount of resistance the muscle must overcome to pump blood out of the chamber.

The *endocardium* is a thin layer of tissue that lines the inner surface of the heart muscle and the heart chambers. Extensions and folds of this tissue form the valves of the heart.

Circulatory system

The circulatory system is required to provide a continuous flow of blood to the body. The circulatory system is a closed system consisting of heart chambers and blood vessels.

The circulatory system consists of two separate circuits, the *systemic circuit* and the *pulmonary circuit*. The systemic circuit is a large circuit and includes the left side of the heart and blood vessels, which carry oxygenated blood to the body and deoxygenated blood back to the right heart. The pulmonary circuit is a small circuit and includes the right side of the heart and blood vessels, which carry deoxygenated blood to the lungs and oxygenated blood back to the left heart. The two circuits are designed so that blood flow is pumped from one circuit to the other.

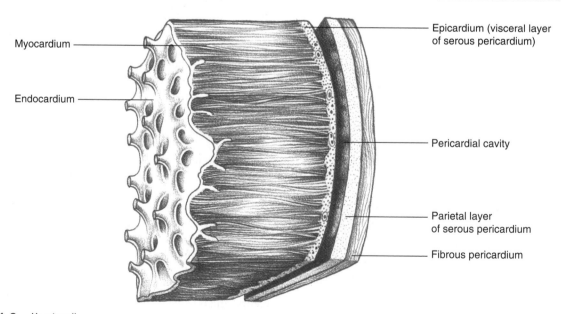

Figure 1-3.   Heart wall.

Heart chambers

The interior of the heart consists of four hollow chambers (Figure 1-4). The two upper chambers, the *right atrium* and the *left atrium*, are divided by a wall called the *interatrial septum*. The two lower chambers, the *right ventricle* and the *left ventricle*, are divided by a thicker wall called the *interventricular septum*. The two septa divide the heart into two pumping systems — a right heart and a left heart.

The right heart pumps venous (deoxygenated) blood through the pulmonary arteries to the lungs (Figure 1-5). Oxygen and carbon dioxide exchange takes place in the alveoli and arterial (oxygenated) blood returns via the pulmonary veins to the left heart. The left heart then pumps arterial blood to the systemic circulation, where oxygen and carbon dioxide exchange takes place in the organs, tissues, and cells; then venous blood returns to the right heart. Blood flow within the body is designed so that arteries carry oxygen-rich blood away from the heart and veins carry oxygen-poor blood back to the heart. This role is reversed in pulmonary circulation: pulmonary arteries carry oxygen-poor blood into the lungs, and pulmonary veins bring oxygen-rich blood back to the left heart.

The thickness of the walls in each chamber is related to the workload performed by that chamber. Both atria are low-pressure chambers serving as blood-collecting reservoirs for the ventricles. They add a small amount of force to the moving blood. Therefore, their walls are relatively thin. The right ventricular wall is thicker than the walls of the atria, but much thinner than that of the left ventricle. The right ventricular chamber pumps blood a fairly short distance to the lungs against a relatively low resistance to flow. The left ventricle has the thickest wall, because it must eject blood through the aorta against a much greater resistance to flow (the arterial pressure in the systemic circulation).

Heart valves

There are four valves in the heart: the *tricuspid valve*, separating the right atrium from the right ventricle; the *pulmonic valve*, separating the right ventricle from the pulmonary arteries; the *mitral valve*, separating the left atrium from the left ventricle; and the *aortic valve*, separating the left ventricle from the aorta (Figure 1-5). The primary function of the valves is to allow blood flow in one direction through the heart's chambers and prevent a backflow of blood (regurgitation). Changes in chamber pressure govern the opening and closing of the heart valves.

The tricuspid and mitral valves separate the atria from the ventricles and are referred to as the *atrioventricular* (AV) *valves*. These valves serve as in-flow valves for the ventricles. The tricuspid valve consists of three separate cusps or leaflets and is larger in diameter and thinner than the mitral valve. The tricuspid valve directs blood flow from the right atrium to the right ventricle. The mitral valve (or bicuspid valve) has only two cusps. The mitral valve directs blood flow from the left atrium to the left ventricle. Both valves are encircled by tough, fibrous rings (valve rings). The leaflets of the AV valves are attached to thin strands of fibrous cords called *chordae tendineae* (heart strings) (Figure 1-6). The chordae tendineae are then attached to *papillary muscles*, which arise from the walls and floor of the ventricles. During ventricular filling (diastole) when the AV valves are open, the valve leaflets, the chordae tendineae, and the papillary muscles form a funnel, promoting blood flow into the ventricles. As pressure increases during ventricular contraction (systole), the valve cusps close. Backflow of blood into the atria is prevented by contraction of the papillary muscles and the tension in the chordae tendineae. Dysfunction of the chordae tendineae or a papillary muscle can cause incomplete closure of an AV valve. This may result in a regurgitation of blood from the ventricle into the atrium, leading to cardiac compromise. The first heart sound (S_1) is the product of tricuspid and mitral valve closure. S_1 is best heard at the apex of the heart located on the left side of the chest, fifth intercostal space, midclavicular line.

The aortic and pulmonic valves have three cuplike cusps shaped like a half-moon and are referred to as the *semilunar* (SL) *valves*. These valves serve as out-flow valves for the ventricles. The cusps of the SL valves are smaller and thicker than the AV valves and do not have the support of the chordae tendineae or papillary muscles. Like the AV valves, the rims of the semilunar valves are supported by valve rings. The pulmonary valve directs blood flow from the right ventricle to the pulmonary artery. The aortic valve directs blood flow from the left ventricle to the aorta. As pressure decreases during ventricular

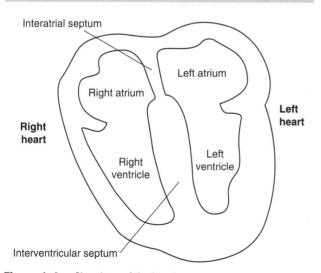

Figure 1-4. Chambers of the heart.

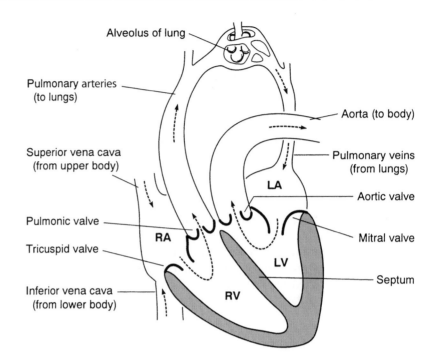

Figure 1-5. Chambers, valves, blood flow. *RA*, right atrium; *RV*, right ventricle; *LA*, left atrium; *LV*, left ventricle.

relaxation (diastole), the valve cusps close. Backflow of blood into the ventricles is prevented because of the cusps' fibrous strength, their close approximation, and their shape. The second heart sound (S$_2$) is produced by closure of the aortic and pulmonic SL valves. It is best heard over the second intercostal space on the left or right side of the sternum.

Blood flow through the heart and lungs

Blood flow through the heart and lungs is traditionally described by tracing the flow as blood returns from the systemic veins to the right side of the heart, to the lungs, back to the left side of the heart, and out to the arterial vessels

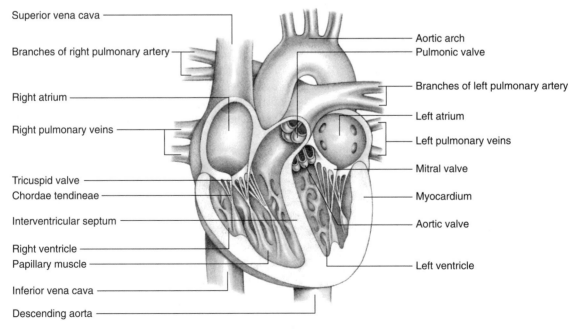

Figure 1-6. Papillary muscles and chordae tendineae.

of the systemic circuit (Figure 1-5). The right atrium receives venous blood from the body via two of the body's largest veins (the superior vena cava and the inferior vena cava) and from the coronary sinus. The superior vena cava returns venous blood from the upper body. The inferior vena cava returns venous blood from the lower body. The coronary sinus returns venous blood from the heart itself.

As the right atrium fills with blood, the pressure in the chamber increases. When pressure in the right atrium exceeds that of the right ventricle, the tricuspid valve opens, allowing blood to flow into the right ventricle. As the right ventricle fills with blood, the pressure in that chamber increases, forcing the tricuspid valve shut and the pulmonic valve open, ejecting blood into the pulmonary arteries and on to the lungs. In the lungs, the blood picks up oxygen and excretes carbon dioxide.

The left atrium receives arterial blood from the pulmonary circulation via the pulmonary veins. As the left atrium fills with blood, the pressure in the chamber increases. When pressure in the left atrium exceeds that of the left ventricle, the mitral valve opens, allowing blood to flow into the left ventricle. As the left ventricle fills with blood, the pressure in that chamber increases, forcing the mitral valve shut and the aortic valve open, ejecting blood into the aorta and systemic circuit, where the blood releases oxygen to the organs, tissues, and cells and picks up carbon dioxide.

Although blood flow can be traced from the right side of the heart to the left side of the heart, it is important to realize that the heart works as two pumps (the right heart and the left heart) working simultaneously. As the right atrium receives venous blood from the systemic circulation, the left atrium receives arterial blood from the pulmonary circulation. As the atria fill with blood, pressure in the atria exceeds that of the ventricles, forcing the AV valves open and allowing blood to flow into the ventricles. Toward the end of ventricular filling, the two atria contract, pumping the remaining blood into the ventricles. Contraction of the atria during the final phase of diastole to complete ventricular filling is called the *atrial kick*. The ventricles are 70% filled before the atria contract. The atrial kick adds another 30% to ventricular capacity. In normal heart rhythms, the atria contract before the ventricles. In abnormal heart rhythms, the loss of the atrial kick results in incomplete filling of the ventricles, causing a reduction in cardiac output (the amount of blood pumped out of the heart). Once the ventricles are filled with blood, pressure in the ventricles increases, forcing the AV valves shut and the SL valves open. The ventricles contract simultaneously, ejecting blood through the pulmonary artery into the lungs and through the aortic valve into the aorta.

Coronary circulation

The blood supply to the heart is supplied by the right coronary artery, the left coronary artery, and their branches (Figure 1-7). There is some individual variation in the pattern of coronary artery branching, but in general, the right coronary artery supplies the right side of the heart and the left coronary artery supplies the left side of the heart.

The right coronary artery arises from the right side of the aorta and consists of one long artery that travels downward and then posteriorly. The major branches of the right coronary artery are:

- conus artery
- sinoatrial (SA) node artery (in 55% of population)
- anterior right ventricular arteries
- acute marginal artery
- AV node artery (in 90% of population)
- posterior descending artery with septal branches (in 90% of population)
- posterior left ventricular arteries (in 90% of population).

Dominance is a term commonly used to describe coronary vasculature and refers to the distribution of the terminal portion of the arteries. The artery that gives rise to both the posterior descending artery with its septal branches and the posterior left ventricular arteries is considered to be a "dominant" system. In approximately 90% of the population, the right coronary artery (RCA) is dominant. The term can be confusing because in most people the left coronary artery is of wider caliber and perfuses the largest percentage of the myocardium. Thus, the dominant artery usually does not perfuse the largest proportion of the myocardium. The left coronary artery arises from the left side of the aorta and consists of the left main coronary artery, a short stem, which divides into the left anterior descending artery and the circumflex artery. The left anterior descending (LAD) travels downward over the anterior surface of the left ventricle, circles the apex, and ends behind it. The major branches of the LAD are:

- diagonal arteries
- right ventricular arteries
- septal perforator arteries.

The circumflex artery travels along the lateral aspect of the left ventricle and ends posteriorly. The major branches of the circumflex are:

- SA node artery (in 45% of population)
- anterolateral marginal artery
- posterolateral marginal artery
- distal left circumflex artery.

In 10% of the population, the circumflex artery gives rise to the posterior descending artery with its septal branches, terminating as the posterior left ventricular arteries. A left coronary artery with a circumflex that gives rise to both the posterior descending artery and the posterior left ventricular arteries is considered a "dominant" left system. When the left coronary artery is dominant, the entire interventricular septum is supplied by this artery. Table 1-1 summarizes the coronary artery distribution to the myocardium and the conduction system.

The right and left coronary artery branches are interconnected by an extensive network of small arteries that provide the potential for cross flow from one artery to the other. These small arteries are commonly called *collateral vessels* or *collateral circulation*. Collateral circulation exists at birth

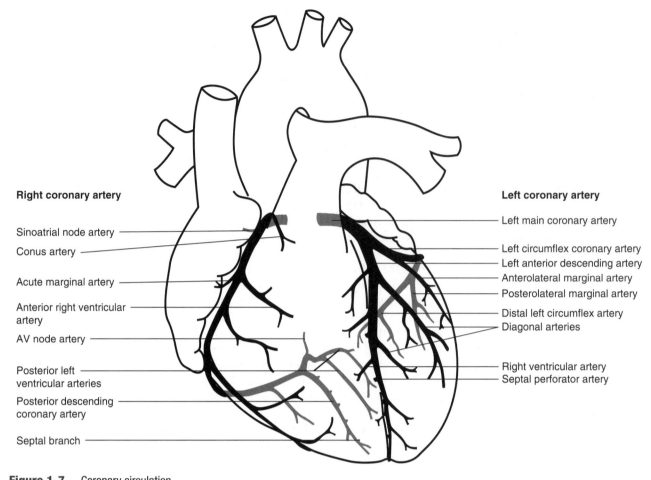

Right coronary artery

Sinoatrial node artery

Conus artery

Acute marginal artery

Anterior right ventricular artery

AV node artery

Posterior left ventricular arteries

Posterior descending coronary artery

Septal branch

Left coronary artery

Left main coronary artery

Left circumflex coronary artery

Left anterior descending artery

Anterolateral marginal artery

Posterolateral marginal artery

Distal left circumflex artery

Diagonal arteries

Right ventricular artery

Septal perforator artery

Figure 1-7.   Coronary circulation.

Table 1-1.
Coronary arteries

Coronary artery and its branches	Portion of myocardium supplied	Portion of conduction system supplied
Right coronary artery		
	Right atrium	Sinotrial (SA) node (55%)*
	Right ventricle	Atrioventricular (AV) node and bundle of His (90%)*
	Inferior wall of left ventricle (90%)*	
	Posterior one-third of interventricular septum (90%)*	
Left coronary artery		
Left anterior descending (LAD)	Anterior wall of left ventricle	Right and left bundle branches
	Anterolateral wall of left ventricle	
	Anterior two-thirds of interventricular septum	
Circumflex	Left atrium	SA node (45%)*
	Anterolateral wall of left ventricle	AV node and bundle of His (10%)*
	Posterolateral wall of left ventricle	
	Posterior wall of left ventricle	
	Inferior wall of left ventricle (10%)*	
	Posterior one-third of interventricular septum (10%)*	

* = of population

but the vessels do not become functionally significant until the myocardium experiences an ischemic insult. If a blockage occurs in a major coronary artery, the collateral vessels enlarge and provide additional blood flow to those areas of reduced blood supply. However, blood flow through the collateral vessels isn't sufficient to meet the total needs of the myocardium in most cases. In other vascular beds of the body, arterial blood flow reaches a peak during ventricular contraction (systole). However, myocardial blood flow is greatest during ventricular diastole (when the ventricular muscle mass is relaxed) than it is during systole (when the heart's blood vessels are compressed). The blood that has passed through the capillaries of the myocardium is drained by branches of the cardiac veins whose path runs parallel to those of the coronary arteries. Some of these veins empty directly into the right atrium and right ventricle, but the majority feed into the coronary sinus, which empties into the right atrium.

Cardiac innervation

The heart is under the control of the autonomic nervous system located in the medulla oblongata, a part of the brain stem. The autonomic nervous system regulates functions of the body that are involuntary, or not under conscious control, such as blood pressure and heart rate. It includes the *sympathetic nervous system* and the *parasympathetic nervous system*, each producing opposite effects when stimulated. Stimulation of the sympathetic nervous system results in the release of norepinephrine, a neurotransmitter, which accelerates the heart rate, speeds conduction through the AV node, and increases the force of ventricular contraction. This system prepares the body to function under stress ("fight-or-flight" response). Stimulation of the parasympathetic nervous system results in the release of acetylcholine, a neurotransmitter, which slows the heart rate, decreases conduction through the AV node, and causes a small decrease in the force of ventricular contraction. This system regulates the calmer functions of the body ("rest-and-digest" response). Normally a balance is maintained between the accelerator effects of the sympathetic system and the inhibitory effects of the parasympathetic system.

2 Electrophysiology

Cardiac cells

The heart is composed of thousands of cardiac cells. The cardiac cells are long and narrow, and divide at their ends into branches. These branches connect with branches of adjacent cells, forming a branching and anastomosing network of cells. At the junctions where the branches join together is a specialized cellular membrane of low electrical resistance, which permits rapid conduction of electrical impulses from one cell to another throughout the cell network. Stimulation of one cardiac cell initiates stimulation of adjacent cells and ultimately leads to cardiac muscle contraction.

There are two basic kinds of cardiac cells in the heart: the *myocardial cells* (or "working" cells) and the *pacemaker cells*. The myocardial cells are contained in the muscular layer of the walls of the atria and ventricles. The myocardial "working" cells are permeated by contractile filaments which, when electrically stimulated, produce myocardial muscle contraction. The primary function of the myocardial cells is cardiac muscle contraction, followed by relaxation. The pacemaker cells are found in the electrical conduction system of the heart and are primarily responsible for the spontaneous generation of electrical impulses.

Cardiac cells have four primary cell characteristics:
- *automaticity* — the ability of the pacemaker cells to generate their own electrical impulses spontaneously; this characteristic is specific to the pacemaker cells.
- *excitability* — the ability of the cardiac cells to respond to an electrical impulse; this characteristic is shared by all cardiac cells.
- *conductivity* — the ability of cardiac cells to conduct an electrical impulse; this characteristic is shared by all cardiac cells.
- *contractility* — the ability of cardiac cells to cause cardiac muscle contraction; this characteristic is specific to myocardial cells.

Depolarization and repolarization

Cardiac cells are surrounded and filled with an electrolyte solution. An *electrolyte* is a substance whose molecules dissociate into charged particles (ions) when placed in water, producing positively and negatively charged ions. An ion with a positive charge is called a *cation*. An ion with a negative charge is called an *anion*. Potassium (K^+) is the primary ion inside the cell and sodium (Na^+) is the primary ion outside the cell.

A membrane separates the inside of the cardiac cell (intracellular) from the outside (extracellular). There is a constant movement of ions across the cardiac cell membrane. Differences in concentrations of these ions determine the cell's electric charge. The distribution of ions on either side of the membrane is determined by several factors:
- Membrane channels (pores) — The cell membrane has openings through which ions pass back and forth between the extracellular and intracellular spaces. Some channels are always open; others can be opened or closed; still others can be selective, allowing one kind of ion to pass through and excluding all others. Membrane channels open and close in response to a stimulus.
- Concentration gradient — Particles in solution move, or diffuse, from areas of higher concentration to areas of lower concentration. In the case of uncharged particles, movement proceeds until the particles are uniformly distributed within the solution.
- Electrical gradient — Charged particles also diffuse, but the diffusion of charged particles is influenced not only by the concentration gradient, but also by an electrical gradient. Like charges repel; opposite charges attract. Therefore, positively charged particles tend to flow toward negatively charged particles and negatively charged particles toward positively charged particles.
- Sodium-potassium pump — The sodium-potassium pump is a mechanism that actively transports ions across the cell membrane against its electrochemical gradient. This pump helps to reestablish the resting concentrations of sodium and potassium after cardiac depolarization.

Electrical impulses are the result of the flow of ions (primarily sodium and potassium) back and forth across the cardiac cell membrane (Figure 2-1). Normally there is an ionic difference between the two sides. In the resting cardiac cell, there are more negative ions inside the cell than outside the cell. When the ions are so aligned, the resting cell is called polarized. During this time, no electrical

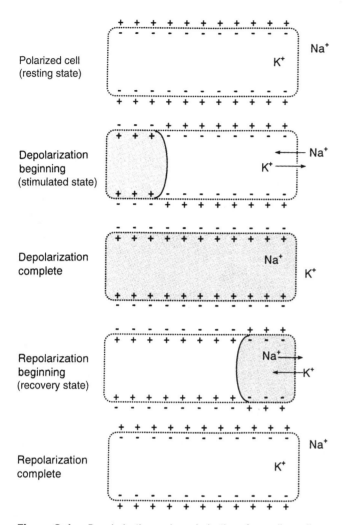

Polarized cell
(resting state)

Na⁺
K⁺

Depolarization
beginning
(stimulated state)

← Na⁺
K⁺ →

Depolarization
complete

Na⁺
K⁺

Repolarization
beginning
(recovery state)

Na⁺ →
← K⁺

Repolarization
complete

Na⁺
K⁺

Figure 2-1.   Depolarization and repolarization of a cardiac cell.

activity is occurring and a straight line (isoelectric line) is recorded on the ECG (Figure 2-5).

Once a cell is stimulated, the membrane permeability changes. Potassium begins to leave the cell, increasing cell permeability to sodium. Sodium rushes into the cell, causing the inside of the cell to become more positive than negative (cell is depolarized). Muscle contraction follows depolarization. Depolarization and muscle contraction are not the same. Depolarization is an electrical event that results in muscle contraction, a mechanical event.

After depolarization, the cardiac cell begins to recover. The sodium-potassium pump is activated to actively transport sodium out of the cell and move potassium back into the cell. The inside of the cell becomes more negative than positive (cell is repolarized) and returns to its resting state.

Depolarization of one cardiac cell acts as a stimulus on adjacent cells and causes them to depolarize. Propagation of the electrical impulses from cell to cell produces an electric current that can be detected by skin electrodes and recorded as waves or deflections onto graph paper, called the *ECG*.

Electrical conduction system of the heart

The heart is supplied with an electrical conduction system that generates and conducts electrical impulses along specialized pathways to the atria and ventricles, causing them to contract (Figure 2-2). The system consists of the sinoatrial node (*SA node*), the *interatrial tract* (Bachmann's bundle), the *internodal tracts*, the atrioventricular node (*AV node*), the *bundle of His*, the *right bundle branch*, the *left bundle branch*, and the *Purkinje fibers*.

The SA node is located in the wall of the upper right atrium near the inlet of the superior vena cava. Specialized electrical cells, called pacemaker cells, in the SA node discharge impulses at a rate of 60 to 100 times per minute. Pacemaker cells are located at other sites along the conduction system, but the SA node is normally in control and is called the pacemaker of the heart because it possesses the highest level of automaticity (its inherent firing rate is greater than that of the other pacemaker sites). If the SA node fails to generate electrical impulses at its normal rate or stops functioning entirely, or if the conduction of these impulses is blocked, pacemaker cells in secondary pacemaker sites can assume control as pacemaker of the heart, but at a much slower rate. Such a pacemaker is called an escape pacemaker because it usually only appears ("escapes") when the faster firing pacemaker (usually the SA node) fails to function. Pacemaker cells in the AV junction generate electrical impulses at 40 to 60 times per minute. Pacemaker cells in the ventricles generate electrical impulses at a much slower rate (30 to 40 times per minute or less). In general, the farther away the impulse originates from the SA node, the slower the rate. A beat or series of beats arising from an escape pacemaker is called an *escape beat* or *escape rhythm* and is identified according to its site of origin (for example, junctional, ventricular).

As the electrical impulse leaves the SA node, it is conducted through the left atria by way of Bachmann's bundle and through the right atria via the internodal tracts, causing electrical stimulation (depolarization) and contraction of the atria. The impulse is then conducted to the AV node located in the lower right atrium near the interatrial septum. The AV node relays the electrical impulses from the atria to the ventricles. It provides the only normal conduction pathway between the atria and the ventricles. The AV node has three main functions:

■ To slow conduction of the electrical impulse through the AV node to allow time for the atria to contract and empty its contents into the ventricles (atrial kick) before the ventricles contract. This delay in the AV node is represented on the ECG tracing as the flat line of the PR interval.

■ To serve as a backup pacemaker, if the SA node fails, at a rate of 40 to 60 beats per minute

■ To block some of the impulses from being conducted to the ventricles when the atrial rate is rapid, thus protecting the ventricles from dangerously fast rates.

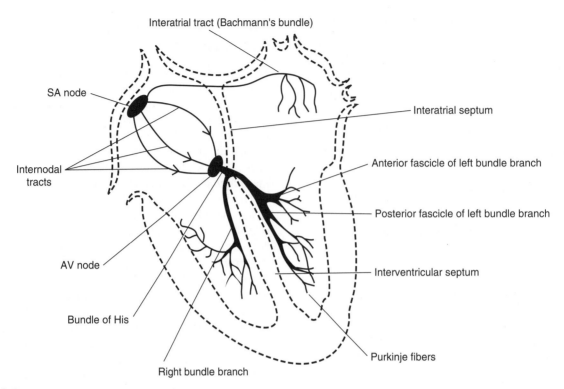

Figure 2-2.   Electrical conduction system of the heart.

After the delay in the AV node, the impulse moves through the bundle of His. The bundle of His divides into two important conducting pathways called the right bundle branch and the left bundle branch. The right bundle branch conducts the electrical impulse to the right ventricle. The left bundle branch divides into two divisions: the anterior fascicle, which carries the electrical impulse to the anterior wall of the left ventricle, and the posterior fascicle, which carries the electrical impulse to the posterior wall of the left ventricle. Both bundle branches terminate in a network of conduction fibers called Purkinje fibers. These fibers make up an elaborate web that carry the electrical impulses directly to the ventricular muscle cells. The ventricles are capable of serving as a backup pacemaker at a rate of 30 to 40 beats per minute (sometimes less). Transmission of the electrical impulses through the conduction system is slowest in the AV node and fastest in the His-Purkinje system (bundle of His, bundle branches, and Purkinje fibers).

The heart's electrical activity is represented on the monitor or ECG tracing by three basic waveforms: the *P wave*, the *QRS complex*, and the *T wave* (Figure 2-3). A U wave is sometimes present. Between the waveforms are the following segments and intervals: the PR interval, the PR segment, the ST segment, and the QT interval. Although the letters themselves have no special significance, each component represents a particular event in the depolarization–repolarization cycle. The P wave depicts atrial depolarization, or the spread of the impulse from the SA node throughout the atria. A waveform representing atrial repolarization is usually not seen on the ECG

because atrial repolarization occurs during ventricular depolarization and is hidden in the QRS complex. The PR interval represents the time from the onset of atrial depolarization to the onset of ventricular depolarization. The PR segment, a part of the PR interval, is the short isoelectric line between the end of the P wave to the beginning of the QRS complex. It is used as a baseline to evaluate elevation or depression of the ST segment. The QRS complex depicts ventricular depolarization, or the spread of the impulse throughout the ventricles. The ST segment represents early ventricular repolarization. The T wave represents

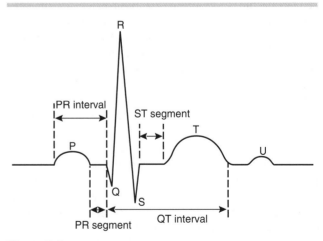

Figure 2-3.   Relationship of the electrical conduction system to the ECG.

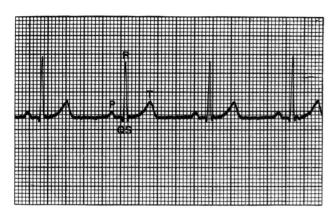

Figure 2-4.   The cardiac cycle.

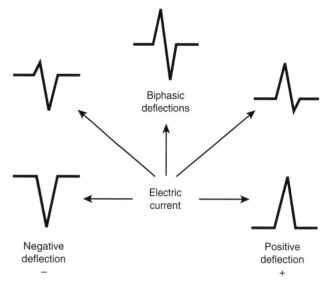

Figure 2-6.   Relationship between current flow and waveform deflections.

ventricular repolarization. The U wave, which isn't always present, represents late ventricular repolarization. The QT interval represents total ventricular activity (the time from the onset of ventricular depolarization to the end of ventricular repolarization).

The cardiac cycle

A cardiac cycle consists of one heartbeat or one *PQRST sequence*. It represents a sequence of atrial contraction and relaxation followed by ventricular contraction and relaxation. The basic cycle repeats itself again and again (Figure 2-4). Regularity of the cardiac rhythm can be assessed by measuring from one heartbeat to the next (from one R wave to the next R wave, also called the R-R interval). Between cardiac cycles, the monitor or ECG recorder returns to the isoelectric line (baseline), the flat line in the ECG during which electrical activity is absent (Figure 2-5). Any waveform above the isoelectric line is considered a positive (upright) deflection and any waveform below this line a negative (downward) deflection. A deflection having both a positive and negative component is called a biphasic deflection. This basic concept

can be applied to the P wave, the QRS complex, and the T wave deflections.

Waveforms and current flow

A monitor lead, or ECG lead, provides a view of the heart's electrical activity between two points or poles (a positive pole and a negative pole). The direction in which the electric current flows determines how the waveforms appear on the ECG tracing (Figure 2-6). An electric current flowing toward the positive pole will produce a *positive deflection*; an electric current traveling toward the negative pole produces a *negative deflection*. Current flowing away from the poles will produce a *biphasic deflection* (both positive and negative). Biphasic deflections may be equally positive and negative, more negative than positive, or more positive than negative (depending on the angle of current flow to the positive or negative pole).

The size of the wave deflection depends on the magnitude of the electrical current flowing toward the individual pole. The magnitude of the electrical current is determined by how much voltage is generated by depolarization of a particular portion of the heart. The QRS complex is normally larger than the P wave because depolarization of the larger muscle mass of the ventricles generates more voltage than does depolarization of the smaller muscle mass of the atria.

Refractory and supernormal periods of the cardiac cycle

There is a period of time in the cardiac cycle during which the cardiac cells may be refractory, or unable to respond, to a stimulus. Refractoriness is divided into three phases (Figure 2-7):

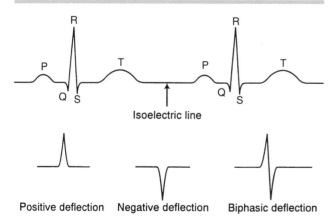

Figure 2-5.   Relationship between waveforms and the isoelectric line.

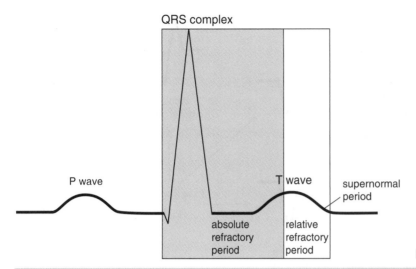

Figure 2-7. Refractory and supernormal periods.

■ *Absolute refractory period* — During this period the cells absolutely cannot respond to a stimulus. This period extends from the onset of the QRS complex to the peak of the T wave. During this time the cardiac cells have depolarized and are in the process of repolarizing. Because the cardiac cells have not repolarized to their threshold potential (the level at which a cell must be repolarized before it can be depolarized again) they cannot be stimulated to depolarize. In other words, the myocardial cells cannot contract, and the cells of the electrical conduction system cannot conduct an electrical impulse during the absolute refractory period.

■ *Relative refractory period* — During this period the cardiac cells have repolarized sufficiently to respond to a strong stimulus. This period begins at the peak of the T wave and ends with the end of the T wave. The relative refractory period is also called the *vulnerable period of repolarization*. A strong stimulus occurring during the vulnerable period may usurp the primary pacemaker of the heart (usually the SA node) and take over pacemaker control. An example might be a premature ventricular contraction (PVC) that falls during the vulnerable period and takes over control of the heart in the form of ventricular tachycardia.

■ *Supernormal period* — During this period the cardiac cells will respond to a weaker than normal stimulus. This period occurs during a short portion near the end of the T wave, just before the cells have completely repolarized.

ECG graph paper

The PQRST sequence is recorded on special graph paper made up of horizontal and vertical lines (Figure 2-8). The horizontal lines measure the duration of the waveforms in seconds of time. Each small square measured horizontally represents 0.04 second in time. The width of the QRS complex in Figure 2-9 extends across for 2 small squares and represents 0.08 second (0.04 second × 2 squares). The vertical lines measure the voltage or amplitude of the waveform in millimeters (mm). Each small square measured vertically represents 1 mm in height. The height of the QRS complex in Figure 2-9 extends upward from baseline 16 small squares and represents 16 mm voltage (1 mm × 16 squares).

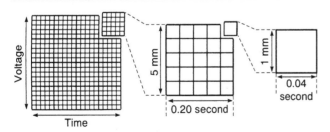

Figure 2-8. Electrocardiographic paper.

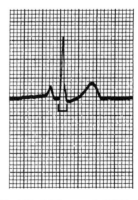

Figure 2-9. QRS width: 0.08 second; QRS height: 16 mm.

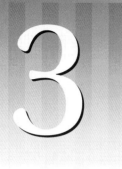

3 Waveforms, intervals, segments, and complexes

Much of the information that the ECG tracing provides is obtained from the examination of the three principal waveforms (the P wave, the QRS complex, and the T wave) and their associated segments and intervals. Assessment of this data provides the facts necessary for an accurate cardiac rhythm interpretation.

P wave

The first deflection of the cardiac cycle, the P wave, is caused by depolarization of the right and left atria (Figure 3-1). The first part of the P wave represents depolarization of the right atrium; the second part represents depolarization of the left atrium. The waveform begins as the deflection leaves baseline and ends when the deflection returns to baseline. A normal sinus P wave originates in the sinus node and travels through normal atria, resulting in normal depolarization. Normal P waves are smooth and round, positive in lead II (a positive lead), 0.5 to 2.5 mm in height, 0.10 second or less in width, with one P wave to each QRS complex. More than one P wave before a QRS complex indicates a conduction disturbance, such as that which occurs in second and third-degree heart block (discussed in Chapter 8).

There are two types of abnormal P waves:

■ *Abnormal sinus P wave* — An abnormal sinus P wave originates in the sinus node and travels through enlarged atria, resulting in abnormal depolarization of the atria. Abnormal atria depolarization results in abnormal-looking P waves.

Impulses traveling through an enlarged right atrium (right atrial hypertrophy) result in P waves that are tall

and peaked. The abnormal P wave in right atrial enlargement is sometimes referred to as *p pulmonale* because the atrial enlargement that it signifies is common with severe pulmonary disease (for example, pulmonary stenosis and insufficiency, chronic obstructive pulmonary disease, acute pulmonary embolism, and pulmonary edema).

Impulses traveling through an enlarged left atrium (left atrial hypertrophy) result in P waves that are wide and notched. The term *p mitrale* is used to describe the abnormal P waves seen in left atrial enlargement because they were first seen in patients with mitral valve stenosis and insufficiency. Left atrial enlargement can also be seen in left heart failure.

■ *Ectopic P wave* — The term *ectopic* means away from its normal location. Therefore, an ectopic P wave arises from a site other than the SA node. Abnormal sites include the atria and the AV junction. P waves from the atria may be positive or negative; some are small, pointed, flat, wavy, or sawtooth in appearance. P waves from the AV junction are always negative (inverted) and may precede or follow the QRS complex or be hidden within the QRS complex and not visible.

Examples of P waves are shown in Figure 3-2.

PR interval

The PR interval (sometimes abbreviated PRI) represents the time from the onset of atrial depolarization to the onset of ventricular depolarization. The PR interval (Figure 3-3) includes a P wave and the short isoelectric line (PR segment) that follows it. The PR interval is measured from the beginning of the P wave as it leaves baseline to the beginning of the QRS complex. The duration of the normal PR interval is 0.12 to 0.20 seconds.

Abnormal PR intervals may be short or prolonged:

■ *Short PR interval* — A short PR interval is less than 0.12 seconds and may be seen if the electrical impulse originates in an ectopic site in the AV junction. A shortened PR interval may also occur if the electrical impulse progresses from the atria to the ventricles through one of several abnormal conduction pathways (called accessory pathways) that bypass a part or all of the AV node. Wolff-Parkinson-White syndrome (WPW) is an example of such an accessory pathway.

■ *Prolonged PR interval* — A prolonged PR interval is greater than 0.20 seconds and indicates that the impulse

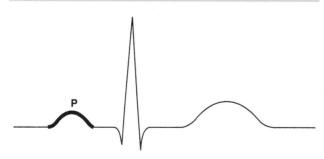

Figure 3-1. The P wave.

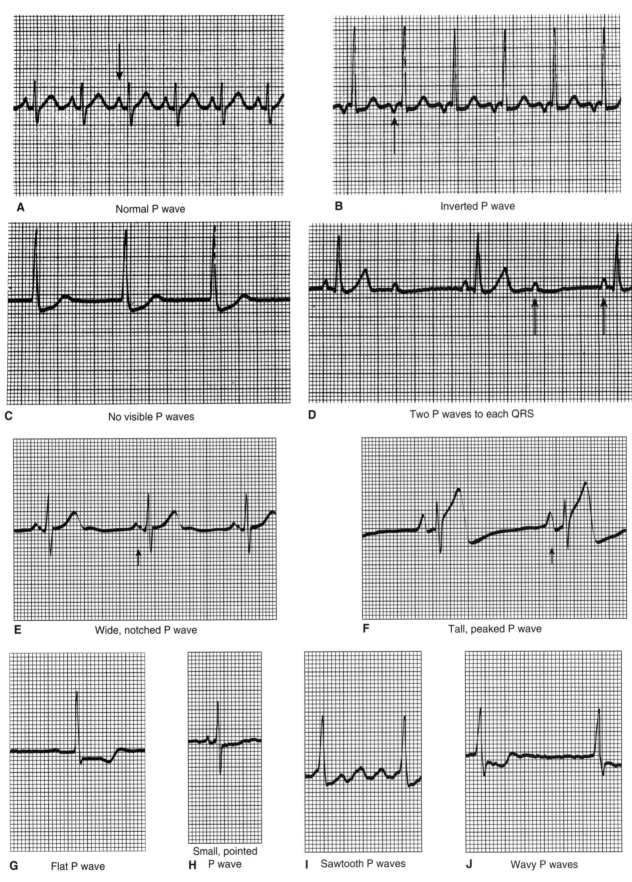

A   Normal P wave

B   Inverted P wave

C   No visible P waves

D   Two P waves to each QRS

E   Wide, notched P wave

F   Tall, peaked P wave

G   Flat P wave

H   Small, pointed P wave

I   Sawtooth P waves

J   Wavy P waves

Figure 3-2.   P wave examples.

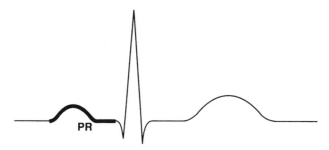

Figure 3-3. The PR interval.

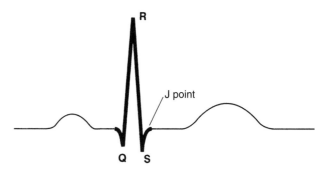

Figure 3-5. The QRS complex.

was delayed longer than normal in the AV node. Prolonged PR intervals are seen in first-degree AV block.

Examples of PR intervals are shown in Figure 3-4.

QRS complex

The QRS complex (Figure 3-5) represents depolarization of the right and left ventricles. The QRS complex is larger than the P wave because depolarization of the ventricles involves a larger muscle mass than depolarization of the atria.

The QRS complex is composed of three wave deflections: the *Q wave*, the *R wave*, and the *S wave*. The R wave is a positive waveform; the Q wave is a negative waveform that precedes the R wave; the S wave is a negative waveform that follows the R wave. The normal QRS complex is predominantly positive in lead II (a positive lead) with a duration of 0.10 second or less.

The QRS complex is measured from the beginning of the QRS complex (as the first wave of the complex leaves baseline) to the end of the QRS complex (when the last wave of the complex begins to level out into the ST segment). The point where the QRS complex meets the ST segment is called the *J point* (junction point).

Finding the beginning of the QRS complex usually isn't difficult. Finding the end of the QRS complex, however, is at times a challenge because of elevation or depression of the ST segment. Remember, the QRS complex ends as soon as the straight line of the ST segment begins, even though the straight line may be above or below baseline.

Although the term QRS complex is used, not every QRS complex contains a Q wave, R wave, and S wave. Many variations exist in the configuration of the QRS complex (Figure 3-6). Whatever the variation, the complex is still called the QRS complex. For example, you might see a QRS complex with a Q and an R wave, but no S wave (Figure 3-6, example B), an R and S wave without a Q wave (Figure 3-6, example C), or an R wave without a Q or an S wave (Figure 3-6, example D). If the entire complex is negative (Figure 3-6, example F), it is termed a *QS complex* (not a negative R wave because R waves are always positive). It's also possible to have more than one R wave (Figure 3-6, example I) and more than one S wave; (Figure 3-6, example J). The second R wave is called *R prime* and is written R'. The second S wave is called *S prime* and is written S'. To be labeled separately, a wave must cross

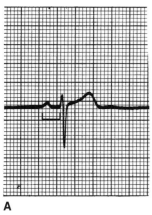

A

Normal PR interval of 0.20 second (0.04 second × 5 squares).

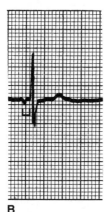

B

Short PR interval of 0.08 second (0.04 second × 2 squares)

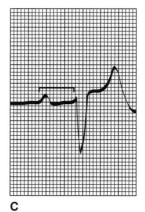

C

Long PR interval of 0.38 second (0.04 second × 9½ squares)

Figure 3-4. PR interval examples.

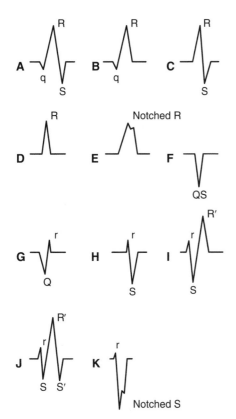

Figure 3-6.   QRS variations.

the baseline. A wave that changes direction but doesn't cross the baseline is called a *notch*. (Figure 3-6, example E, shows a notched R and Figure 3-6, example K, shows a notched S.)

Capital letters are used to designate waves of large amplitude (5 mm or more) and lowercase letters are used to designate waves of small amplitude (less than 5 mm). This allows you to visualize a complex mentioned in a textbook when illustrations aren't available. For example, if a complex is described in a text as having an rS waveform, the reader can easily picture a complex with a small r wave and a big S wave.

An abnormal QRS complex is wide with a duration of 0.12 second or more. An abnormally wide QRS complex may result from:

■ a block in the conduction of impulses through the right or left bundle branch (bundle-branch block)

■ an electrical impulse that has arrived early (as with premature beats) at the bundle branches before repolarization is complete, allowing the electrical impulse to initiate depolarization of the ventricles earlier than usual, resulting in abnormal (aberrant) ventricular conduction and causing a wide QRS complex

■ an electrical impulse that has been conducted from the atria to the ventricles through an abnormal accessory conduction pathway that bypasses the AV node, allowing the electrical impulse to initiate depolarization of

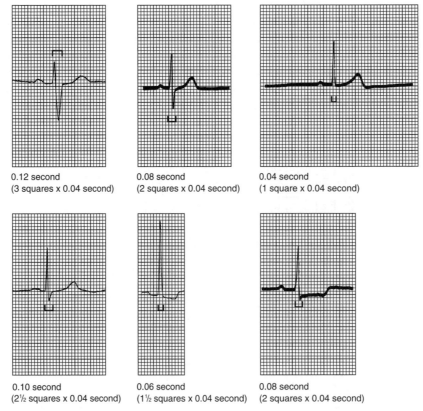

0.12 second
(3 squares x 0.04 second)

0.08 second
(2 squares x 0.04 second)

0.04 second
(1 square x 0.04 second)

0.10 second
(2½ squares x 0.04 second)

0.06 second
(1½ squares x 0.04 second)

0.08 second
(2 squares x 0.04 second)

Figure 3-7.   QRS examples.

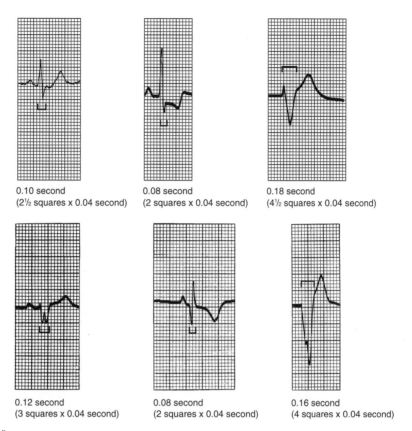

0.10 second
(2½ squares x 0.04 second)

0.08 second
(2 squares x 0.04 second)

0.18 second
(4½ squares x 0.04 second)

0.12 second
(3 squares x 0.04 second)

0.08 second
(2 squares x 0.04 second)

0.16 second
(4 squares x 0.04 second)

Figure 3-7. *(continued)*

the ventricles earlier than usual, resulting in abnormal (aberrant) ventricular conduction and causing a wide QRS complex

■ an electrical impulse that has originated in an ectopic site in the ventricles.

Examples of QRS complexes are shown in Figure 3-7.

ST segment

The ST segment represents early ventricular repolarization. The ST segment is the flat line between the QRS complex and the T wave (Figure 3-8). Normally the ST segment is positioned at baseline (the isoelectric line). The ST seg-

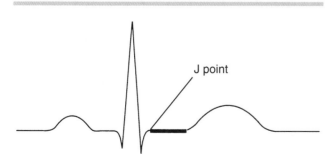

J point

Figure 3-8. The ST segment.

ment may be displaced above baseline (*elevated ST segment*) or below baseline (*depressed ST segment*). The PR segment is normally used as a baseline reference to evaluate the degree of displacement of the ST segment from the isoelectric line. An ST segment is abnormal when it is elevated or depressed 1 mm or more, measured at a point 0.04 second past the J point (the point where the QRS complex and the ST segment meet).

Elevated ST segments may be horizontal (straight across), convex (rounded upward), or concave (rounded inward). Common causes include ST elevation myocardial infarction (STEMI), coronary artery spasm (Prinzmetal's angina), acute pericarditis, ventricular aneurysm, early repolarization pattern (a form of myocardial repolarization seen in normal healthy individuals that produces ST-segment elevation closely mimicking that of acute myocardial infarction [MI] or pericarditis), hyperkalemia, and hypothermia.

Depressed ST segments may be horizontal, downsloping, upsloping, or sagging. Common causes include myocardial ischemia, non-ST elevation MI (non-STEMI), reciprocal ECG changes associated with STEMI, hypokalemia, and digitalis effect. Digitalis causes a sagging ST-segment depression, with a characteristic "scooped-out" appearance. Examples of ST segments are shown in Figure 3-9.

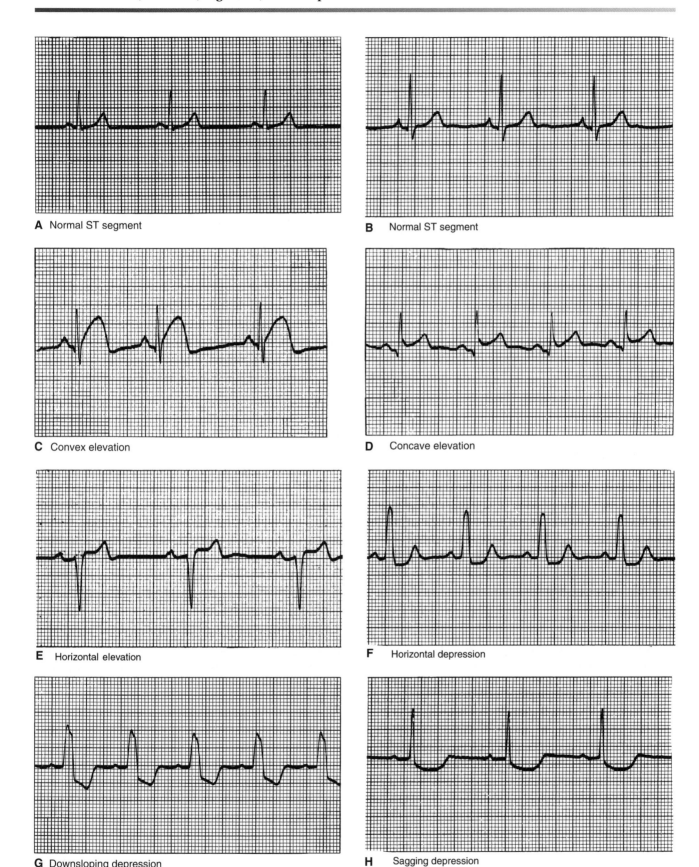

A Normal ST segment

B Normal ST segment

C Convex elevation

D Concave elevation

E Horizontal elevation

F Horizontal depression

G Downsloping depression

H Sagging depression

Figure 3-9. ST segment samples.

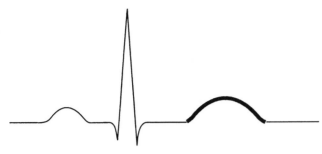

Figure 3-10. The T wave.

T wave

The T wave represents ventricular repolarization. The normal T wave begins as the deflection gradually slopes upward from the ST segment, and ends when the waveform returns to baseline (Figure 3-10). Normal T waves are rounded and slightly asymmetrical (with the first part of the T wave gradually sloping to the peak and returning more abruptly to baseline), positive in lead II (a positive lead), with an amplitude less than 5 mm. The T wave always follows the QRS complex (repolarization always follows depolarization).

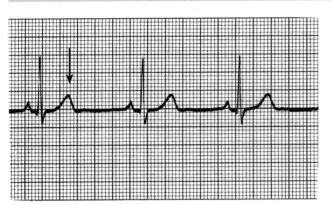

A   Normal T wave

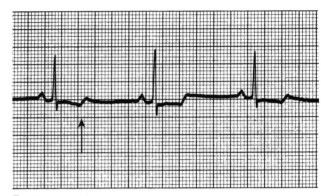

B   Biphasic T wave

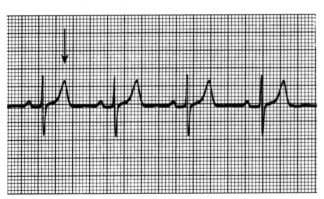

C   Tall, peaked T wave

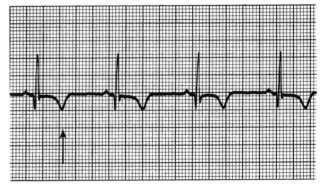

D   Inverted T wave

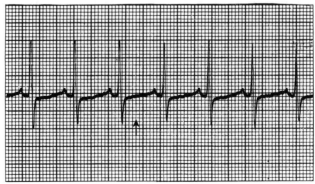

E   Flat T wave

Figure 3-11. T wave examples.

Abnormal T waves may be abnormally tall or low, flattened, biphasic, or inverted. Common causes include myocardial ischemia, acute MI, pericarditis, hyperkalemia, ventricular enlargement, bundle-branch block, and subarachnoid hemorrhage. Significant cerebral disease, such as subarachnoid hemorrhage, may be associated with deeply inverted T waves (called cerebral T waves).

Examples of T waves are shown in Figure 3-11.

QT interval

The QT interval represents the time between the onset of ventricular depolarization and the end of ventricular repolarization. The QT interval is measured from the beginning of the QRS complex to the end of the T wave (Figure 3-12).

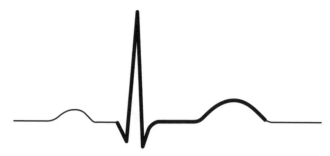

Figure 3-12. QT Interval.

Duration of the QT interval can be determined by multiplying the number of small squares in the QT interval by 0.04 second (Figure 3-13). The length of the QT interval normally

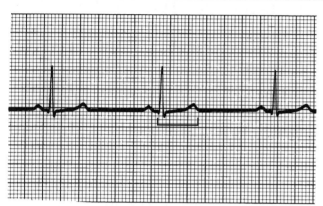

A 1. Number of small squares between R waves = 31. Half of 31 = 15.
2. Number of small squares in QT interval = 11
3. Compare the difference: QT interval is less than half the R-R interval (11 small squares are less than 15 small squares); QT interval is normal for this heart rate. (Duration of QT interval: 11 squares × 0.04 second = 0.44 second.)

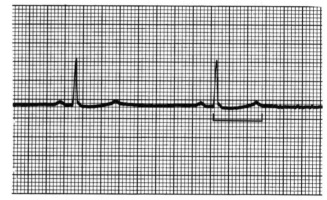

B 1. Number of small squares between R waves = 38. Half of 38 = 19.
2. Number of small squares in QT interval = 13
3. Compare the difference: QT interval is less than half the R-R interval (13 small squares are less than 19 small squares); QT interval is normal for this heart rate. (Duration of QT interval: 13 small squares × 0.04 second = 0.52 second.)

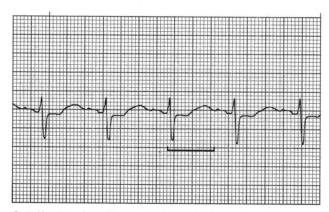

C 1. Number of small squares between R waves = 18. Half of 18 = 9.
2. Number of small squares in QT interval = 13.
3. Compare the difference: QT interval is more than half the R-R interval (13 small squares are more than 9 small squares); QT interval is prolonged for this heart rate. (Duration of QT interval: 13 squares × 0.04 second = 0.52 second.)

Figure 3-13. QT interval examples.

varies according to age, sex, and particularly heart rate. The QT interval is more prolonged with slow heart rates.

Generally speaking, the normal QT interval should be less than half the *R-R interval* (the distance between two consecutive R waves) when the rhythm is regular. The determination of the QT interval should be made in a lead where the T wave is most prominent and shouldn't include the U wave. Accurate measurement of the QT interval can be done only when the rhythm is regular for at least two cardiac cycles before the measurement.

To determine if the QT interval is normal or prolonged:
■ Count the number of small boxes in the R-R interval and divide by two.
■ Count the number of small boxes in the QT interval.
■ Compare the difference. If the QT interval measures less than half the R-R interval, it's probably normal. If the QT interval measures the same as half the R-R interval, it's considered borderline. If the QT interval measures longer than half the R-R interval, it's prolonged.

A prolonged QT interval indicates a delay in ventricular repolarization. The prolongation of the QT interval lengthens the relative refractory period (the vulnerable period of repolarization), allowing more time for an ectopic focus to take control and putting the ventricles at risk for life-threatening arrhythmias such as *torsades de pointes*

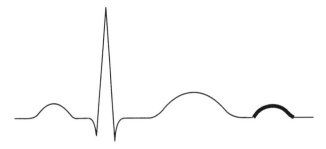

Figure 3-14.   The U wave.

ventricular tachycardia (discussed in Chapter 9). Common causes include electrolyte imbalances (hypokalemia, hypomagnesemia, hypocalcemia), hypothermia, bradyarrhythmias, liquid protein diets, myocardial ischemia, antiarrhythmics, psychotropic agents (phenothiazines, tricyclic antidepressants), and hereditary long-QT syndrome. It can also occur without a known cause (idiopathic).

Examples of QT intervals are shown in Figure 3-13.

U wave

The U wave is a small deflection sometimes seen following the T wave (Figure 3-14). Neither its presence nor its

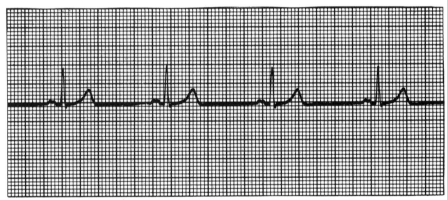

ECG without U wave

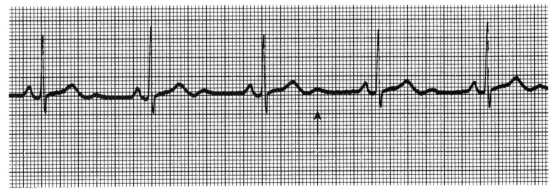

ECG with U wave

Figure 3-15.   U wave examples.

absence is considered abnormal. The U wave represents late repolarization of the ventricles, probably a small segment of the ventricles.

The waveform begins as the deflection leaves baseline and ends when the deflection returns to baseline. Normal U waves are small, rounded, and symmetrical, positive in lead II (a positive lead), and 2 mm or less in amplitude (always smaller than the preceding T wave). The U wave can best be seen when the heart rate is slow.

Abnormal U waves are tall (greater than 2 mm in height). Common causes include hypokalemia, cardiomyopathy, and left ventricular enlargement, among other causes. A large U wave may occasionally be mistaken for a P wave, but usually a comparison of the morphology of both waveforms will help differentiate the U wave from the P wave.

Examples of U waves are shown in Figure 3-15.

Waveform practice: Labeling waves

For each of the following rhythm strips (strips 3-1 through 3-14), label the P, Q, R, S, T, and U waves. Some of the strips may not have all of these waveforms. Check your answers with the answer key in the back of the book.

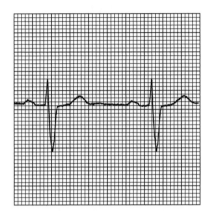

Strip 3-1.

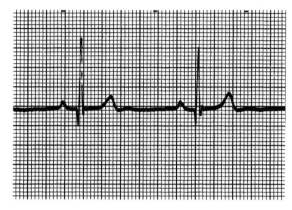

Strip 3-2.

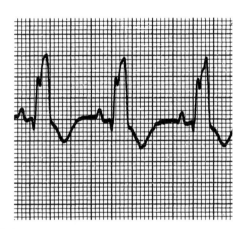

Strip 3-3.

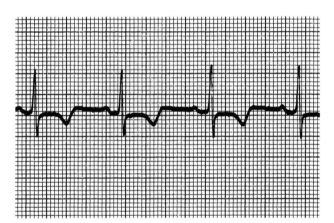

Strip 3-4.

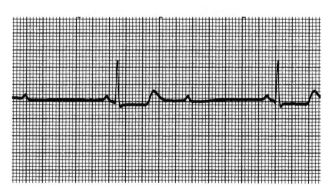

Strip 3-5.

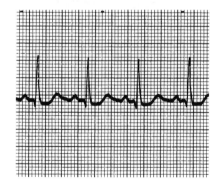

Strip 3-6.

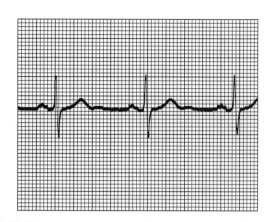

Strip 3-7.

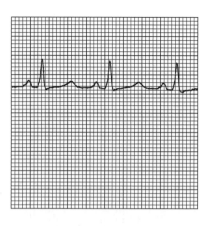

Strip 3-8.

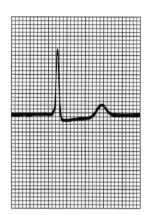

Strip 3-9.

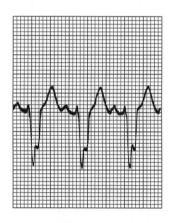

Strip 3-10.

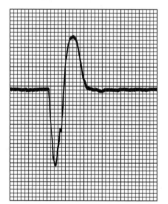

Strip 3-11.

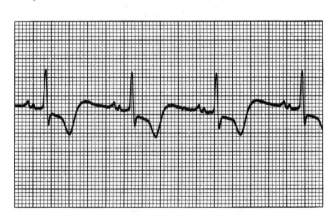

Strip 3-12.

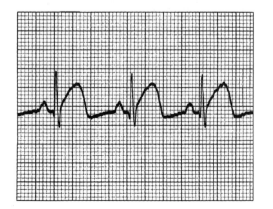

Strip 3-13.

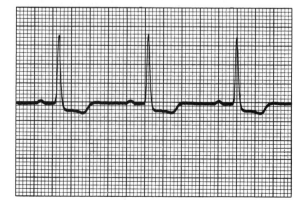

Strip 3-14.

4 Cardiac monitors

Purpose of ECG monitoring

The electrocardiogram (ECG) is a recording of the electrical activity of the heart. The ECG records two basic electrical processes:
- *Depolarization* — the spread of the electrical stimulus through the heart muscle, producing the P wave from the atria and the QRS complex from the ventricles.
- *Repolarization* — the recovery of the stimulated muscle to the resting state, producing the ST segment, the T wave, and the U wave.

The depolarization-repolarization process produces electrical currents that are transmitted to the surface of the body. This electrical activity is detected by electrodes attached to the skin. After the electric current is detected, it's amplified, displayed on a monitor screen (oscilloscope), and recorded on ECG graph paper as waves and complexes. The waveforms can then be analyzed in a systematic manner and the "cardiac rhythm" identified.

Bedside monitoring allows continuous observation of the heart's electrical activity and is used to identify arrhythmias (disturbances in rate, rhythm, or conduction), evaluate pacemaker function, and evaluate the response to medications (for example, antiarrhythmics). Continuous cardiac monitoring is useful in monitoring patients in critical care units, cardiac stepdown units, surgery suites, outpatient surgery departments, emergency departments, and postanesthesia recovery units.

Types of ECG monitoring

There are two types of ECG monitoring: *hardwire* and *telemetry*. With hardwire monitoring (bedside monitoring), electrode pads (conductive gel discs) are placed on the patient's chest and attached to a lead-cable system and then connected to a monitor at the bedside. With telemetry monitoring (portable monitoring), electrode pads are attached to the patient's chest and connected to leads that are attached to a portable monitor transmitter.
- *Hardwire monitoring* — Hardwire monitoring uses either a *five-leadwire* system or a *three-leadwire* system.

With the five-leadwire system (Figure 4-1), five electrode pads and five leadwires are used. One electrode is placed below the right clavicle (2nd interspace, right

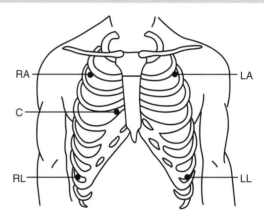

Figure 4-1. Hardwire monitoring — Five leadwire system. This illustration shows you where to place the electrodes and attach leadwires using a five-leadwire system. The leadwires are color-coded as follows:
- white — right arm (RA)
- black — left arm (LA)
- green — right leg (RL)
- red — left leg (LL)
- brown — chest (C).

Leads placed in the arm and leg positions as shown allow you to view leads I, II, III, aVR, aVL, and aVF. To view chest leads V_1–V_6, the chest lead must be placed in the specific chest lead position desired. In this example, the brown chest lead is in V_1 position.

midclavicular line), one below the left clavicle (2nd interspace, left midclavicular line), one on the right lower rib cage (8th interspace, right midclavicular line), one on the left lower rib cage (8th interspace, left midclavicular line), and one in a chest lead position (V_1 to V_6). The six chest lead positions (Figure 4-2) include:
- V_1 – 4th intercostal space, right sternal border
- V_2 – 4th intercostal space, left sternal border
- V_3 – midway between V_2 and V_4
- V_4 – 5th intercostal space, left midclavicular line
- V_5 – 5th intercostal space, left anterior axillary line
- V_6 – 5th intercostal space, left midaxillary line

The right arm (RA) lead is attached to the electrode pad below the right clavicle; the left arm (LA) lead to the electrode pad below the left clavicle; the right leg (RL) lead to the electrode pad on the right lower rib cage; the left

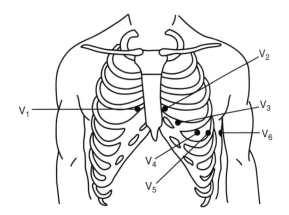

Figure 4-2.   Chest lead positions.

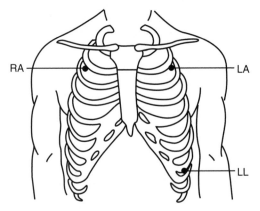

Figure 4-3.   Hardwire monitoring — Three-leadwire system. This illustration shows you where to place the electrodes and attach leadwires using a three-leadwire system. The lead wires are color-coded as follows:
■ white — right arm (RA)
■ black — left arm (LA)
■ red — left leg (LL).
  Leads placed in this position will allow you to monitor leads I, II, or III using the lead selector on the monitor.

leg (LL) lead to the electrode pad on the left lower rib cage; and the chest lead to the electrode pad of the specific chest position desired (V_1 through V_6).

With the five-leadwire system for hardwire monitoring, you can continuously monitor two leads using a lead selector on the monitor. Leads placed in the arm and leg positions allow you to view leads I, II, III, AVR, AVL, and AVF (Figure 4-1). To view chest lead V_1 to V_6, the chest lead must be placed in the specific chest lead position desired. Generally, a limb lead (usually I, II, or III) and a chest lead (usually V_1 or V_6) are chosen to be monitored.

With the three-leadwire system (Figure 4-3), three electrode pads and three leadwires are used. One electrode pad is placed below the right clavicle (2nd interspace, right midclavicular line), one below the left clavicle (2nd interspace, left midclavicular line), and one on the left lower rib cage (8th interspace, left midclavicular line). The RA lead is attached to the electrode pad below the right clavicle,

the LA lead is attached to the electrode pad below the left clavicle, and the LL lead is attached to the electrode pad on the left lower rib cage. You can monitor either limb leads I, II, or III by turning the lead selector on the monitor. Although you can't monitor chest leads (V_1 to V_6) with a three-leadwire system, you can monitor modified chest leads that provide similar information. To monitor any of these leads, reposition the LL lead to the appropriate position for the chest lead you want to monitor, and turn the lead selector on the monitor to lead III. Examples of modified chest lead V_1 (MCL$_1$) and modified chest lead V_6 (MCL$_6$) are shown in Figure 4-4.

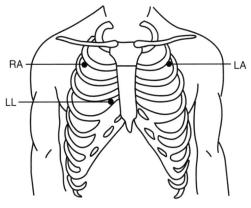

Modified Chest Lead V_1 (MCL$_1$)

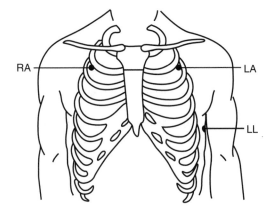

Modified Chest Lead V_6 (MCL$_6$)

Figure 4-4.   Hardwire monitoring — Three-leadwire system: Leads MCL$_1$ and MCL$_6$. Modified chest leads can be monitored with the three-leadwire system by repositioning the left leg (LL) lead to the chest position desired and turning the lead selector on the monitor to lead III.

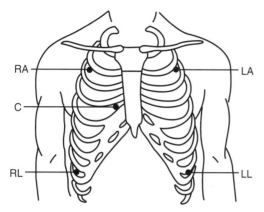

Figure 4-5. Telemetry monitoring — Five-leadwire system. This illustration shows you where to place the electrodes and attach leadwires using a five-leadwire system. The leadwires are color-coded as follows:

- white — right arm (RA)
- black — left arm (LA)
- green — right leg (RL)
- red — left leg (LL)
- brown — chest (C).

With the five-leadwire system for telemetry monitoring you can monitor any one of the 12 leads using a lead selector on the monitor. Leads placed in the conventional limb positions allow you to view leads I, II, III, aVR, aVL, and aVF. To view chest leads V_1–V_6, the chest lead must be placed in the specific chest lead desired.

- *Telemetry monitoring* — Wireless monitoring, or telemetry, gives your patient more freedom than hardwire monitoring. Instead of being connected to a bedside monitor, the patient is connected to a portable monitor transmitter, which can be placed in a pajama pocket or in a telemetry pouch. Telemetry monitoring systems are available in a five-leadwire system and a three-leadwire system.

The five-leadwire system for telemetry (Figure 4-5) is connected in the same manner as the five-leadwire system for hardwire monitoring with the four limb positions (RA, LA, RL, and LL) in the conventional locations and the chest leads placed in the desired V_1 to V_6 location. With this system you can monitor any one of the 12 leads using a lead selector on the monitor. Leads placed in the limb positions as shown in Figure 4-5 allow you to view leads I, II, III, AV_R, AV_L, or AV_F. To view chest leads V_1 through V_6, the chest lead must be placed in the specific chest lead position desired.

The three-leadwire system for telemetry (Figure 4-6) uses three electrodes and three leadwires. The leadwires are connected to positive, negative, and ground connections on the telemetry transmitter and attached to electrode pads placed in specific chest lead positions (leads I, II, III, MCL_1, and MCL_6). Only one lead position can be

monitored at a time, and a lead selector on the monitor isn't available.

Applying electrode pads

Proper attachment of the electrode pads to the skin is the most important step in obtaining a good quality ECG tracing. Unless there is good contact between the skin and the electrode pad, distortions of the ECG tracing (artifacts) may appear. An artifact is any abnormal wave, spike, or movement on the ECG tracing that isn't generated by the electrical activity of the heart. The procedure for attaching the electrodes is as follows:

- Choose monitor lead position. It's helpful to assess the 12-lead ECG to ascertain which lead provides the best QRS complex voltage and P wave identification.
- Prepare the skin. Clip the hair from the skin using a clipper; hair interferes with good contact between the electrode pad and the skin. Using a dry washcloth, wipe site free of loose hair. If the patient is perspiring and the electrodes won't stay adhered to skin, apply a thin coat of tincture of benzoin and allow to dry.
- Attach the electrode pads. Remove pads from packaging and check them for moist conductive gel; dried gel can cause loss of the ECG signal. Place an electrode pad on each prepared site, pressing firmly around periphery of the pad and avoiding bony areas, such as the clavicles or prominent rib markings.
- Connect the leadwires. Attach appropriate leadwires to the electrode pads according to established electrode-lead positions.

Troubleshooting monitor problems

Many problems may be encountered during cardiac monitoring. The most common problems are related to patient movement, interference from equipment in or near the patient's room, weak ECG signals, poor choice of monitor lead or electrode placement, and poor contact between the skin and electrode-lead attachments. Monitor problems can cause artifacts on the ECG tracing, making identification of the cardiac rhythm difficult or triggering false monitor alarms (false high-rate alarms and false low-rate alarms). Some problems are potentially serious and require intervention, whereas others are temporary, non-life-threatening occurrences that will correct themselves. The nurse and monitor technician need to be proficient in recognizing monitoring problems, identifying probable causes, and seeking solutions to correct the problem. The most common monitoring problems are:

- *False high-rate alarms* — High-voltage artifact potentials are commonly interpreted by the monitor as QRS complexes

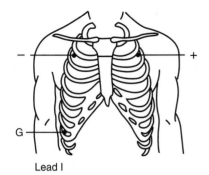

Lead I

Negative lead – 2nd interspace
right midclavicular line

Positive lead – 2nd interspace
left midclavicular line

Ground lead – 8th interspace
right midclavicular line

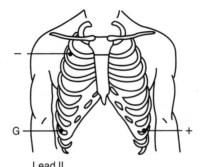

Lead II

Negative lead – 2nd interspace
right midclavicular line

Positive lead – 8th interspace
left midclavicular line

Ground lead – 8th interspace
right midclavicular line

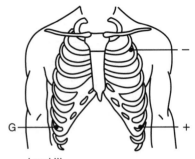

Lead III

Negative lead – 2nd interspace
left midclavicular line

Positive lead – 8th interspace
left midclavicular line

Ground lead – 8th interspace
right midclavicular line

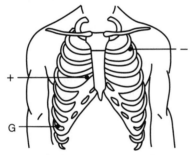

Modified Chest Lead V$_1$ (MCL$_1$)

Negative lead – 2nd interspace
left midclavicular line

Positive lead – 4th interspace
right sternal border

Ground lead – 8th interspace
right midclavicular line

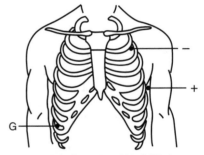

Modified Chest Lead V$_6$ (MCL$_6$)

Negative lead – 2nd interspace
left midclavicular line

Positive lead – 5th interspace
left midaxillary line

Ground lead – 8th interspace
right midclavicular line

Figure 4-6. Telemetry monitoring: Three-leadwire system.
The three-leadwire system uses three electrode pads and three leadwires. The leadwires are connected to positive, negative, or ground connections on the telemetry transmitter and attached to specific lead positions (lead I, lead II, lead III, lead MCL$_1$, or lead MCL$_6$). Only one lead position can be monitored at a time. A lead selector isn't available.

and activate the high-rate alarm. Most high-voltage arti-facts are related to muscle movements from the patient turning in bed or moving the extremities (Figure 4-7). Seizure activity can also produce high-voltage artifact potentials (Figure 4-8).
■ *False low-rate alarms* — Any disturbance in the trans-mission of the electrical signal from the skin electrode to the monitoring system can activate a false low-rate alarm (Figures 4-9, 4-10, 4-11, and 4-12). This problem is usu-ally caused by ineffective contact between the skin and the electrode-leadwire system, resulting from dried conductive gel, a loose electrode, or a disconnected leadwire. Low-voltage QRS complexes can also activate the low-rate alarm; if the ventricular waveforms aren't tall enough, the monitor detects no electrical activity and will sound the low-rate alarm.
■ *Muscle tremors* — Muscle tremors (Figures 4-13 and 4-14) can occur in tense, nervous patients or those shiver-ing from cold or having a chill. The ECG baseline has an uneven, coarsely jagged appearance, obscuring the wave-forms on the ECG tracing. The problem may be continuous or intermittent.

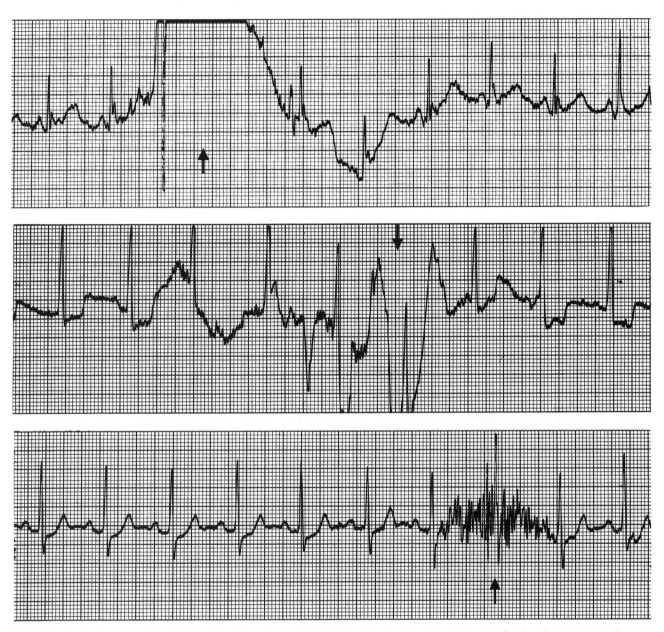

Figure 4-7. Patient movement. *Cause:* Strips above show patient turning in bed or extremity movement. *Solution:* Problem is usually intermittent and no correction is necessary. Movement artifact can be reduced by avoiding placement of electrode pads in areas where extremity movement is greatest (bony areas such as the clavicles).

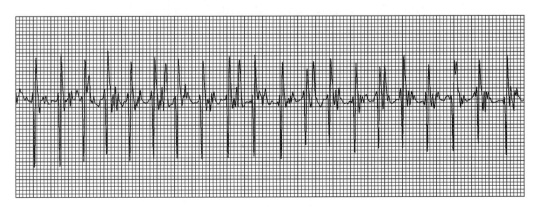

Figure 4-8. Seizure activity can activate the high-rate alarm on the monitor.

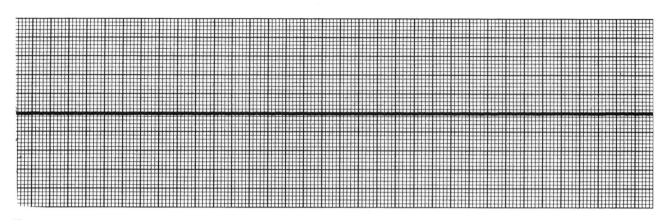

Figure 4-9.   Continuous straight line. *Cause:* Dried conductive gel, disconnected lead wire, or disconnected electrode pad. *Solution:* Check electrode-lead system; re-prep and re-attach electrodes and leads as necessary. *Note:* A straight line may also indicate the absence of electrical activity in the heart; the patient must be evaluated immediately for the presence of a pulse.

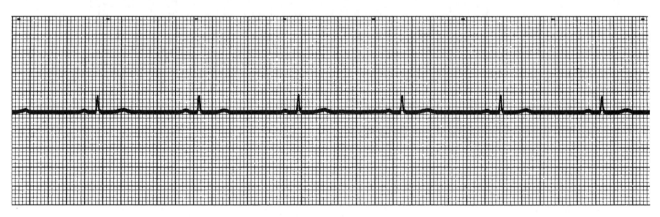

Figure 4-10.   Intermittent straight line. *Cause:* Ineffective contact between skin and electrode pad. *Solution:* Make sure hair is clipped and electrode pad is placed on clean, dry skin; if diaphoresis is a problem, prep skin surface with tincture of benzoin solution.

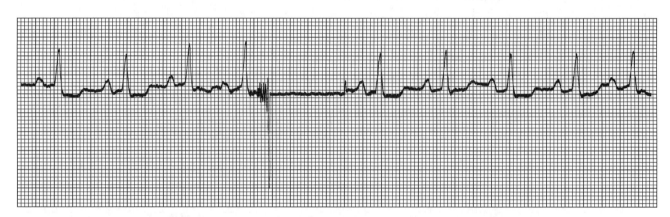

Figure 4-11.   Continuous low waveform voltage. *Cause:* Low-voltage QRS complexes. *Solution:* Turn up amplitude (gain) knob on monitor or change lead positions.

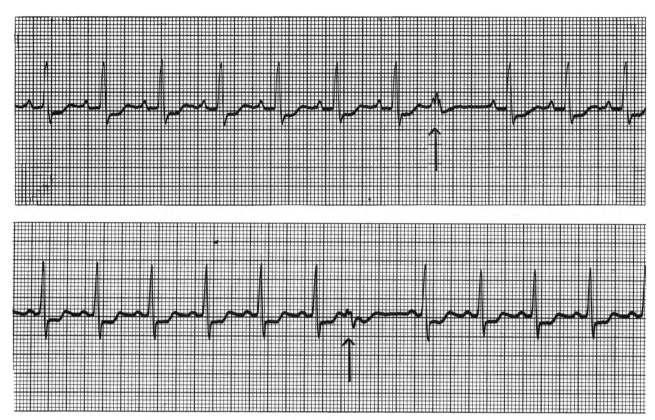

Figure 4-12.   Intermittent low waveform voltage. *Cause:* Intermittent low-voltage QRS complexes are seen in both strips above. *Solution:* If the problem is frequent and activates the low-rate alarm, change lead positions.

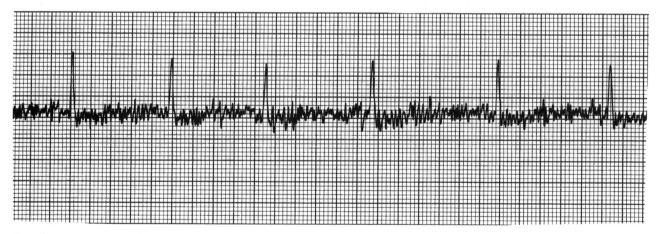

Figure 4-13.   Continuous muscle tremor. *Cause:* Muscle tremors are usually related to tense or nervous patients or those shivering from cold or a chill. *Solution:* Treat cause.

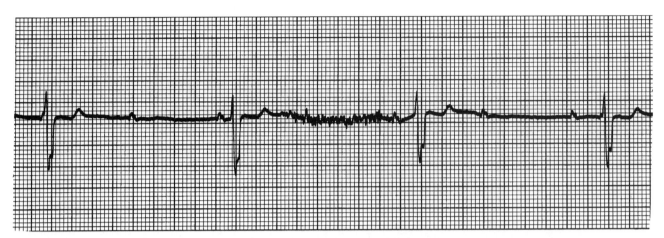

Figure 4-14. Intermittent muscle tremor. *Cause:* Muscle tremors that occur intermittently. *Solution:* Correction is usually unnecessary. *Note:* In this strip, the patient has two P waves preceding each QRS complex (second-degree atrioventricular block, Mobitz II). If the muscle tremors were continuous (as in Figure 4-13), you would be unable to identify this serious arrhythmia.

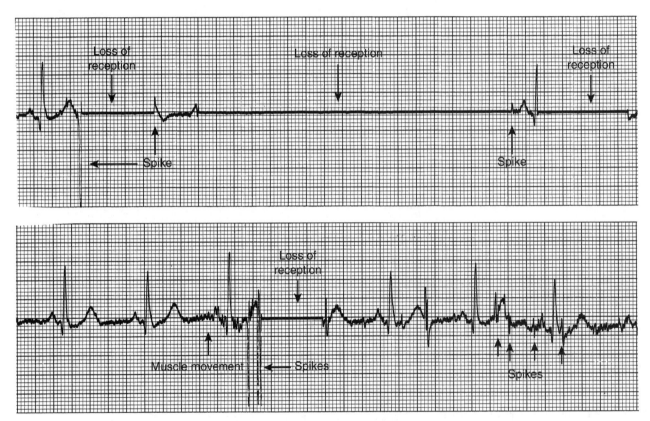

Figure 4-15. Telemetry-related interference. *Cause:* ECG signals are poorly received over the telemetry system causing sharp spikes and sometimes loss of signal reception. This problem is usually related to weak batteries or the transmitter being used in the outer fringes of the reception area for the base station receiver. *Solution:* Change batteries; keep patient in reception area of base station receivers.

■ *Telemetry-related interference* — Telemetry-related artifacts occur when the ECG signals are poorly received over a telemetry monitoring system (Figure 4-15). Weak ECG signals are caused by weak batteries or by the transmitter being used in the outer fringes of the reception area of the base station receiver, resulting in sharp spikes or straight lines on the ECG tracing.

■ *Electrical interference (AC interference)* — Electrical interference (Figure 4-16) can occur when multiple pieces of electrical equipment are in use in the patient's room;

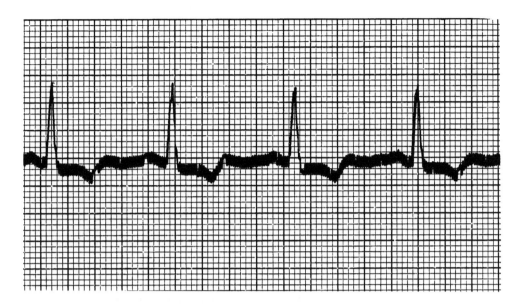

Figure 4-16. Electrical interference (AC interference). *Cause:* Patient using electrical equipment (electric razor, hair dryer); multiple electrical equipment in use in room; improperly grounded equipment; loose electrical connections or exposed wiring. *Solution:* If patient is using electrical equipment, problem is transient and will correct itself. If patient is not using electrical equipment, unplug all equipment not in continuous use, remove from service and report any equipment with breaks or wires showing, and ask the electrical engineer to check the wiring.

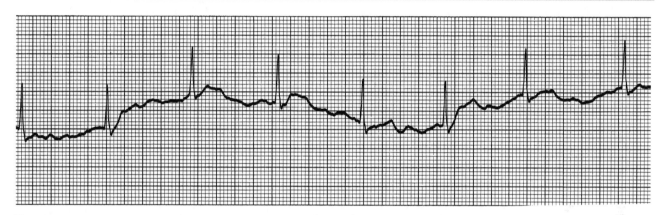

Figure 4-17. Wandering baseline. *Cause:* Exaggerated respiratory movements usually seen in patients in respiratory distress (patients with chronic obstructive pulmonary disease). *Solution:* Avoid placing electrode pads in areas where movements of the accessory muscles are most exaggerated (which can be anywhere on the anterior chest wall). Place the pads on the upper back or top of the shoulders if necessary.

when the patient is using an electrical appliance (such as an electric razor or hair dryer); when improperly grounded equipment is in use; or when loose or exposed wiring is present. This type of interference results in an artifact with a wide baseline consisting of a continuous series of fine, even, rapid spikes, which can obscure the waveforms on the ECG tracing.

■ *Wandering baseline* — A wandering baseline (Figure 4-17) is a monitor pattern that wanders up and down on the monitor screen or ECG tracing and is caused by exaggerative respiratory movements commonly seen in patients with severe pulmonary disease (for example, chronic obstructive pulmonary disease). This type of artifact makes it difficult to identify the cardiac rhythm as well as changes in the ST segment and T wave.

5 Analyzing a rhythm strip

There are five basic steps to be followed in analyzing a rhythm strip. Each step should be followed in sequence. Eventually this will become a habit and will enable you to identify a strip quickly and accurately.

Step 1: Determine the regularity (rhythm) of the R waves

Starting at the left side of the rhythm strip, place an index card above the first two R waves (Figure 5-1). Using a sharp pencil, mark on the index card above the two R waves. Measure from R wave to R wave across the rhythm strip, marking on the index card any variation in R wave regularity. If the rhythm varies by 0.12 second (3 small squares) or more between the shortest and longest R wave variation marked on the index card, the rhythm is irregular. If the rhythm doesn't vary or varies by less than 0.12 second, the rhythm is considered regular.

Calipers may also be used, instead of an index card, to determine regularity of the rhythm strip. R wave regularity is assessed in the same manner as with the index card, by placing the two caliper points on top of two consecutive R waves and proceeding left to right across the rhythm strip, noting any variation in the R-R regularity

The author prefers the index card method, because each R wave variation (however slight) can be marked and measured to determine if a 0.12-second or greater variance exists between the shorter and longer R-wave variations. With calipers, a variation in the R-wave regularity may be noted, but without marking and measuring between the shortest and longest R-wave variation, there is no way to determine how irregular the rhythm is. Examples of rhythm measurement are shown in Figures 5-2, 5-3, and 5-4.

Step 2: Calculate the heart rate

This measurement will always refer to the ventricular rate unless the atrial and ventricular rates differ, in which case both will be given. The ventricular rate is usually determined by looking at a 6-second rhythm strip. The top of the electrocardiogram paper is marked at 3-second intervals; two intervals equal 6 seconds (Figure 5-5). Several methods can be used to calculate heart rate. These methods differ according to the regularity or irregularity of the rhythm.

Regular rhythms

Two methods can be used to calculate heart rate in regular rhythms:

■ *Rapid rate calculation* — Count the number of R waves in a 6-second strip and multiply by 10 (6 seconds × 10 = 60 seconds, or the heart rate per minute). This method provides an approximate heart rate in beats per minute, is fast and simple, and can be used with both regular and irregular rhythms.

■ *Precise rate calculation* — Count the number of small squares between two consecutive R waves (Figure 5-6) and refer to the conversion table printed on the inside back cover of the book. A removable conversion table is also provided. Although this method is accurate, it can be used only for regular rhythms. If a conversion table isn't available, divide the number of small squares between the two consecutive R waves into 1500 (the number of small squares in a 1-minute rhythm strip). The heart rates for regular rhythms in the answer keys were determined by the precise rate calculation method.

Irregular rhythms

Only rapid rate calculation is used to calculate heart rate in irregular rhythms. Count the number of R waves in a 6-second strip and multiple by 10 (Figure 5-7), or count the number of R waves in a 3-second strip and multiply by 20 (3 seconds × 20 = 60 seconds, or the heart rate per minute).

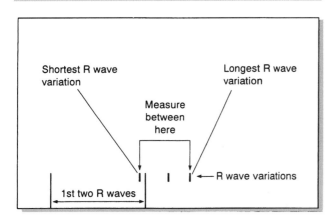

Figure 5-1. Index card.

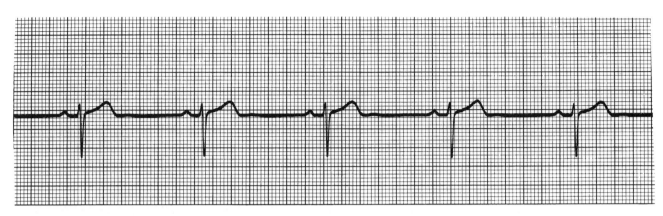

Figure 5-2. Regular rhythm; R-R intervals do not vary.

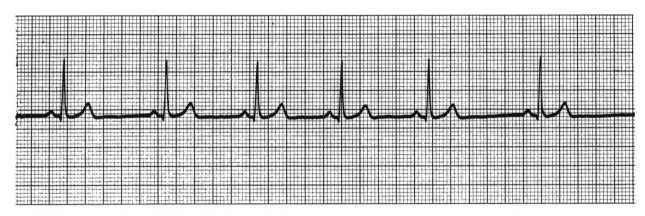

Figure 5-3. Irregular rhythm; R-R intervals vary by 0.32 second.

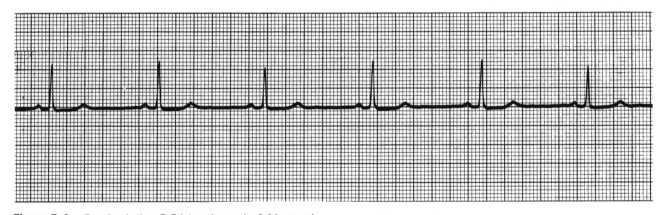

Figure 5-4. Regular rhythm; R-R intervals vary by 0.04 second.

Other hints

When rhythm strips have a premature beat (Figure 5-8), the premature beat isn't included in the calculation of the rate. In this example the first rhythm is regular and the heart rate is 68 beats per minute (22 small squares between R waves = 68).

When rhythm strips have more than one rhythm on a 6-second strip (Figure 5-9), rates must be calculated for each rhythm. This will aid in the identification of each rhythm. In the example, the first rhythm is irregular and the heart rate is 140 beats per minute (7 R waves in 3 seconds × 20 = 140). The second rhythm is regular and the heart rate is 250 beats per minute (6 small squares between R waves = 250).

When a rhythm covers less than 3 seconds on a rhythm strip (Figure 5-10), rate calculation is difficult, but not impossible. In the example, the first rhythm takes up half of a 3-second interval. There are only two R waves.

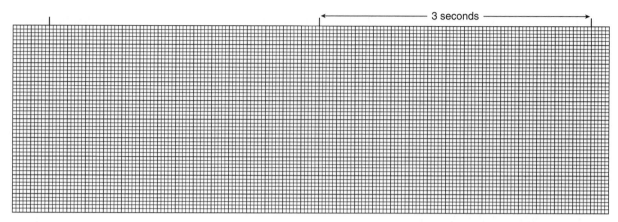

Figure 5-5. ECG graph paper.

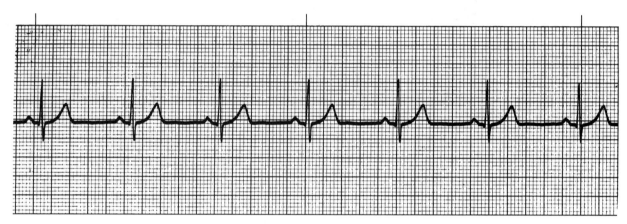

Figure 5-6. Regular rhythm; 25 small squares between R waves = 60 heart rate.

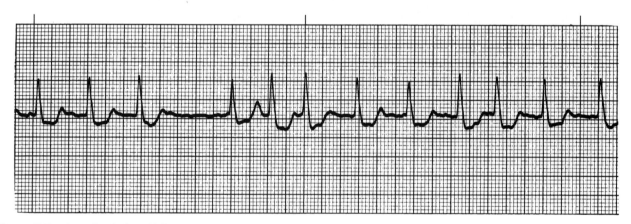

Figure 5-7. Irregular rhythm; 11 R waves × 10 = 110 heart rate.

Therefore, you can't determine if the rhythm is regular or irregular. In this situation, multiply the two R waves by 40 (1½ second × 40 = 60 seconds, or the heart rate per minute) to obtain an approximate heart rate of 80 beats per minute. The second rhythm is regular, with a heart rate of 167 beats per minute (9 small squares between R waves = 167).

As you have seen, rhythm strips may have one rhythm or several rhythms. Therefore, each rhythm strip may have one answer or several answers. Figures 5-8, 5-9, and 5-10 have two different rhythms and thus two different answers. Each rhythm on the strip must be analyzed separately. When interpreting a rhythm strip, describe the basic underlying rhythm first, then add additional information,

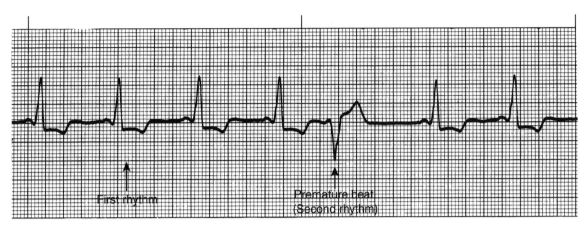

Figure 5-8.   Rhythm with premature beat.

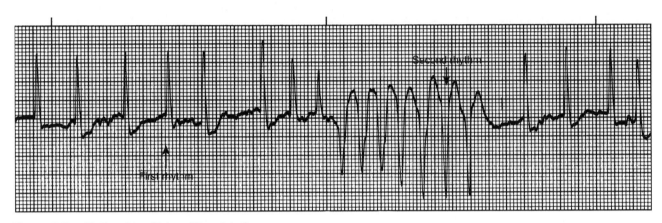

Figure 5-9.   Rhythm strip with two different rhythms.

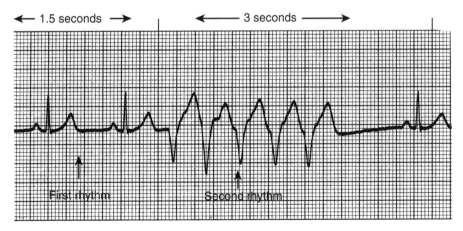

Figure 5-10.   Calculating rate when a rhythm covers less than 3 seconds.

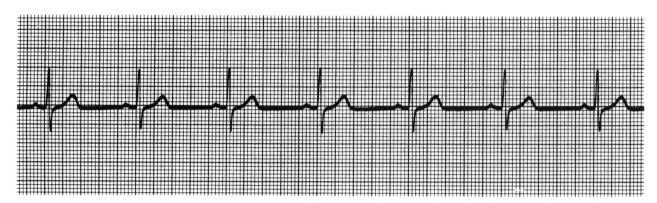

Figure 5-11.   Normal P waves.

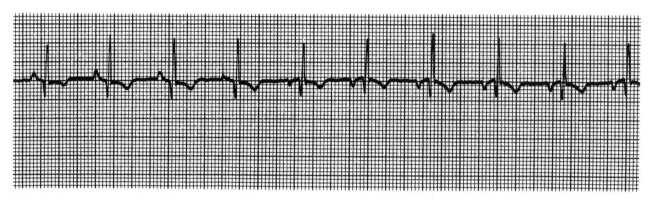

Figure 5-12.   Abnormal P waves.

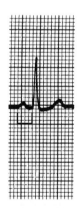

Figure 5-13.   PR interval 0.16 second.

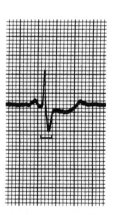

Figure 5-14.   QRS complex 0.12 second.

Box 5-1.
Rhythm strip analysis

1. Determine regularity (rhythm).
2. Calculate rate.
3. Examine P waves.
4. Measure PR interval.
5. Measure QRS complex.

such as normal sinus rhythm with one premature ventricular contraction (PVC) (Figure 5-8).

Step 3: Identify and examine P waves

Analyze the P waves; one P wave should precede each QRS complex. All P waves should be identical (or near identical) in size, shape, and position. In Figure 5-11

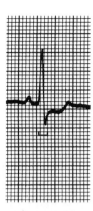

Figure 5-15.   QRS complex 0.10 second.

there is one P wave to each QRS complex, and all P waves are the same in size, shape, and position. In Figure 5-12 there is one P wave to each QRS complex, but the P waves vary in size, shape, and position across the rhythm strip.

Step 4: Measure the PR interval

Measure from the beginning of the P wave as it leaves baseline to the beginning of the QRS complex. Count the number of small squares contained in this interval and multiply by 0.04 second. In Figure 5-13 the PR interval is 0.16 second (4 small squares × 0.04 second = 0.16 second).

Step 5: Measure the QRS complex

Measure from the beginning of the QRS complex as it leaves baseline until the end of the QRS complex when the ST segment begins. Count the number of small squares in this measurement and multiply by 0.04 second. In Figure 5-14 the QRS complex takes up 3 small squares and represents 0.12 second (3 small squares × 0.04 second = 0.12 second). In Figure 5-15 the QRS complex takes up 2½ small squares and represents 0.10 second (2½ small squares x 0.04 second = 0.10 second).

If rhythm strips are analyzed using a systematic step-by-step approach (Box 5-1), accurate interpretation will be achieved most of the time.

Rhythm strip practice: Analyzing rhythm strips

Analyze the following rhythm strips using the five-step process discussed in this chapter. Check your answers with the answer key in the appendix.

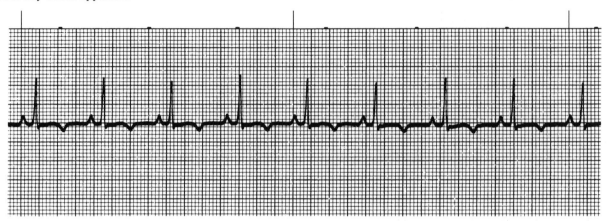

Strip 5-1. Rhythm: _____ Rate: _____ P wave: _____

PR interval: _____ QRS complex: _____

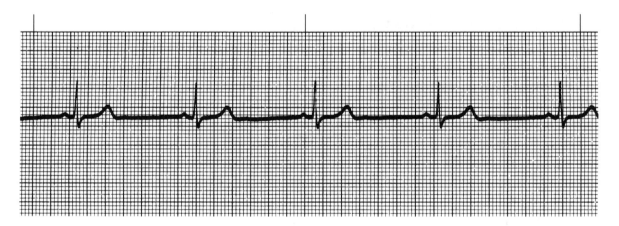

Strip 5-2. Rhythm: _____ Rate: _____ P wave: _____

PR interval: _____ QRS complex: _____

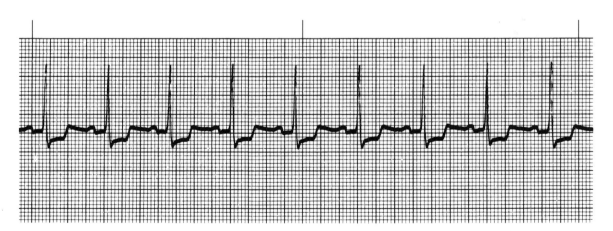

Strip 5-3. Rhythm: _____ Rate: _____ P wave: _____

PR interval: _____ QRS complex: _____

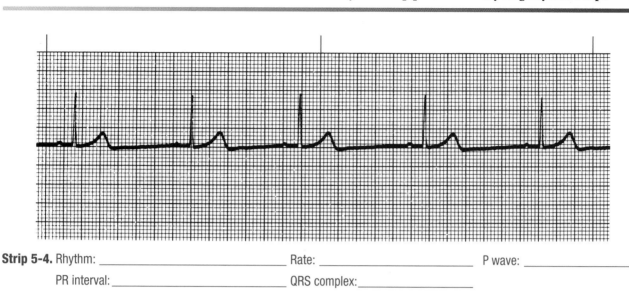

Strip 5-4. Rhythm: _____ Rate: _____ P wave: _____

PR interval: _____ QRS complex: _____

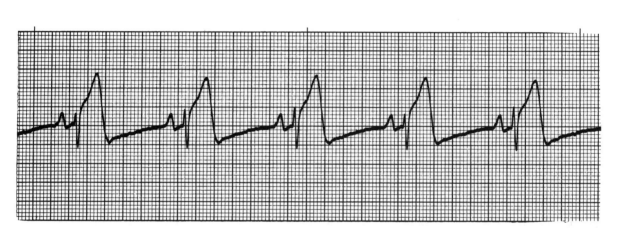

Strip 5-5. Rhythm: _____ Rate: _____ P wave: _____

PR interval: _____ QRS complex: _____

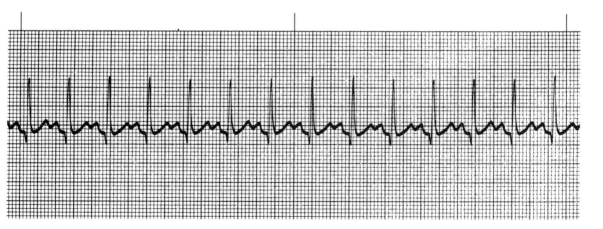

Strip 5-6. Rhythm: _____ Rate: _____ P wave: _____

PR interval: _____ QRS complex: _____

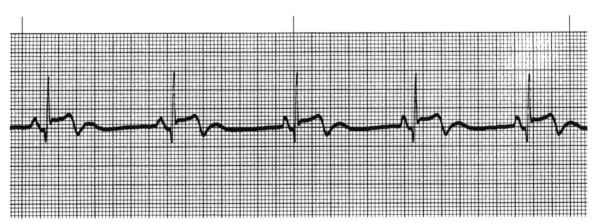

Strip 5-7. Rhythm: _____ Rate: _____ P wave: _____

PR interval: _____ QRS complex: _____

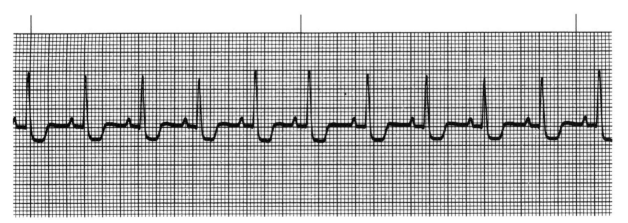

Strip 5-8. Rhythm: _____ Rate: _____ P wave: _____

PR interval: _____ QRS complex: _____

Strip 5-9. Rhythm: _____ Rate: _____ P wave: _____

PR interval: _____ QRS complex: _____

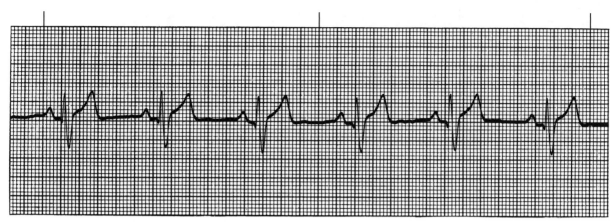

Strip 5-10. Rhythm: _____ Rate: _____ P wave: _____

PR interval: _____ QRS complex: _____

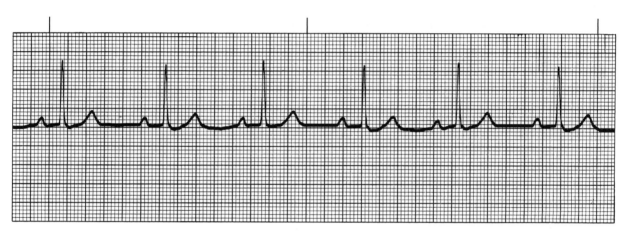

Strip 5-11. Rhythm: _____ Rate: _____ P wave: _____

PR interval: _____ QRS complex: _____

6 Sinus arrhythmias

Overview

The term *arrhythmia* (also called *dysrhythmia*) is very general, referring to all rhythms other than the normal rhythm of the heart (normal sinus rhythm). Sinus arrhythmias (Figure 6-1) result from disturbances in impulse discharge or impulse conduction from the sinus node. The sinus node retains its role as pacemaker of the heart, but discharges impulses too fast (sinus tachycardia) or too slow (sinus bradycardia); discharges impulses irregularly (sinus arrhythmia); fails to discharge an impulse (sinus arrest); or the impulse discharged is blocked as it exits the sinoatrial (SA) node (SA exit block). Sinus bradycardia, sinus tachycardia, sinus arrhythmia, sinus arrest, and sinus block are all considered arrhythmias. However, sinus bradycardia at rest, sinus tachycardia with exercise, and sinus arrhythmia associated with the phases of respiration are considered normal responses of the heart.

Normal sinus rhythm

Normal sinus rhythm (Figure 6-2 and Box 6-1) reflects the heart's normal electrical activity. The SA node normally initiates impulses at a rate of 60 to 100 beats per minute.

Since this rate is faster than other pacemaker sites in the conduction system, the SA node retains control as the primary pacemaker of the heart. Sinus rhythm originates in the SA node and the impulse follows the normal conduction pathway through the atria, the AV node, the bundle branches, and the ventricles, resulting in normal atrial and ventricular depolarization.

Box 6-1.

Normal sinus rhythm: Identifying ECG features

Rhythm:	Regular
Rate:	60 to 100 beats/minute
P waves:	Normal in size, shape, and direction; positive in lead II; one P wave precedes each QRS complex
PR interval:	Normal (0.12 to 0.20 second)
QRS complex:	Normal (0.10 second or less)

Normal sinus rhythm is regular with a heart rate between 60 and 100 beats per minute. The P waves are normal in size, shape, and direction; positive in lead II (a positive lead), with one P wave preceding each QRS complex. The duration of the PR interval and the QRS complex is within

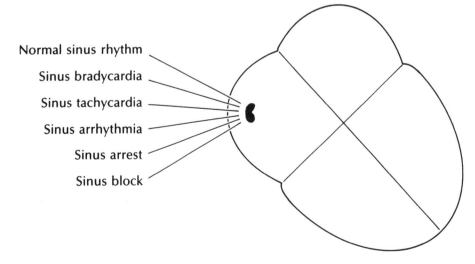

Normal sinus rhythm
Sinus bradycardia
Sinus tachycardia
Sinus arrhythmia
Sinus arrest
Sinus block

Figure 6-1. Sinus arrhythmias.

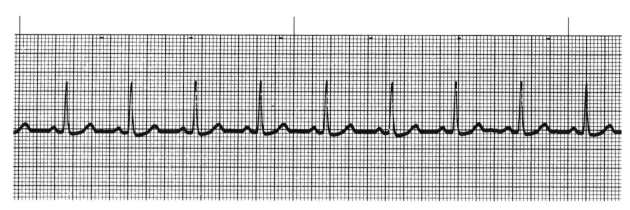

Figure 6-2.   Normal sinus rhythm.
Rhythm: Regular
Rate: 84 beats/minute
P waves: Normal and precede each QRS
PR interval: 0.14 to 0.16 second
QRS complex: 0.06 to 0.08 second.

normal limits. Normal sinus rhythm is the normal rhythm of the heart. No treatment is indicated.

Sinus tachycardia

Sinus tachycardia (Figure 6-3 and Box 6-2) is a rhythm that originates in the sinus node and discharges impulses regularly at a rate between 100 and 160 beats per minute. The P waves are normal in size, shape, and direction; positive in lead II (a positive lead), with one P wave preceding each QRS complex. The duration of the PR interval and the QRS complex is within normal limits. The distinguishing feature of this rhythm is the sinus origin and the rate between 100 and 160 beats per minute.

Box 6-2.

Sinus tachycardia: Identifying ECG features

Rhythm:	Regular
Rate:	100 to 160 beats/minute
P waves:	Normal in size, shape, and direction; positive in lead II; one P wave precedes each QRS complex
PR interval:	Normal (0.12 to 0.20 second)
QRS complex:	Normal (0.10 second or less)

Sinus tachycardia is the normal response of the heart to the body's demand for an increase in blood flow (for example, exercise). The sinus node increases its rate in response to an increased need. When needs decrease, the

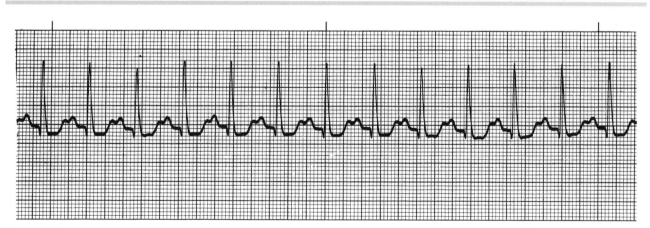

Figure 6-3.   Sinus tachycardia.
Rhythm: Regular
Rate: 115 beats/minute
P waves: Sinus
PR interval: 0.16 to 0.18 second
QRS complex: 0.08 to 0.10 second.

heart rate slows down. Sinus tachycardia begins and ends gradually in contrast to other tachycardias, which begin and end suddenly.

Sinus tachycardia can be caused by anything that increases sympathetic tone or anything that decreases parasympathetic tone. Factors commonly associated with sinus tachycardia are:

- anxiety, excitement, stress, exertion, exercise
- fever, anemia, shock
- hypoxia, hypovolemia, hypotension, heart failure, hyperthyroidism
- pain, pulmonary embolism (sinus tachycardia is the most common arrhythmia seen with pulmonary embolism)
- myocardial ischemia, myocardial infarction (MI) (sinus tachycardia persisting after an acute infarct implies extensive heart damage and is generally a bad prognostic sign)
- drugs that increase sympathetic tone (epinephrine, norepinephrine, dopamine, dobutamine, tricyclic antidepressants, isoproterenol, and nitroprusside)
- drugs that decrease parasympathetic tone (atropine)
- use of substances such as caffeine, cocaine, and nicotine.

Sinus tachycardia is usually a benign arrhythmia and treatment is directed at correcting the underlying cause (relief of pain, fluid replacement, removal of offending medications or substances, and reducing fever or anxiety). However, persistent sinus tachycardia should never be ignored in any patient, especially the cardiac patient. A rapid heart rate increases the workload of the heart and its oxygen requirements and may cause a decreased stroke volume leading to a decrease in cardiac output. In addition, heart rates higher than normal decrease the amount of time the heart spends in diastole, leading to a decrease in coronary artery perfusion (coronary arteries are perfused during diastole). Sinus tachycardia that persists may be one of the first signs of early heart failure.

Sinus bradycardia

Sinus bradycardia (Figure 6-4 and Box 6-3) is a rhythm that originates in the SA node and discharges impulses regularly at a rate between 40 and 60 beats per minute. The P waves are normal in size, shape, and direction; positive in lead II (a positive lead), with one P wave preceding each QRS complex. The duration of the PR interval and the QRS complex is within normal limits. The distinguishing feature of this rhythm is the sinus origin and a heart rate between 40 and 60 beats per minute.

Box 6-3.

Sinus bradycardia: Identifying ECG features

Rhythm:	Regular
Rate:	40 to 60 beats/minute
P waves:	Normal in size, shape, and direction; positive in lead II; one P wave precedes each QRS complex
PR interval:	Normal (0.12 to 0.20 second)
QRS complex:	Normal (0.10 second or less)

Sinus bradycardia is the normal response of the heart to relaxation or sleeping when the parasympathetic effect on cardiac automaticity dominates over the sympathetic effect. It's common among trained athletes who may have a resting or sleeping pulse rate as low as 35 beats per minute. Mild bradycardia may actually be beneficial in some patients (for example, acute MI) because of the decrease in workload on the heart.

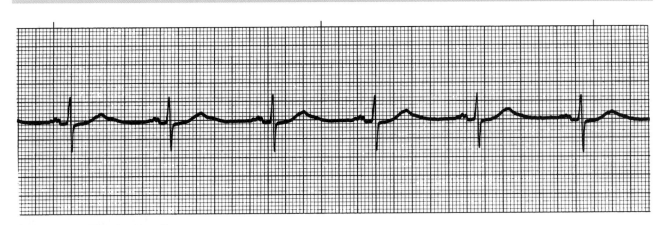

Figure 6-4.   Sinus bradycardia.

Rhythm:	Regular
Rate:	54 beats/minute
P waves:	Sinus
PR interval:	0.20 second
QRS complex:	0.06 to 0.08 second
Note:	A notched P wave is usually indicative of left atrial hypertrophy.

Sinus bradycardia can be caused by anything that increases parasympathetic tone or anything that decreases sympathetic tone. It commonly occurs with the following:

- during sleep and in athletes
- in acute inferior wall MI involving the right coronary artery, which usually supplies blood to the SA node
- as a reperfusion rhythm after coronary angioplasty or after treatment with thrombolytics
- vagal stimulation from vomiting, bearing down (Valsalva's maneuver), or carotid sinus pressure
- as a vasovagal reaction. A vasovagal reaction is an extreme body response that causes a marked decrease in heart rate (due to vagal stimulation) and a marked decrease in blood pressure (due to vasodilation). This reaction may occur with pain, nausea, vomiting, fright, or sudden stressful situations. The combination of extreme bradycardia and hypotension may result in fainting (vasovagal syncope). The situation is usually reversed when the individual is placed into a recumbent position, thereby increasing venous return to the heart. If fainting occurs with the individual in a recumbent position, it can usually be reversed with leg elevation.
- carotid sinus hypersensitivity syndrome, sleep apnea
- decreased metabolic rate (hypothyroidism, hypothermia); hyperkalemia
- sudden movement from recumbent to an upright position (common in the elderly)
- increased intracranial pressure (a sudden appearance of sinus bradycardia in a patient with cerebral edema or subdural hematoma is an important clinical observation)
- drugs such as digoxin, calcium channel blockers, and beta blockers
- degenerative disease of the sinus node (sick sinus syndrome). Persistent sinus bradycardia is the most common and often the earliest manifestation of sick sinus syndrome. Sick sinus syndrome is a dysfunctioning sinus node, which is manifested on the ECG by marked bradyarrhythmias alternating with episodes of tachyarrhythmias and is commonly accompanied by symptoms such as dizziness, fainting episodes, chest pain, shortness of breath, and heart failure. This syndrome has also been called *tachy-brady syndrome*. Permanent pacemaker implantation is recommended once patients become symptomatic.

Sinus bradycardia doesn't require treatment unless the patient becomes symptomatic. Some clinical signs and symptoms requiring treatment include cold, clammy skin; hypotension; shortness of breath, chest pain, changes in mental status, decrease in urine output, and heart failure. If sinus bradycardia persists, the treatment of choice is atropine, a drug that increases the heart rate by decreasing parasympathetic tone. The usual dose is 0.5 mg IV push every 5 minutes until the bradycardia is resolved or a maximum dose of 3 mg is given. Atropine must be administered correctly; atropine administered too slowly or in doses less than 0.5 mg can further decrease the heart rate instead of increasing it. If the rhythm still doesn't resolve after the atropine is administered, a transcutaneous (external) or transvenous pacemaker may be needed. All medications that cause a decrease in heart rate should be reviewed and discontinued if indicated. For chronic bradycardia, permanent pacing may be indicated.

Sinus arrhythmia

Sinus arrhythmia (Figure 6-5 and Box 6-4) is a rhythm that originates in the sinus node and discharges impulses irregularly. The heart rate may be normal (60 to 100 beats per minute) or slow (commonly associated with a bradycardic

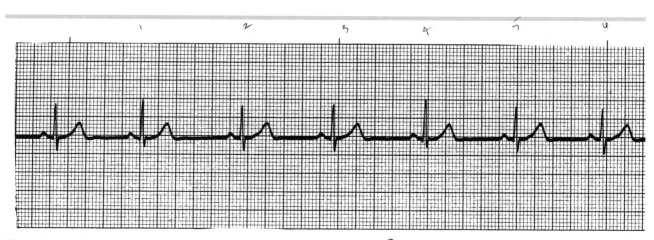

Figure 6-5.   Sinus arrhythmia

Rhythm:	Irregular
Rate:	60 beats/minute
P waves:	Normal in configuration; precede each QRS
PR interval:	0.12 to 0.14 second
QRS complex:	0.06 to 0.08 second

Box 6-4.
Sinus arrhythmia: Identifying ECG features

Rhythm:	Irregular
Rate:	Normal (60 to 100 beats/minute) or slow (less than 60 beats/minute)
P waves:	Normal in size, shape, and direction; positive in lead II; one P wave precedes each QRS complex
PR interval:	Normal (0.12 to 0.20 second)
QRS complex:	Normal (0.10 second or less)

rate). The P waves are normal in size, shape, and direction; positive in lead II (a positive lead), with one P wave preceding each QRS complex. The duration of the PR interval and the QRS complex is within normal limits. The distinguishing feature of this rhythm is the sinus origin and the rhythm irregularity.

Sinus arrhythmia is commonly associated with the phases of respiration. During inspiration, the sinus node fires faster; during expiration, it slows down. This rhythm is an extremely common finding among infants, children, and young adults, but may occur in any age-group. Sinus arrhythmia is a normal phenomenon that usually doesn't require treatment unless it is accompanied by a bradycardia rate that causes symptoms.

Sinus pause (sinus arrest and sinus exit block)

Sinus pause is a broad term used to describe rhythms in which there is a sudden failure of the SA node to initiate or conduct an impulse. Two rhythms fall under this category:

sinus arrest and *sinus exit block*. Sinus arrest and sinus exit block, two separate arrhythmias with different pathophysiologies (Figures 6-6, 6-7, and 6-8 and Box 6-5), are discussed together because distinguishing between them is at times difficult, and because their treatment and clinical significance are the same.

Box 6-5.
Sinus arrest and sinus exit block: Identifying ECG features

Rhythm:	Basic rhythm usually regular; there is a sudden pause in the basic rhythm (causing irregularity) with one or more missing beats; heart rate may slow down for several beats after pause (temporary rate suppression) but returns to basic rate
Rate:	That of underlying rhythm, usually sinus
P waves:	Sinus P waves with basic rhythm; absent during pause
PR interval:	Normal (0.12 to 0.20 second) with basic rhythm; absent during pause
QRS complex:	Normal (0.10 second or less) with basic rhythm; absent during pause

Differentiating features

Sinus block:	Basic rhythm (R-R regularity) resumes on time after pause
Sinus arrest:	Basic rhythm (R-R regularity) doesn't resume on time after pause

Both sinus arrest and sinus exit block originate in the sinus node and are characterized by a sudden pause in the sinus rhythm in which one or more beats (cardiac cycles)

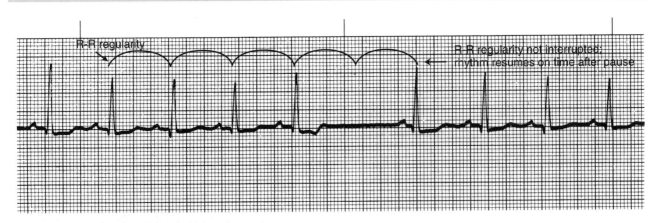

Figure 6-6.   Normal sinus rhythm with sinus block.

Rhythm:	Basic rhythm regular; irregular during pause
Rate:	Basic rhythm 84 beats/minute
P waves:	Normal in basic rhythm; absent during pause
PR interval:	0.16 to 0.18 second in basic rhythm; absent during pause
QRS complex:	0.08 to 0.10 second in basic rhythm; absent during pause
Comment:	ST-segment depression is present.

R-R regularity

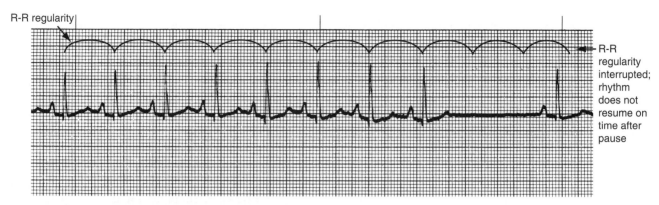

R-R regularity interrupted; rhythm does not resume on time after pause

Figure 6-7.   Normal sinus rhythm with sinus arrest.
Rhythm: Basic rhythm regular, irregular during pause
Rate: Basic rhythm 94 beats/minute
P waves: Normal in basic rhythm; absent during pause
PR interval: 0.16 to 0.18 second in basic rhythm; absent during pause
QRS complex: 0.06 to 0.08 second in basic rhythm; absent during pause.

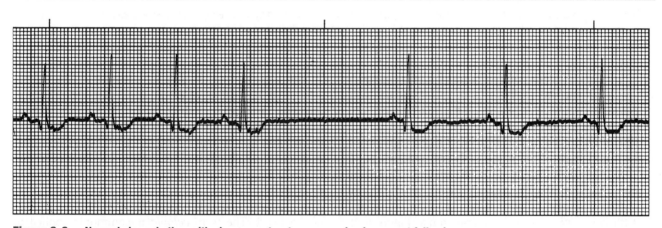

Figure 6-8.   Normal sinus rhythm with sinus arrest; rate suppression is present following pause.
Rhythm: Basic rhythm regular; irregular during pause
Rate: Basic rhythm rate 84 beats/minute; rate slows to 56 beats/minute following pause (temporary rate suppression may occur
                   following a pause in the basic rhythm)
P waves: Sinus in basic rhythm; absent during pause
PR interval: 0.16 to 0.18 second in basic rhythm; absent during pause
QRS complex: 0.08 to 0.10 second in basic rhythm; absent during pause.

are missing. The P waves in the underlying rhythm will be normal in size, shape, and direction; positive in lead II (a positive lead), with one P wave preceding each QRS complex. The duration of the PR interval and the QRS complex in the underlying rhythm is within normal limits. The distinguishing feature of both rhythms is the abrupt pause in the underlying sinus rhythm in which one or more beats are missing, followed by a resumption of the basic rhythm after the pause.

Sinus arrest is caused by a failure of the SA node to initiate an impulse and is therefore a disorder of automaticity. This failure in the automaticity of the SA node upsets

the timing of the sinus node discharge, and the underlying rhythm won't resume on time after the pause.

With sinus exit block, an electrical impulse is initiated by the SA node, but is blocked as it exits the sinus node, preventing conduction of the impulse to the atria. Thus, SA exit block is a disorder of conductivity. Because the regularity of the sinus node discharge isn't interrupted (just blocked), the underlying rhythm will resume on time after the pause. Once the rhythm resumes after the pause (in both sinus arrest and sinus exit block) it's common for the rate to be slower for several cycles (*rate suppression*). Rate

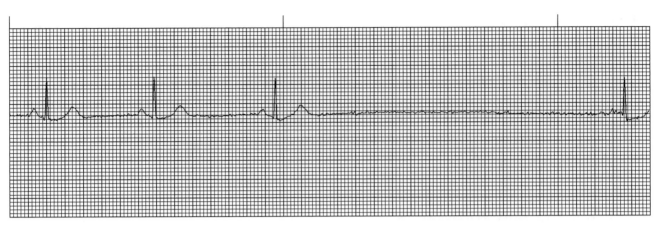

Figure 6-9. **Sinus arrhythmia with sinus pause.**

Rhythm: Basic rhythm irregular

Rate: 60 beats/minute

P waves: Normal in basic rhythm; absent during pause

PR interval: 0.14 to 0.16 second in basic rhythm; absent during pause

QRS complex: 0.06 to 0.08 second in basic rhythm; absent during pause

Comment: Because of the irregularity of the basic rhythm, sinus arrest can't be differentiated from sinus block, and the rhythm is interpreted using the broad term *sinus pause,* indicating that either rhythm could be present.

suppression is temporary and will cause a brief irregularity in the underlying rhythm, but after several cycles the basic rate and rhythm will return. An example of rate suppression is shown in Figure 6-8.

Differentiating between the two rhythms involves comparing the length of the pause with the underlying P-P or R-R interval to determine if the underlying rhythm resumes on time after the pause. This can be determined only if the underlying rhythm is regular. If the underlying rhythm is irregular, as in sinus arrhythmia (Figure 6-9), it's impossible to distinguish sinus arrest from sinus exit block. In this case, the rhythm would best be interpreted using the broad term *sinus pause*, indicating that either rhythm could be present. From a clinical viewpoint, distinguishing between sinus arrest and sinus exit block usually isn't essential.

Sinus arrest or sinus exit block can be caused by numerous factors, including:
- increase in vagal (parasympathetic) tone on the SA node
- myocardial ischemia or infarction
- use of certain drugs such as digoxin, beta blockers, or calcium channel blockers.

The patient may become symptomatic if the pauses associated with sinus arrest or sinus exit block are frequent or prolonged. Another danger is that the SA node may lose pacemaker control. When the sinus node slows down below its minimum firing rate of 60 beats per minute because of bradycardia or a pause in the underlying rhythm, an opportunity is provided for pacemaker cells in other areas of the conduction system to usurp control from the sinus node and become the dominant pacemaker of the heart. The term *ectopic* is commonly applied to rhythms that originate from any site other than the SA node. Ectopic sites in the atria, AV node, or ventricles may assume pacemaker control for one beat, several beats, or continuously.

If symptomatic, the rhythm is treated the same as in symptomatic sinus bradycardia. In addition, all medications that depress sinus node discharge or conduction should be stopped.

A summary of the identifying ECG features of sinus arrhythmias can be found in Table 6-1.

Table 6-1.

Sinus arrhythmias: Summary of identifying ECG features

	Rhythm	Rate (beats/minute)	P waves (lead II)	PR interval	QRS complex
Normal sinus rhythm	Regular	60 to 100	Positive in lead II; normal in size, shape, and direction; one P wave precedes each QRS complex	Normal (0.12 to 0.20 second)	Normal (0.10 second or less)
Sinus bradycardia	Regular	40 to 60	Positive in lead II; normal in size, shape, and direction; one P wave precedes each QRS complex	Normal (0.12 to 0.20 second)	Normal (0.10 second or less)
Sinus tachycardia	Regular	100 to 160	Positive in lead II; normal in size, shape, and direction; one P wave precedes each QRS complex	Normal (0.12 to 0.20 second)	Normal (0.10 second or less)
Sinus arrhythmia	Irregular	60 to 100 (normal) or < 60 (slow)	Positive in lead II; normal in size, shape, and direction; one P wave precedes each QRS complex	Normal (0.12 to 0.20 second)	Normal (0.10 second or less)
Sinus block and sinus arrest	Basic rhythm usually regular; there is a sudden pause in the basic rhythm (causing irregularity) with one or more missing beats; temporary rate suppression common following pause	That of underlying rhythm, usually sinus	Sinus P waves with basic rhythm; absent during pause	Normal (0.12 to 0.20 second) with basic rhythm; absent during pause	Normal (0.10 second or less) with basic rhythm; absent during pause
Differentiating features Sinus block:	Basic rhythm resumes on time after pause				
Sinus arrest:	Basic rhythm does not resume on time after pause				

Note: If the basic rhythm is irregular (sinus arrhythmia), sinus arrest can't be differentiated from sinus block, and the rhythm is interpreted as sinus arrhythmia with sinus pause.

Rhythm strip practice: Sinus arrhythmias

Analyze the following rhythm strips by following the five basic steps:

■ Determine *rhythm regularity.*
■ Calculate *heart rate* (this usually refers to the ventricular rate, but if atrial rate differs you need to calculate both).
■ Identify and examine *P waves.*

■ Measure *PR interval.*
■ Measure *QRS complex.*

Interpret the rhythm by comparing this data with the ECG characteristics for each rhythm. All rhythm strips are lead II, a positive lead, unless otherwise noted. Check your answers with the answer keys in the appendix.

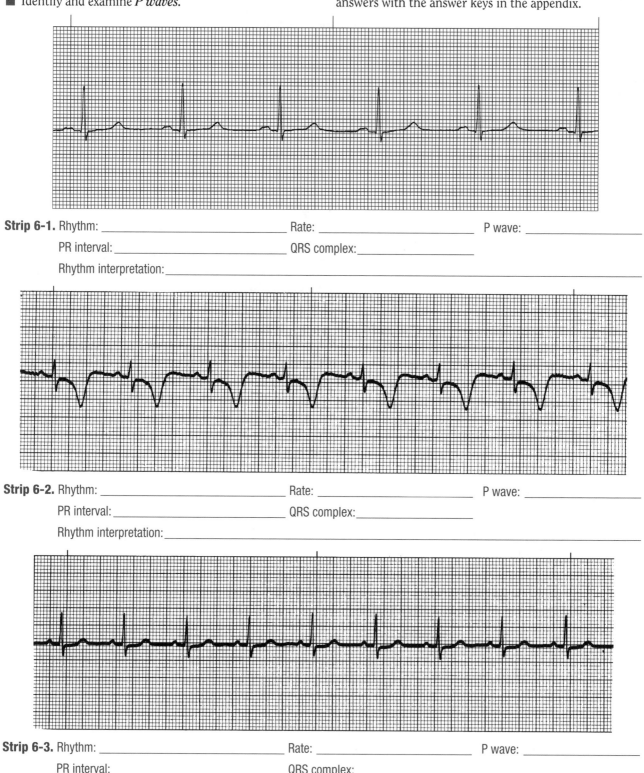

Strip 6-1. Rhythm: _____ Rate: _____ P wave: _____

PR interval: _____ QRS complex: _____

Rhythm interpretation: _____

Strip 6-2. Rhythm: _____ Rate: _____ P wave: _____

PR interval: _____ QRS complex: _____

Rhythm interpretation: _____

Strip 6-3. Rhythm: _____ Rate: _____ P wave: _____

PR interval: _____ QRS complex: _____

Rhythm interpretation: _____

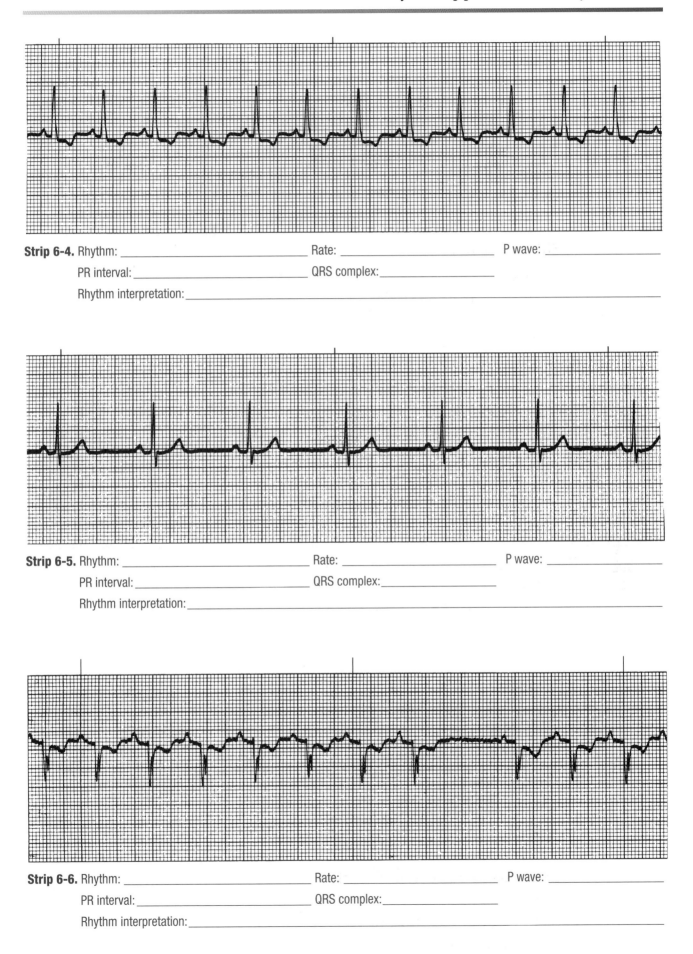

Strip 6-4. Rhythm: _____ Rate: _____ P wave: _____

PR interval: _____ QRS complex: _____

Rhythm interpretation: _____

Strip 6-5. Rhythm: _____ Rate: _____ P wave: _____

PR interval: _____ QRS complex: _____

Rhythm interpretation: _____

Strip 6-6. Rhythm: _____ Rate: _____ P wave: _____

PR interval: _____ QRS complex: _____

Rhythm interpretation: _____

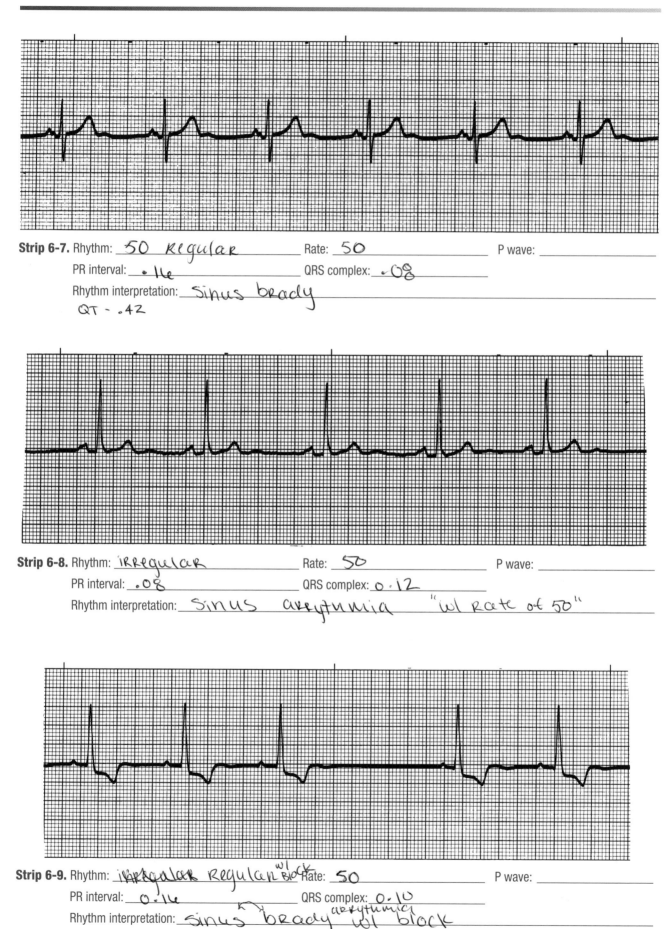

Strip 6-7. Rhythm: _50 Regular_   Rate: _50_   P wave: _____
PR interval: _.16_   QRS complex: _.08_
Rhythm interpretation: _Sinus brady_
QT - .42

Strip 6-8. Rhythm: _irregular_   Rate: _50_   P wave: _____
PR interval: _.08_   QRS complex: _0.12_
Rhythm interpretation: _Sinus arrythmia   "w/ rate of 50"_

Strip 6-9. Rhythm: _irregular Regular w/ Block_   Rate: _50_   P wave: _____
PR interval: _0.16_   QRS complex: _0.10_
Rhythm interpretation: _Sinus brady arrythmia w/ block_
ST depressions

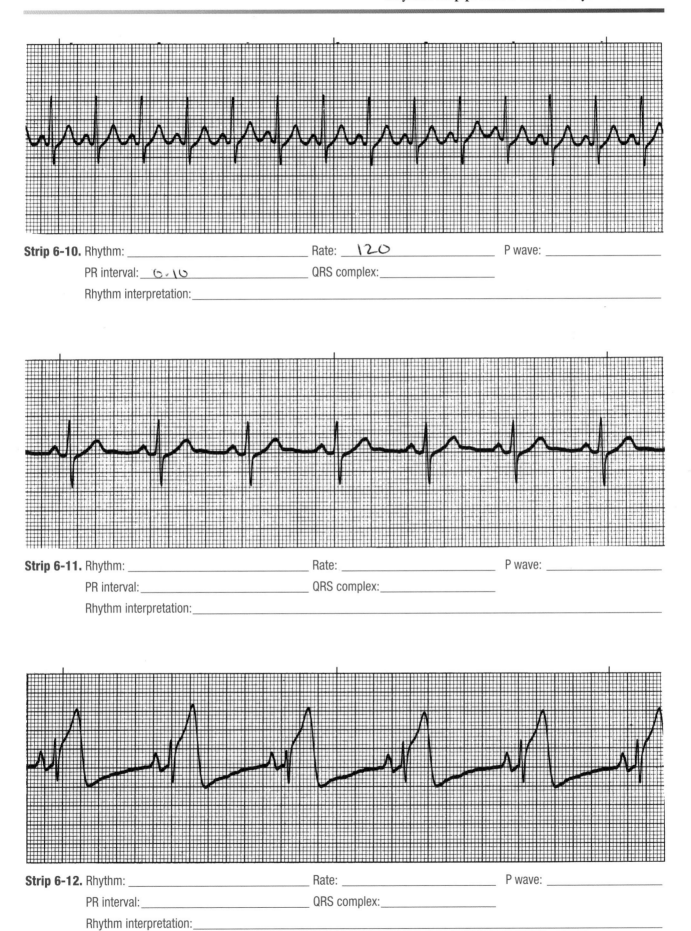

Strip 6-10. Rhythm: _____ Rate: ___120_____ P wave: _____

PR interval: ___6.16_____ QRS complex:_____

Rhythm interpretation:_____

Strip 6-11. Rhythm: _____ Rate: _____ P wave: _____

PR interval:_____ QRS complex:_____

Rhythm interpretation:_____

Strip 6-12. Rhythm: _____ Rate: _____ P wave: _____

PR interval:_____ QRS complex:_____

Rhythm interpretation:_____

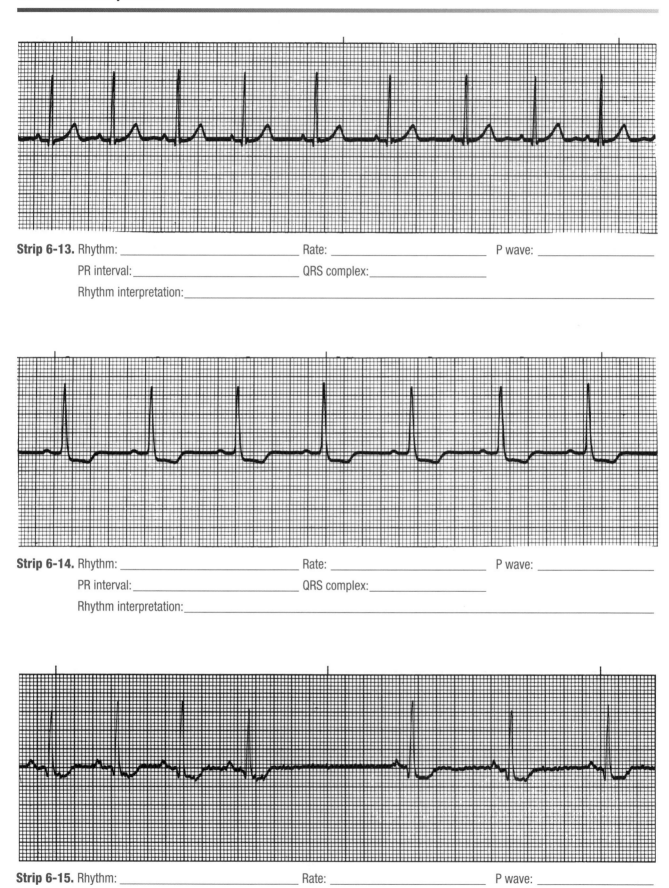

Strip 6-13. Rhythm: _____ Rate: _____ P wave: _____

PR interval: _____ QRS complex: _____

Rhythm interpretation: _____

Strip 6-14. Rhythm: _____ Rate: _____ P wave: _____

PR interval: _____ QRS complex: _____

Rhythm interpretation: _____

Strip 6-15. Rhythm: _____ Rate: _____ P wave: _____

PR interval: _____ QRS complex: _____

Rhythm interpretation: _____

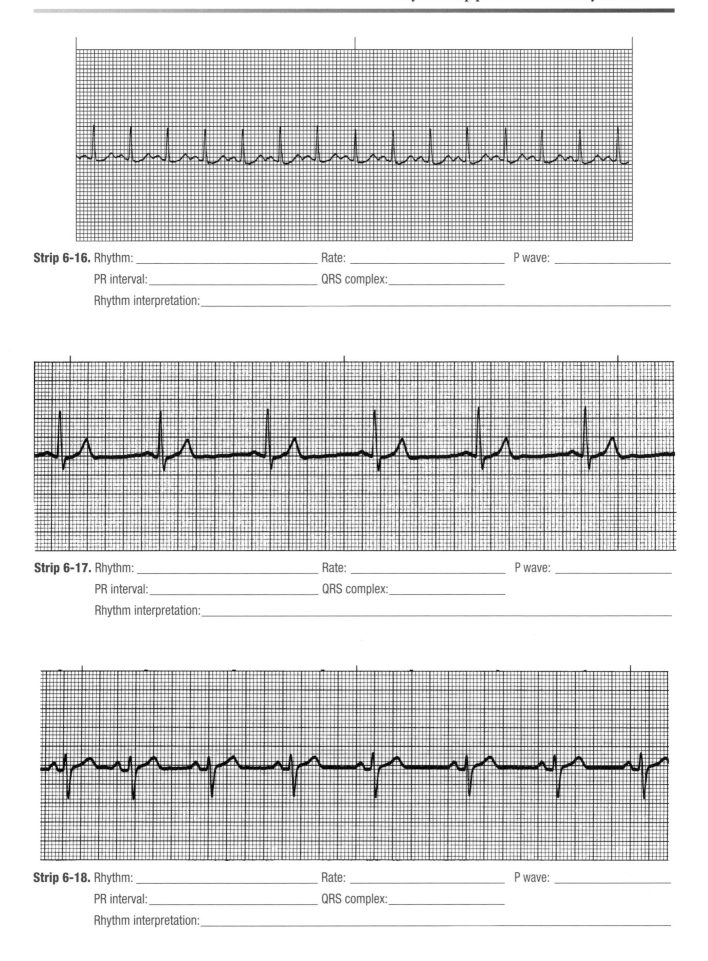

Strip 6-16. Rhythm: _____ Rate: _____ P wave: _____

PR interval: _____ QRS complex: _____

Rhythm interpretation: _____

Strip 6-17. Rhythm: _____ Rate: _____ P wave: _____

PR interval: _____ QRS complex: _____

Rhythm interpretation: _____

Strip 6-18. Rhythm: _____ Rate: _____ P wave: _____

PR interval: _____ QRS complex: _____

Rhythm interpretation: _____

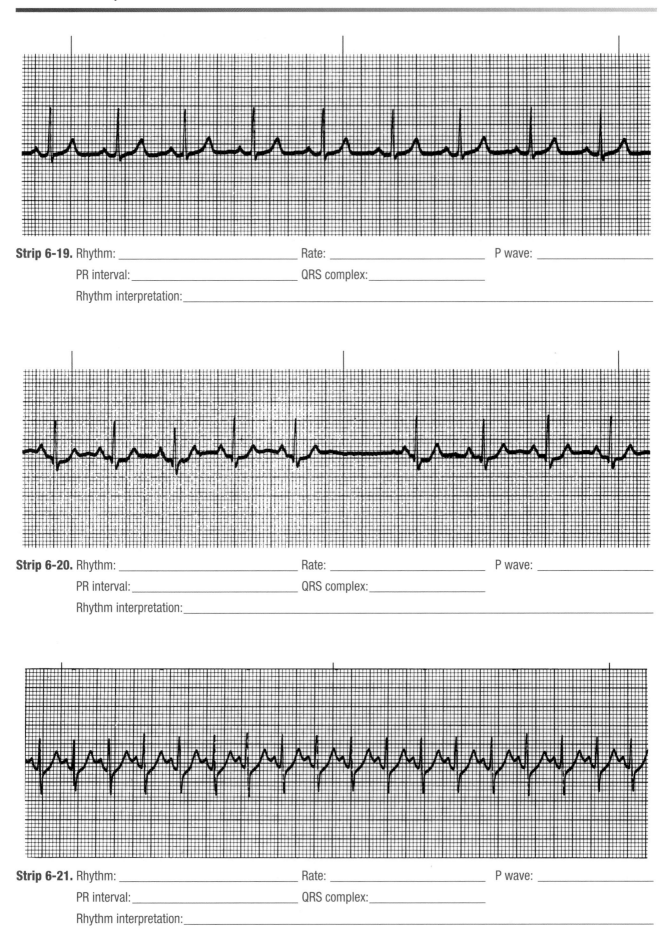

Strip 6-19. Rhythm: _____ Rate: _____ P wave: _____

PR interval: _____ QRS complex: _____

Rhythm interpretation: _____

Strip 6-20. Rhythm: _____ Rate: _____ P wave: _____

PR interval: _____ QRS complex: _____

Rhythm interpretation: _____

Strip 6-21. Rhythm: _____ Rate: _____ P wave: _____

PR interval: _____ QRS complex: _____

Rhythm interpretation: _____

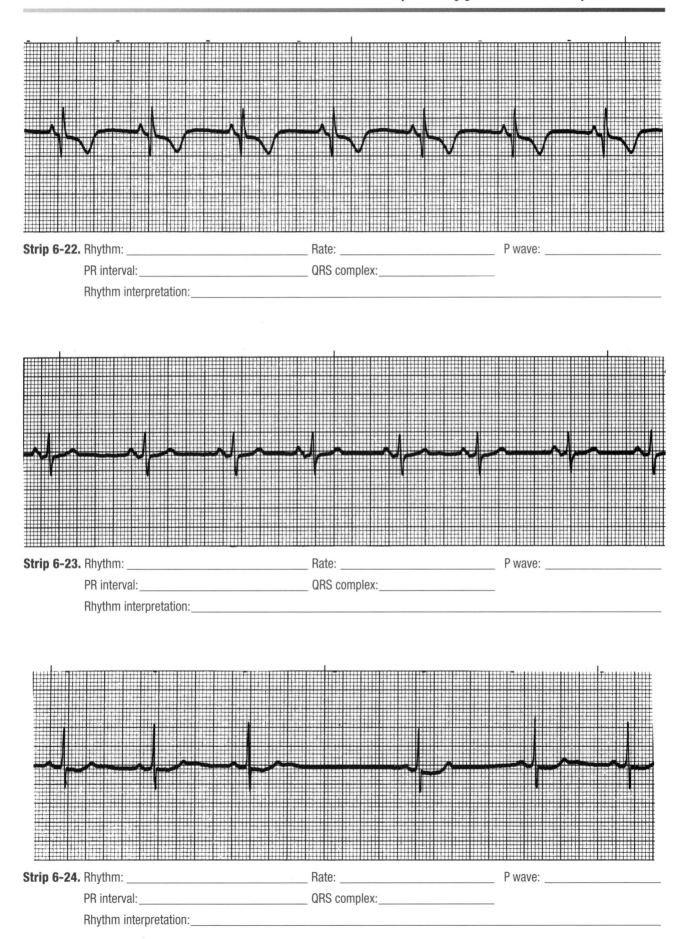

Strip 6-22. Rhythm: _____ Rate: _____ P wave: _____

PR interval: _____ QRS complex: _____

Rhythm interpretation: _____

Strip 6-23. Rhythm: _____ Rate: _____ P wave: _____

PR interval: _____ QRS complex: _____

Rhythm interpretation: _____

Strip 6-24. Rhythm: _____ Rate: _____ P wave: _____

PR interval: _____ QRS complex: _____

Rhythm interpretation: _____

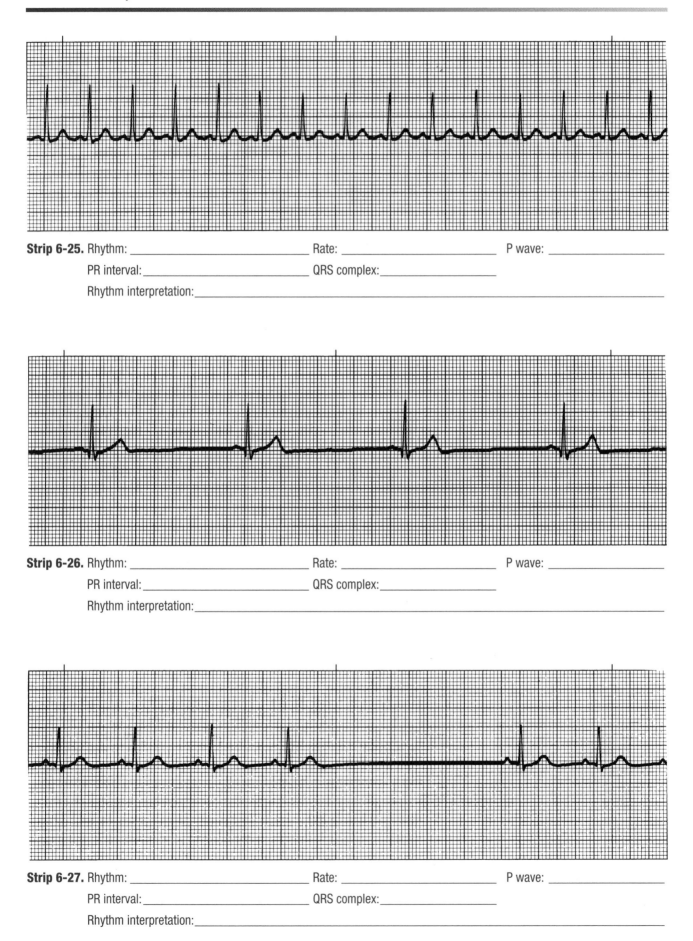

Strip 6-25. Rhythm: _____ Rate: _____ P wave: _____

PR interval: _____ QRS complex: _____

Rhythm interpretation: _____

Strip 6-26. Rhythm: _____ Rate: _____ P wave: _____

PR interval: _____ QRS complex: _____

Rhythm interpretation: _____

Strip 6-27. Rhythm: _____ Rate: _____ P wave: _____

PR interval: _____ QRS complex: _____

Rhythm interpretation: _____

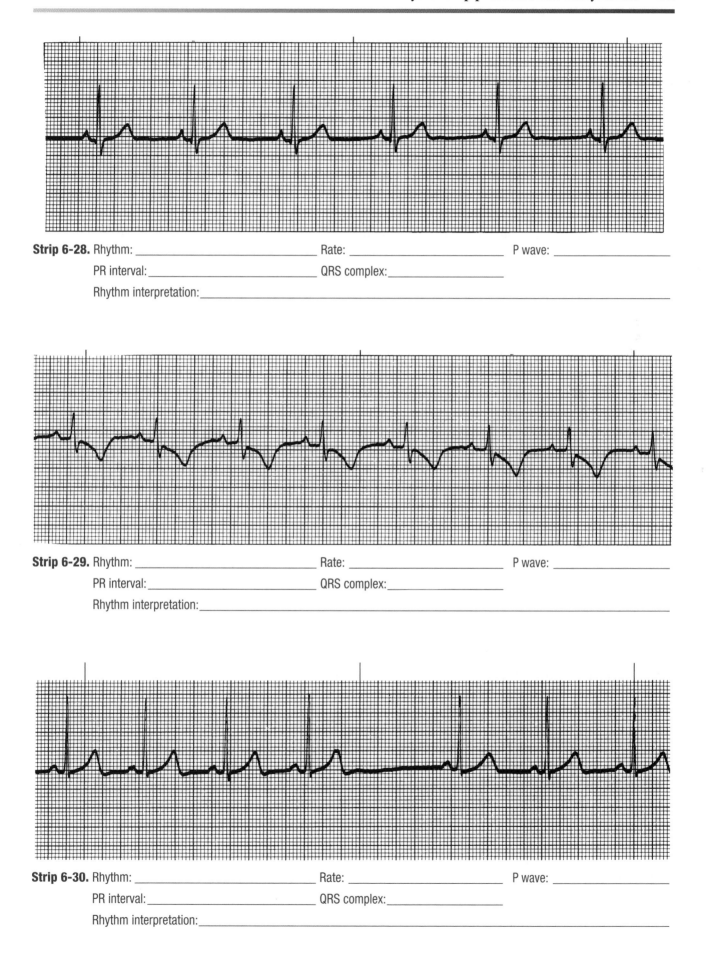

Strip 6-28. Rhythm: _____ Rate: _____ P wave: _____

PR interval: _____ QRS complex: _____

Rhythm interpretation: _____

Strip 6-29. Rhythm: _____ Rate: _____ P wave: _____

PR interval: _____ QRS complex: _____

Rhythm interpretation: _____

Strip 6-30. Rhythm: _____ Rate: _____ P wave: _____

PR interval: _____ QRS complex: _____

Rhythm interpretation: _____

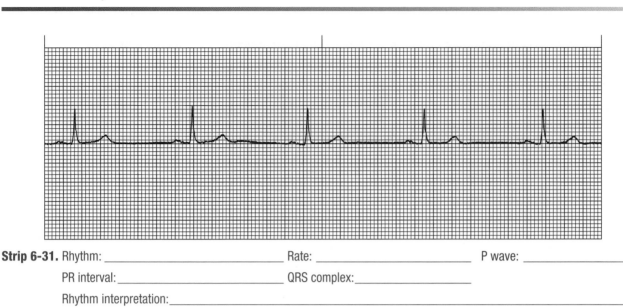

Strip 6-31. Rhythm: _____ Rate: _____ P wave: _____

PR interval: _____ QRS complex: _____

Rhythm interpretation: _____

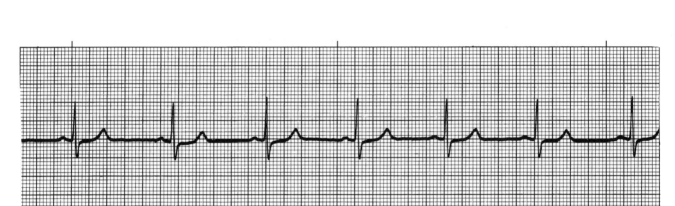

Strip 6-32. Rhythm: _____ Rate: _____ P wave: _____

PR interval: _____ QRS complex: _____

Rhythm interpretation: _____

Strip 6-33. Rhythm: _____ Rate: _____ P wave: _____

PR interval: _____ QRS complex: _____

Rhythm interpretation: _____

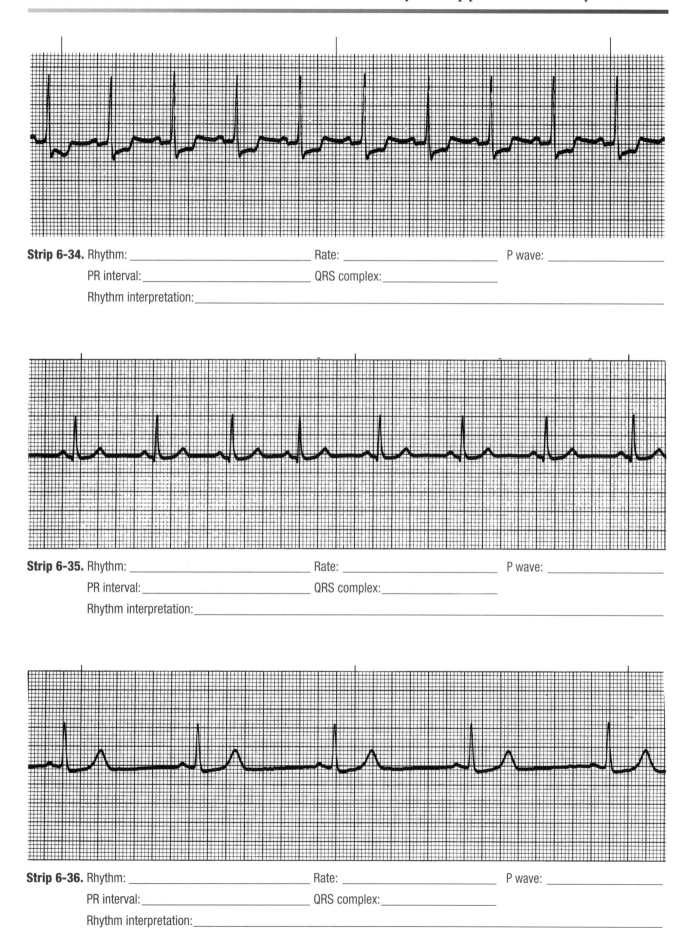

Strip 6-34. Rhythm: _____ Rate: _____ P wave: _____

PR interval: _____ QRS complex: _____

Rhythm interpretation: _____

Strip 6-35. Rhythm: _____ Rate: _____ P wave: _____

PR interval: _____ QRS complex: _____

Rhythm interpretation: _____

Strip 6-36. Rhythm: _____ Rate: _____ P wave: _____

PR interval: _____ QRS complex: _____

Rhythm interpretation: _____

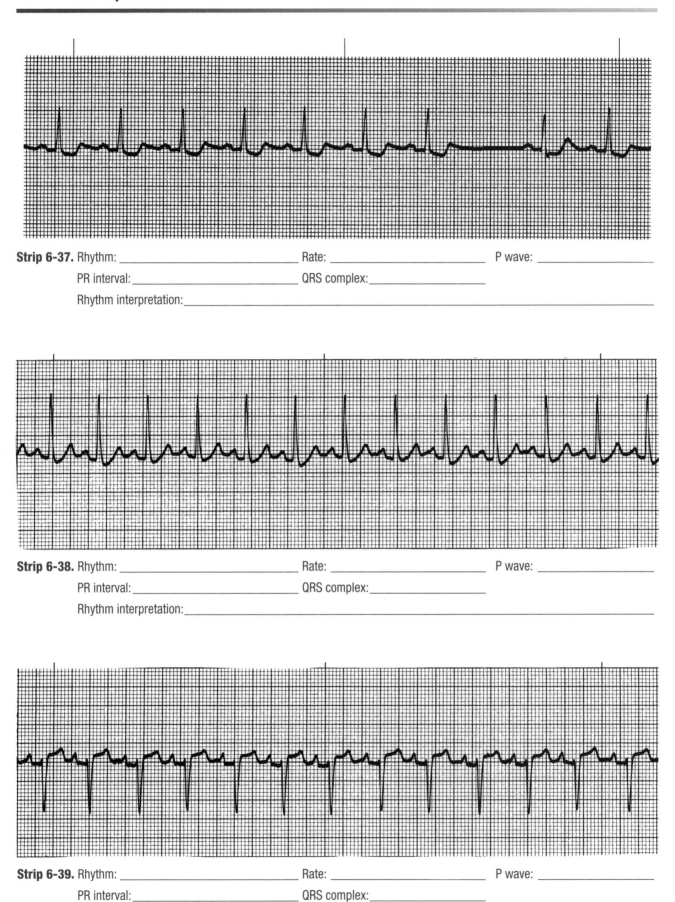

Strip 6-37. Rhythm: _____ Rate: _____ P wave: _____

PR interval: _____ QRS complex: _____

Rhythm interpretation: _____

Strip 6-38. Rhythm: _____ Rate: _____ P wave: _____

PR interval: _____ QRS complex: _____

Rhythm interpretation: _____

Strip 6-39. Rhythm: _____ Rate: _____ P wave: _____

PR interval: _____ QRS complex: _____

Rhythm interpretation: _____

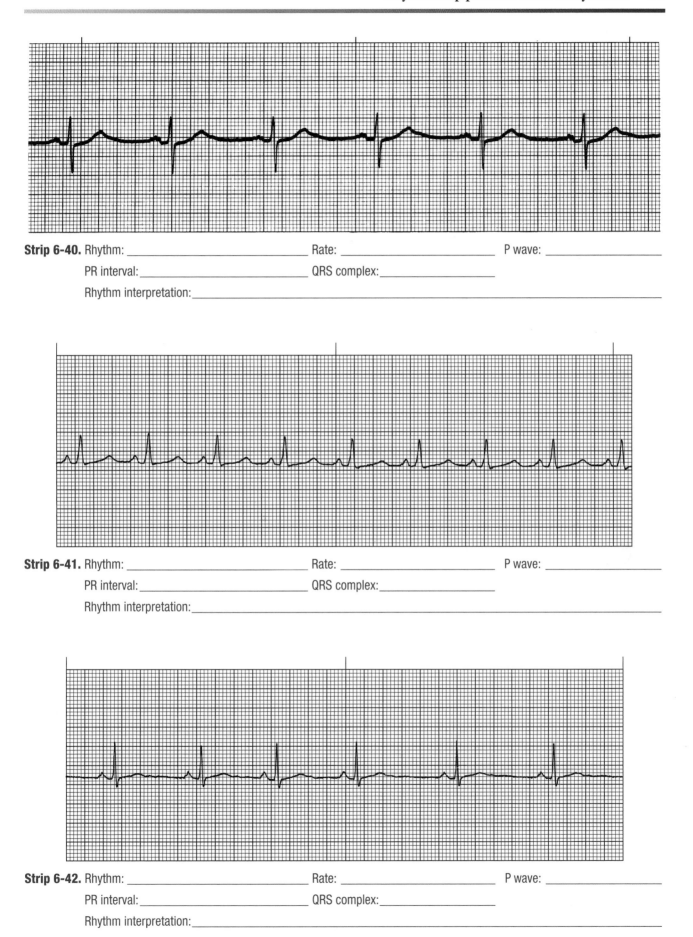

Strip 6-40. Rhythm: _____ Rate: _____ P wave: _____

PR interval: _____ QRS complex: _____

Rhythm interpretation: _____

Strip 6-41. Rhythm: _____ Rate: _____ P wave: _____

PR interval: _____ QRS complex: _____

Rhythm interpretation: _____

Strip 6-42. Rhythm: _____ Rate: _____ P wave: _____

PR interval: _____ QRS complex: _____

Rhythm interpretation: _____

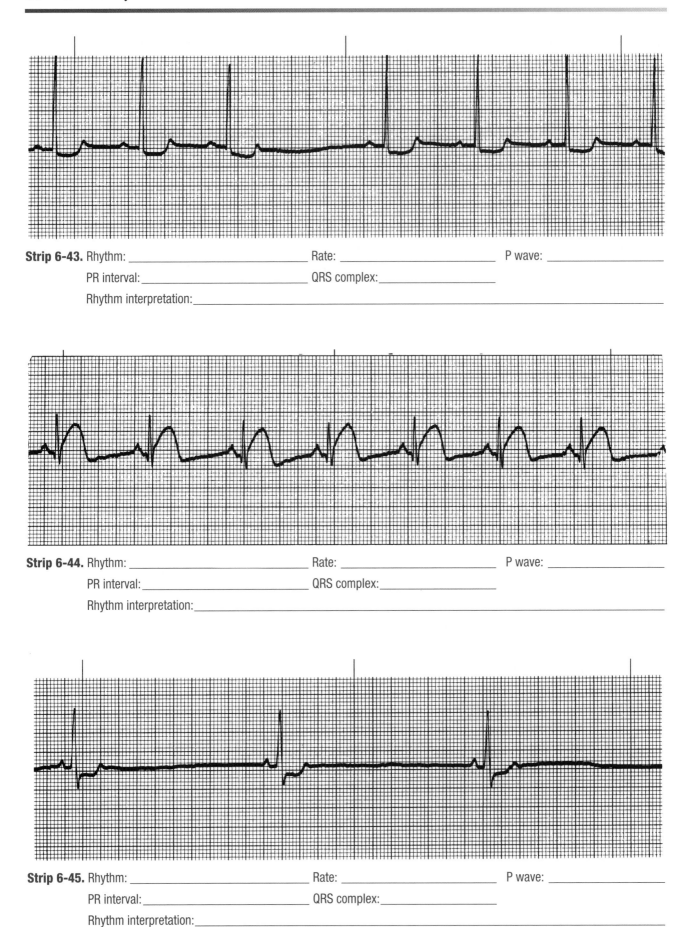

Strip 6-43. Rhythm: _____ Rate: _____ P wave: _____

PR interval: _____ QRS complex: _____

Rhythm interpretation: _____

Strip 6-44. Rhythm: _____ Rate: _____ P wave: _____

PR interval: _____ QRS complex: _____

Rhythm interpretation: _____

Strip 6-45. Rhythm: _____ Rate: _____ P wave: _____

PR interval: _____ QRS complex: _____

Rhythm interpretation: _____

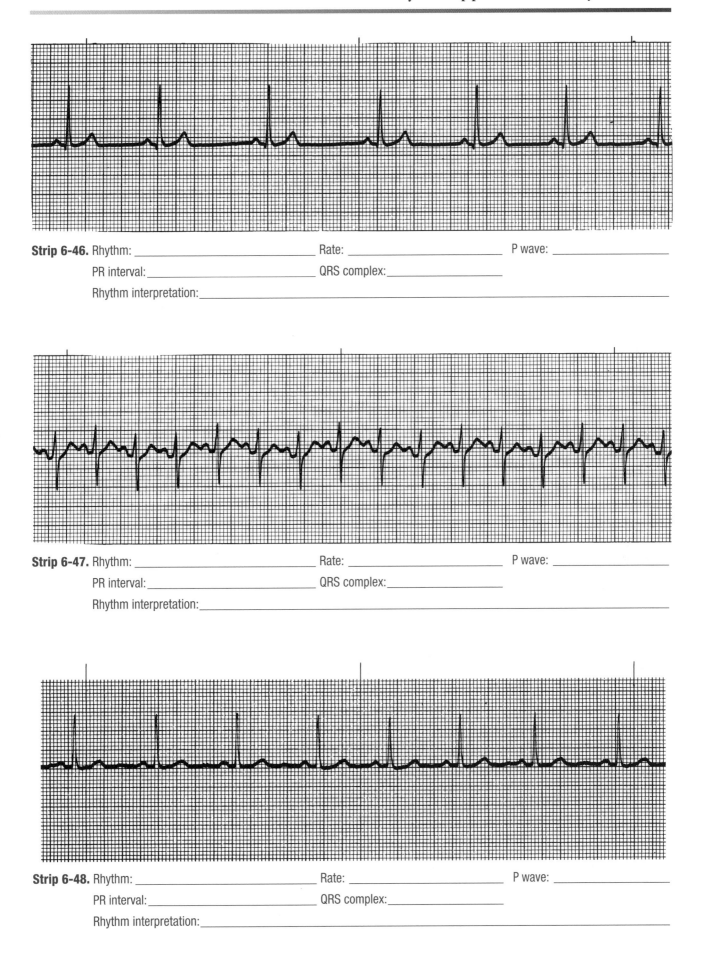

Strip 6-46. Rhythm: _____ Rate: _____ P wave: _____

PR interval: _____ QRS complex: _____

Rhythm interpretation: _____

Strip 6-47. Rhythm: _____ Rate: _____ P wave: _____

PR interval: _____ QRS complex: _____

Rhythm interpretation: _____

Strip 6-48. Rhythm: _____ Rate: _____ P wave: _____

PR interval: _____ QRS complex: _____

Rhythm interpretation: _____

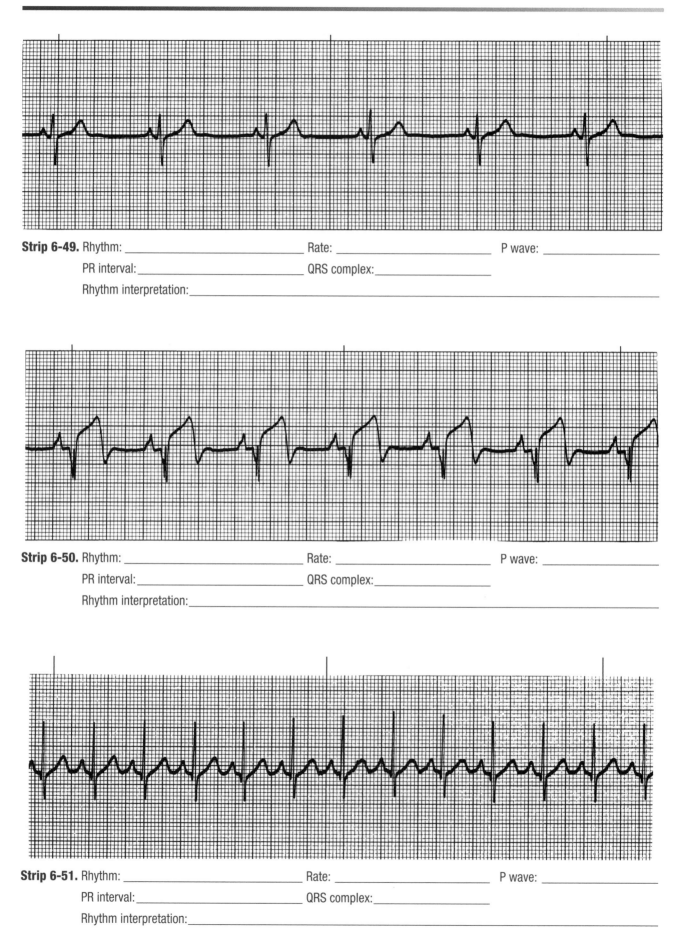

Strip 6-49. Rhythm: _____ Rate: _____ P wave: _____

PR interval: _____ QRS complex: _____

Rhythm interpretation: _____

Strip 6-50. Rhythm: _____ Rate: _____ P wave: _____

PR interval: _____ QRS complex: _____

Rhythm interpretation: _____

Strip 6-51. Rhythm: _____ Rate: _____ P wave: _____

PR interval: _____ QRS complex: _____

Rhythm interpretation: _____

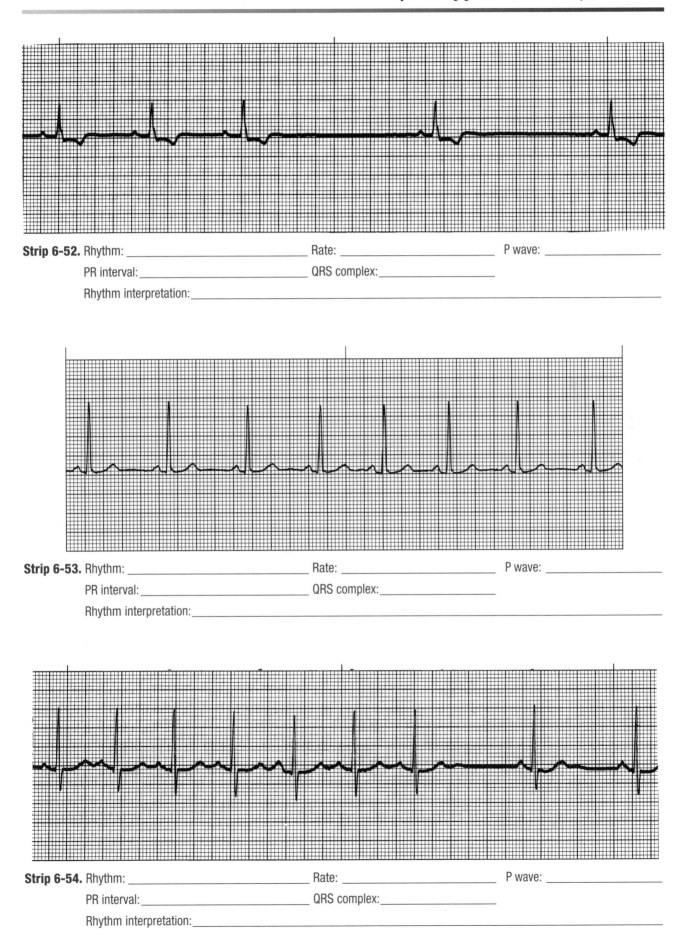

Strip 6-52. Rhythm: _____ Rate: _____ P wave: _____

PR interval: _____ QRS complex: _____

Rhythm interpretation: _____

Strip 6-53. Rhythm: _____ Rate: _____ P wave: _____

PR interval: _____ QRS complex: _____

Rhythm interpretation: _____

Strip 6-54. Rhythm: _____ Rate: _____ P wave: _____

PR interval: _____ QRS complex: _____

Rhythm interpretation: _____

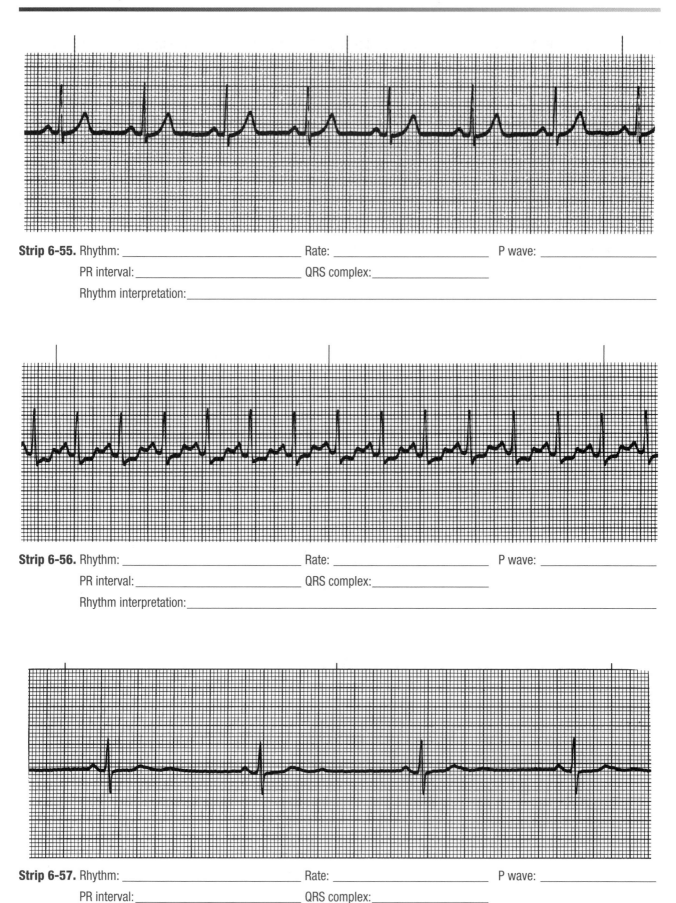

Strip 6-55. Rhythm: _____ Rate: _____ P wave: _____

PR interval: _____ QRS complex: _____

Rhythm interpretation: _____

Strip 6-56. Rhythm: _____ Rate: _____ P wave: _____

PR interval: _____ QRS complex: _____

Rhythm interpretation: _____

Strip 6-57. Rhythm: _____ Rate: _____ P wave: _____

PR interval: _____ QRS complex: _____

Rhythm interpretation: _____

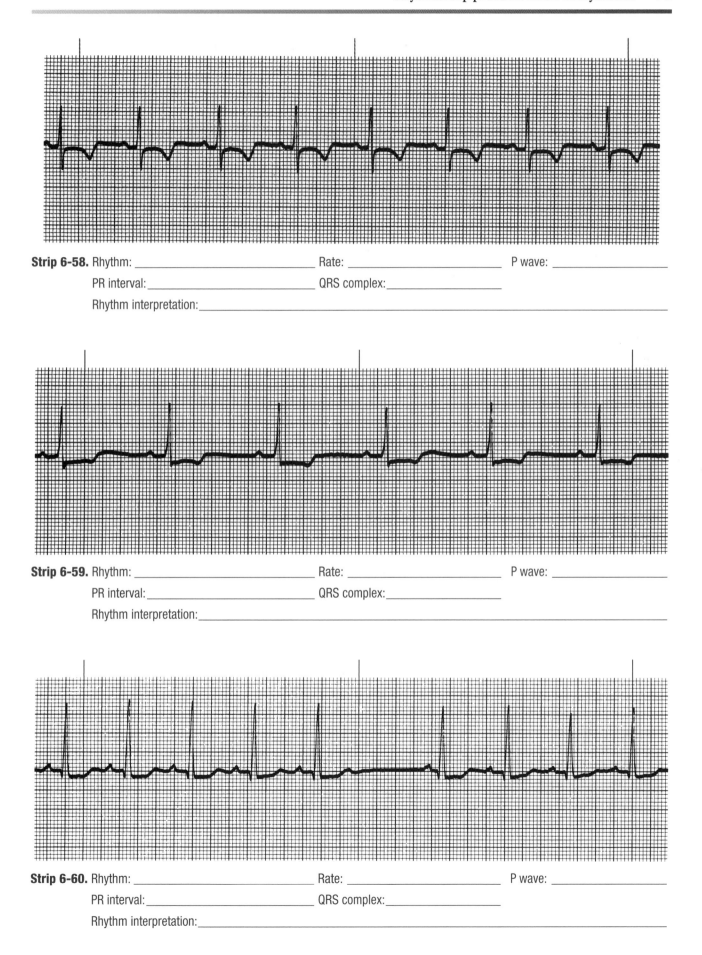

Strip 6-58. Rhythm: _____ Rate: _____ P wave: _____

PR interval:_____ QRS complex:_____

Rhythm interpretation:_____

Strip 6-59. Rhythm: _____ Rate: _____ P wave: _____

PR interval:_____ QRS complex:_____

Rhythm interpretation:_____

Strip 6-60. Rhythm: _____ Rate: _____ P wave: _____

PR interval:_____ QRS complex:_____

Rhythm interpretation:_____

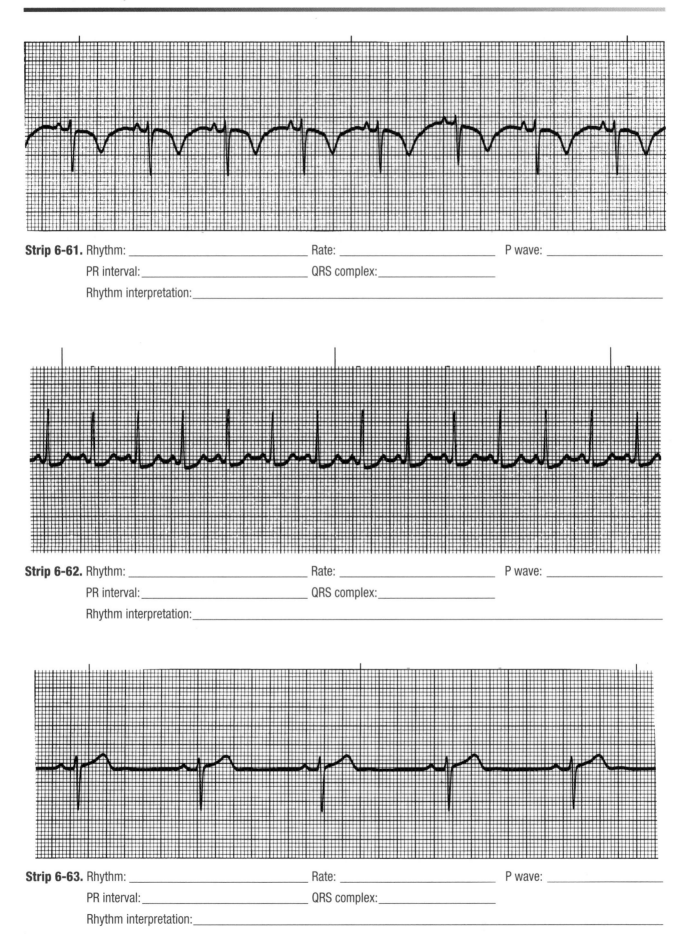

Strip 6-61. Rhythm: _____ Rate: _____ P wave: _____

PR interval: _____ QRS complex: _____

Rhythm interpretation: _____

Strip 6-62. Rhythm: _____ Rate: _____ P wave: _____

PR interval: _____ QRS complex: _____

Rhythm interpretation: _____

Strip 6-63. Rhythm: _____ Rate: _____ P wave: _____

PR interval: _____ QRS complex: _____

Rhythm interpretation: _____

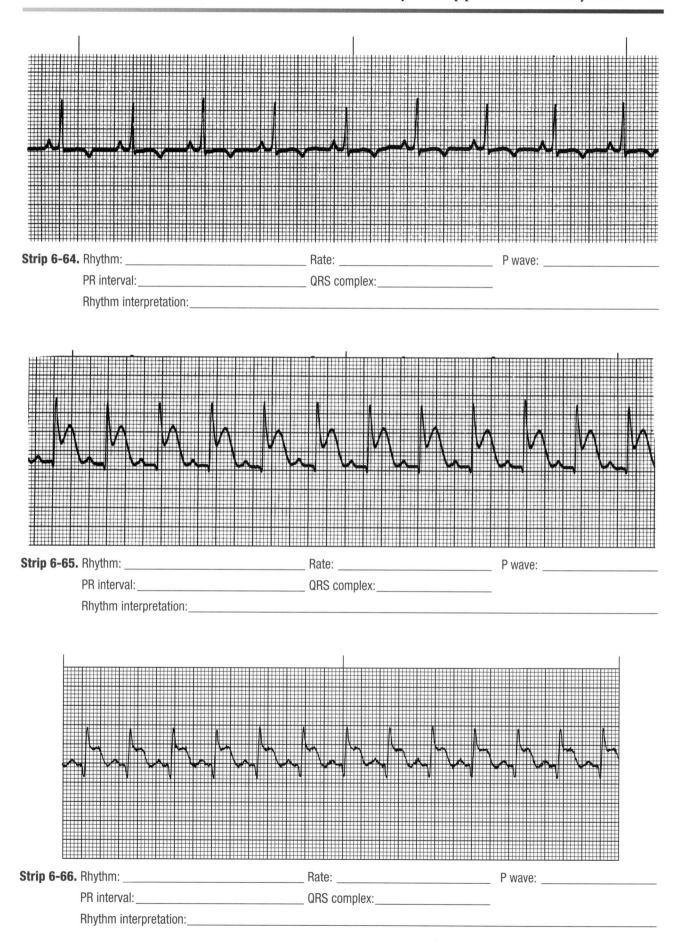

Strip 6-64. Rhythm: _____ Rate: _____ P wave: _____

PR interval: _____ QRS complex: _____

Rhythm interpretation: _____

Strip 6-65. Rhythm: _____ Rate: _____ P wave: _____

PR interval: _____ QRS complex: _____

Rhythm interpretation: _____

Strip 6-66. Rhythm: _____ Rate: _____ P wave: _____

PR interval: _____ QRS complex: _____

Rhythm interpretation: _____

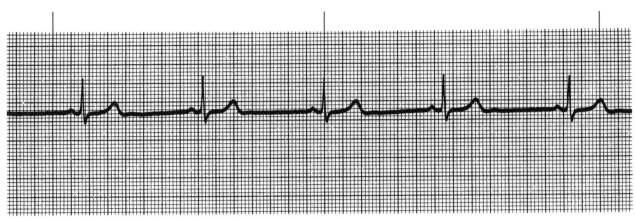

Strip 6-67. Rhythm: _____ Rate: _____ P wave: _____

PR interval: _____ QRS complex: _____

Rhythm interpretation: _____

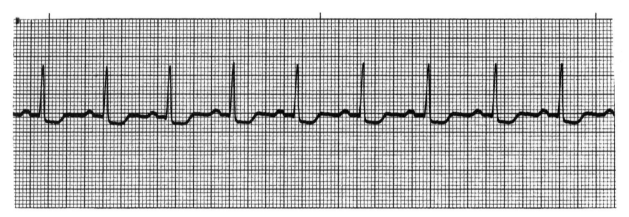

Strip 6-68. Rhythm: _____ Rate: _____ P wave: _____

PR interval: _____ QRS complex: _____

Rhythm interpretation: _____

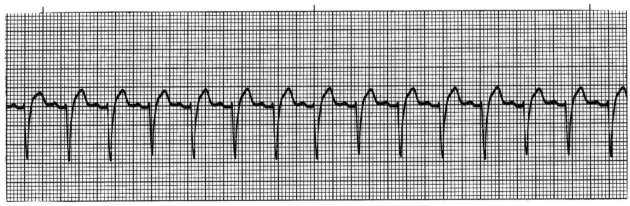

Strip 6-69. Rhythm: _____ Rate: _____ P wave: _____

PR interval: _____ QRS complex: _____

Rhythm interpretation: _____

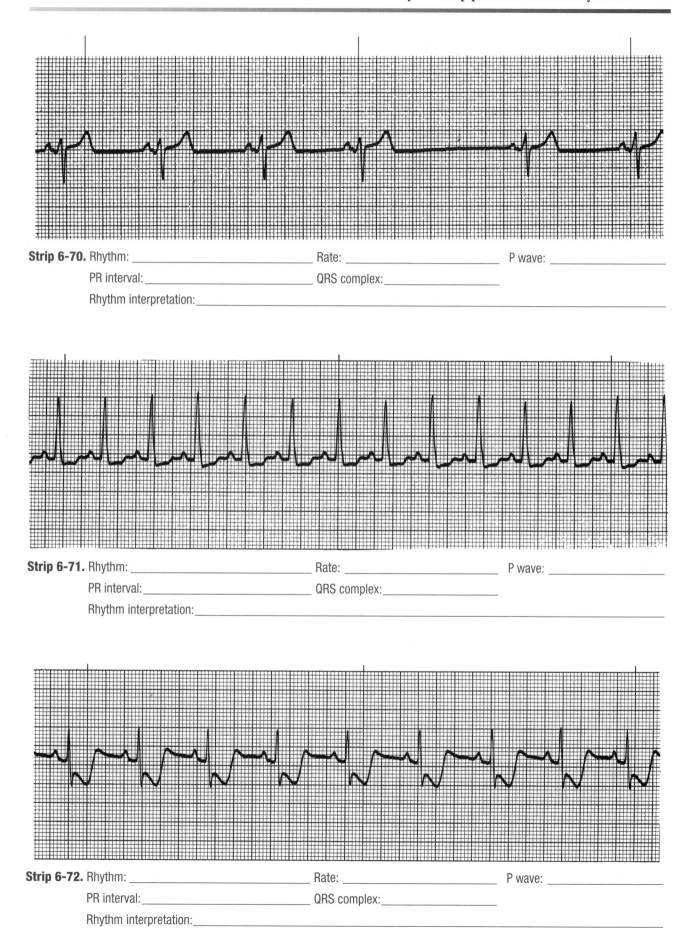

Strip 6-70. Rhythm: _____ Rate: _____ P wave: _____

PR interval: _____ QRS complex: _____

Rhythm interpretation: _____

Strip 6-71. Rhythm: _____ Rate: _____ P wave: _____

PR interval: _____ QRS complex: _____

Rhythm interpretation: _____

Strip 6-72. Rhythm: _____ Rate: _____ P wave: _____

PR interval: _____ QRS complex: _____

Rhythm interpretation: _____

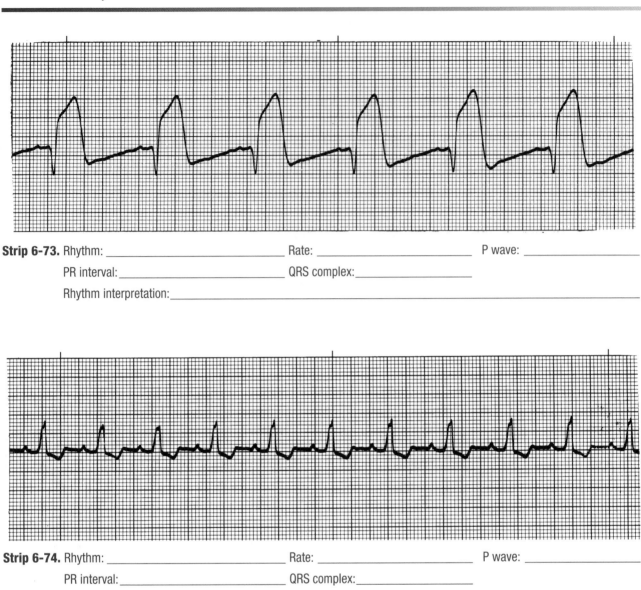

Strip 6-73. Rhythm: _____ Rate: _____ P wave: _____

PR interval: _____ QRS complex: _____

Rhythm interpretation: _____

Strip 6-74. Rhythm: _____ Rate: _____ P wave: _____

PR interval: _____ QRS complex: _____

Rhythm interpretation: _____

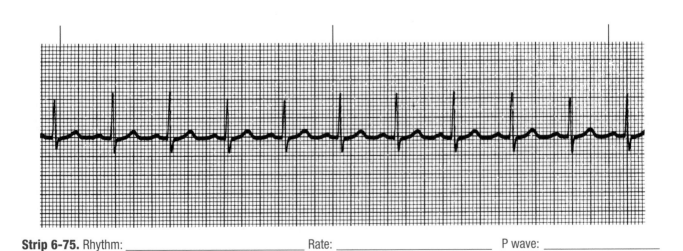

Strip 6-75. Rhythm: _____ Rate: _____ P wave: _____

PR interval: _____ QRS complex: _____

Rhythm interpretation: _____

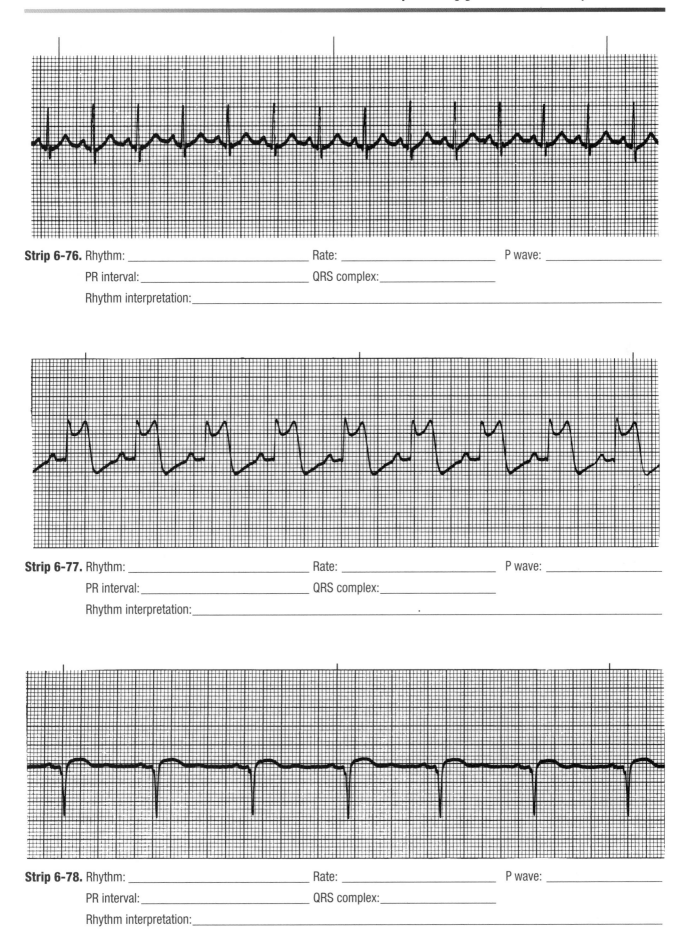

Strip 6-76. Rhythm: _____ Rate: _____ P wave: _____

PR interval: _____ QRS complex: _____

Rhythm interpretation: _____

Strip 6-77. Rhythm: _____ Rate: _____ P wave: _____

PR interval: _____ QRS complex: _____

Rhythm interpretation: _____

Strip 6-78. Rhythm: _____ Rate: _____ P wave: _____

PR interval: _____ QRS complex: _____

Rhythm interpretation: _____

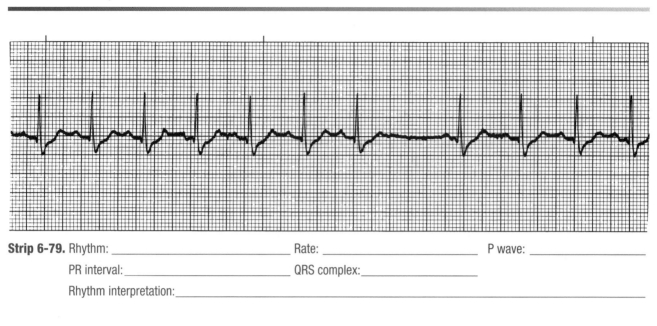

Strip 6-79. Rhythm: _____ Rate: _____ P wave: _____

PR interval: _____ QRS complex: _____

Rhythm interpretation: _____

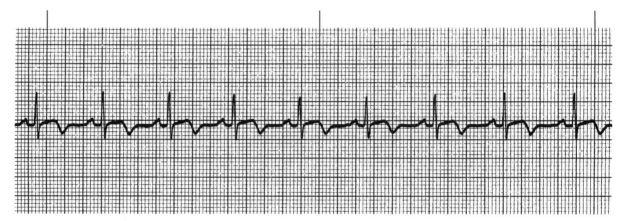

Strip 6-80. Rhythm: _____ Rate: _____ P wave: _____

PR interval: _____ QRS complex: _____

Rhythm interpretation: _____

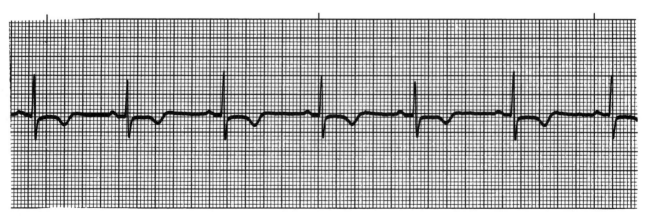

Strip 6-81. Rhythm: _____ Rate: _____ P wave: _____

PR interval: _____ QRS complex: _____

Rhythm interpretation: _____

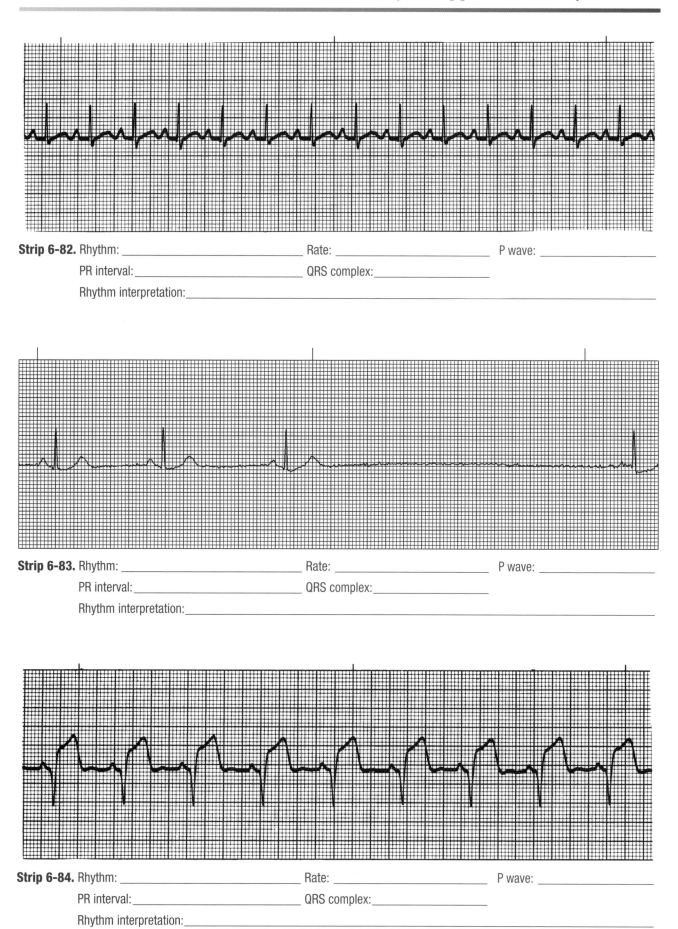

Strip 6-82. Rhythm: _____ Rate: _____ P wave: _____

PR interval:_____ QRS complex:_____

Rhythm interpretation:_____

Strip 6-83. Rhythm: _____ Rate: _____ P wave: _____

PR interval:_____ QRS complex:_____

Rhythm interpretation:_____

Strip 6-84. Rhythm: _____ Rate: _____ P wave: _____

PR interval:_____ QRS complex:_____

Rhythm interpretation:_____

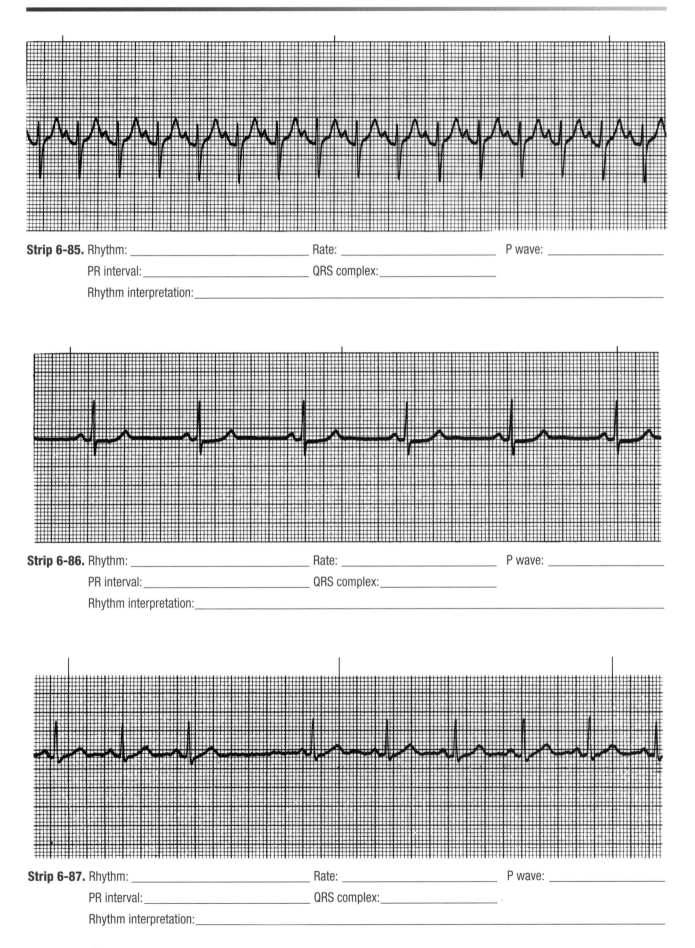

Strip 6-85. Rhythm: _____ Rate: _____ P wave: _____

PR interval: _____ QRS complex: _____

Rhythm interpretation: _____

Strip 6-86. Rhythm: _____ Rate: _____ P wave: _____

PR interval: _____ QRS complex: _____

Rhythm interpretation: _____

Strip 6-87. Rhythm: _____ Rate: _____ P wave: _____

PR interval: _____ QRS complex: _____

Rhythm interpretation: _____

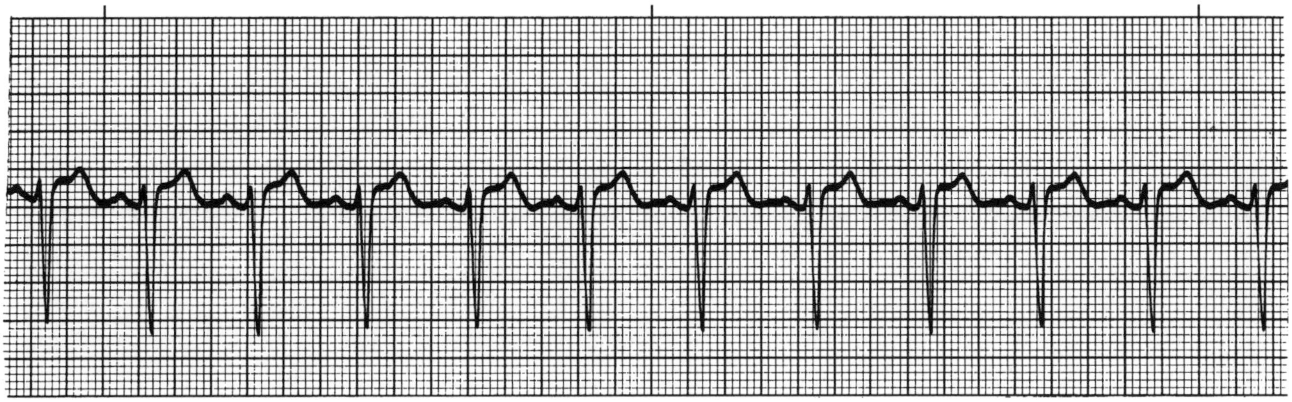

Strip 6-88. Rhythm: _____ Rate: _____ P wave: _____

PR interval: _____ QRS complex: _____

Rhythm interpretation: _____

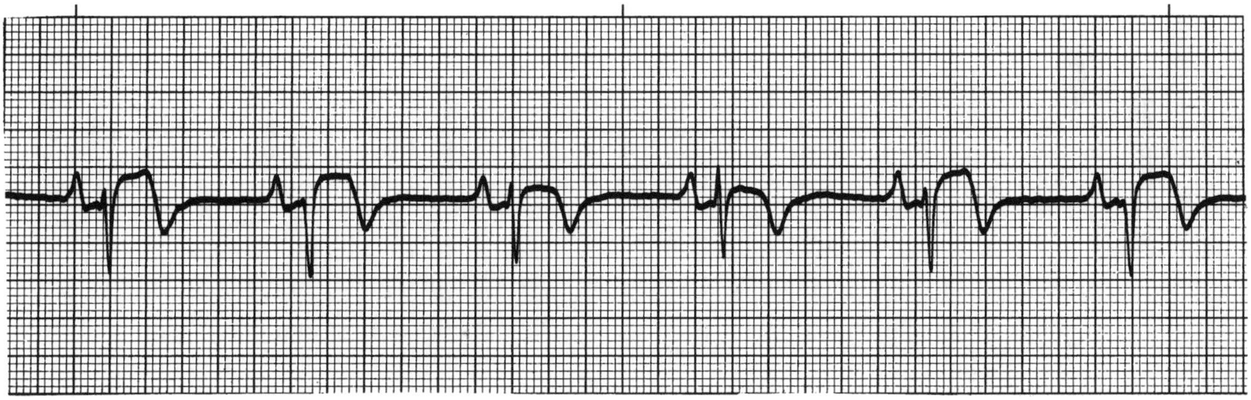

Strip 6-89. Rhythm: _____ Rate: _____ P wave: _____

PR interval: _____ QRS complex: _____

Rhythm interpretation: _____

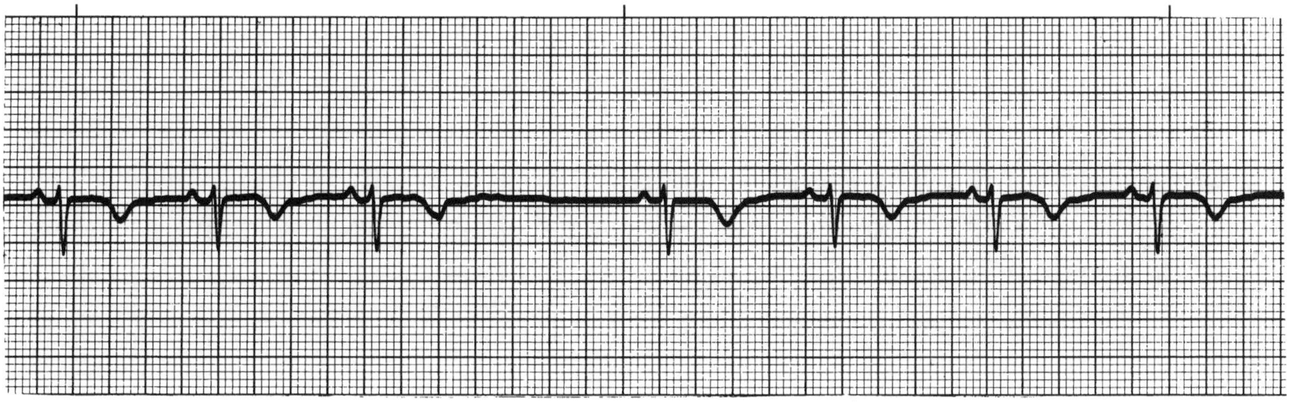

Strip 6-90. Rhythm: _____ Rate: _____ P wave: _____

PR interval: _____ QRS complex: _____

Rhythm interpretation: _____

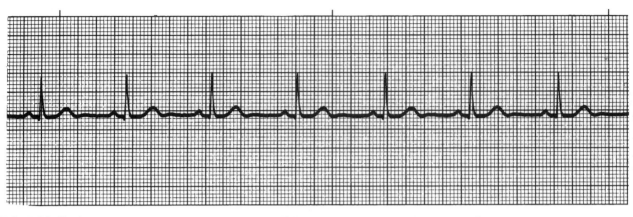

Strip 6-91. Rhythm: _____ Rate: _____ P wave: _____

PR interval:_____ QRS complex:_____

Rhythm interpretation:_____

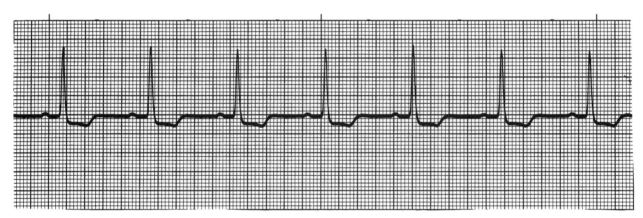

Strip 6-92. Rhythm: _____ Rate: _____ P wave: _____

PR interval:_____ QRS complex:_____

Rhythm interpretation:_____

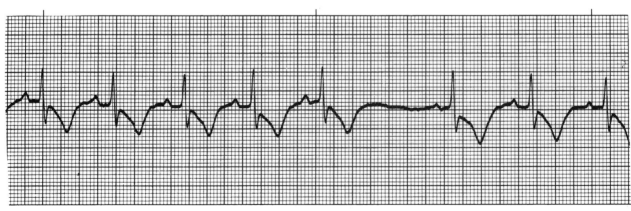

Strip 6-93. Rhythm: _____ Rate: _____ P wave: _____

PR interval:_____ QRS complex:_____

Rhythm interpretation:_____

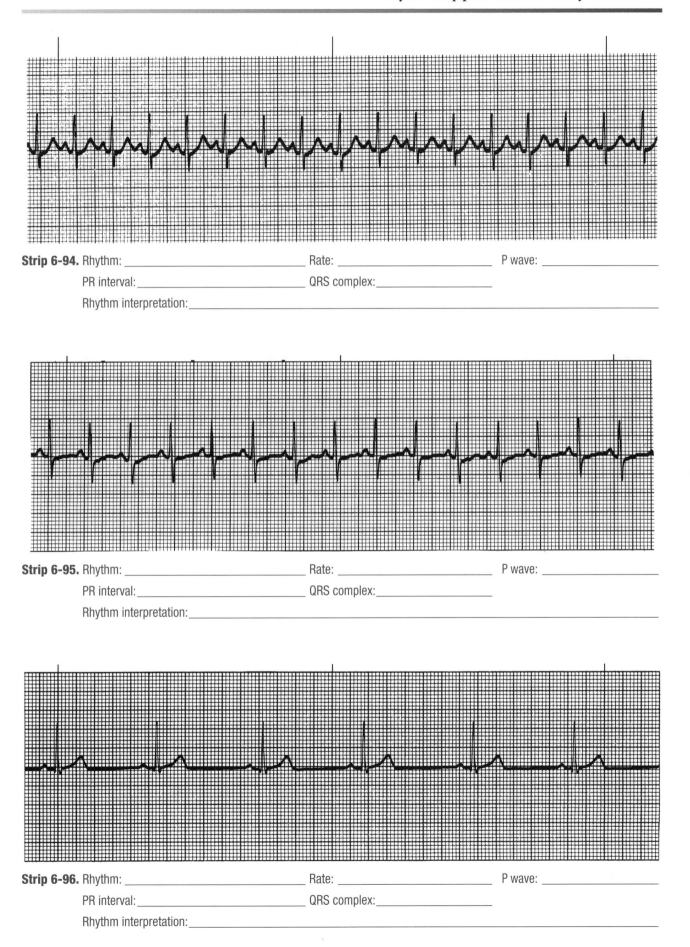

Strip 6-94. Rhythm: _____ Rate: _____ P wave: _____

PR interval: _____ QRS complex: _____

Rhythm interpretation: _____

Strip 6-95. Rhythm: _____ Rate: _____ P wave: _____

PR interval: _____ QRS complex: _____

Rhythm interpretation: _____

Strip 6-96. Rhythm: _____ Rate: _____ P wave: _____

PR interval: _____ QRS complex: _____

Rhythm interpretation: _____

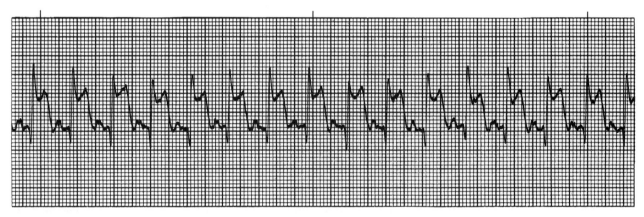

Strip 6-97. Rhythm: _____ Rate: _____ P wave: _____

PR interval: _____ QRS complex: _____

Rhythm interpretation: _____

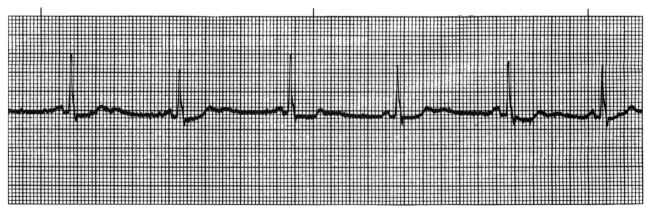

Strip 6-98. Rhythm: _____ Rate: _____ P wave: _____

PR interval: _____ QRS complex: _____

Rhythm interpretation: _____

Strip 6-99. Rhythm: _____ Rate: _____ P wave: _____

PR interval: _____ QRS complex: _____

Rhythm interpretation: _____

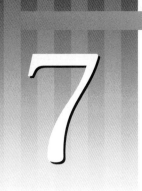

Atrial arrhythmias

Mechanisms of arrhythmias

Under certain circumstances cardiac cells in any part of the heart may take on the role of pacemaker of the heart. Such a pacemaker is called an ectopic pacemaker (a pacemaker other than the sinus node). The result can be ectopic beats or rhythms. These rhythms are identified according to the location of the ectopic pacemaker (for example, atrial, junctional, or ventricular). The three basic mechanisms that are responsible for ectopic beats and rhythms are *altered automaticity*, *triggered activity*, and *reentry*:

■ Altered automaticity — Normally the automaticity of the sinus node exceeds that of all other parts of the conduction system, allowing it to control the heart rate and rhythm. Pacemaker cells in other areas of the heart also have the property of automaticity, including cells in the atria, atrioventricular (AV) junction, and the ventricles. The rates of these other pacemaker sites are slower. Therefore, they're suppressed by the sinus node under normal circumstances. Because the inherent firing rate of the pacemaker cells of the sinus node is faster than the other pacemaker sites, it is the dominant and primary pacemaker of the heart. An ectopic pacemaker site can take over the role of pacemaker either because it usurps control from the sinus node by accelerating its own automaticity (enhanced automaticity) or because the sinus node relinquishes its role by decreasing its automaticity. Conditions that may predispose cardiac cells to altered automaticity include myocardial ischemia or injury, hypoxia, an increase in sympathetic tone, digitalis toxicity, hypokalemia, and hypocalcemia.

■ Triggered activity — Triggered activity results from abnormal electrical impulses that occur during repolarization when cells are normally quiet. The ectopic pacemaker cells may depolarize more than once after stimulation by a single electrical impulse. Triggered activity may result in atrial, junctional, or ventricular beats occurring singly, in pairs, in runs (3 or more beats), or as a sustained ectopic rhythm. Causes of triggered activity may include myocardial ischemia or injury, hypoxia, an increase in sympathetic tone, and digitalis toxicity.

■ Reentry — Normally an impulse spreads through the heart only once. With reentry, an impulse can travel through an area of myocardium, depolarize it, and then reenter that same area to depolarize it again. Reentry involves a circular movement of the impulse, which continues as long as it encounters receptive cells. Reentry (like triggered activity) may result in atrial, junctional, or ventricular beats occurring singly, in pairs, in runs, or as a sustained ectopic rhythm. Common causes of reentry include myocardial ischemia or injury, hyperkalemia, and the presence of an accessory conduction pathway between the atria and the ventricles.

Atrial arrhythmias (Figure 7-1) originate from ectopic sites in the atria. Ectopic P waves from the atrium differ in *morphology* (shape) from the normal sinus P waves (Figure 7-2). For example, in slower atrial rhythms (premature atrial contractions, wandering atrial pacemaker) the P wave may appear as a small, pointed, and upright waveform; a small squiggle that is barely visible; or it may be inverted if the impulse originates from a site in the lower atrium near the AV junction. In faster atrial rhythms, the ectopic P wave is either superimposed on the preceding T wave (PA T), appears in a sawtooth pattern (atrial flutter), or is seen as a wavy baseline (atrial fibrillation).

Some atrial arrhythmias may be associated with rapid ventricular rates. Increases in heart rate decrease the length of time spent in diastole. If diastole is shortened, there is less time for coronary artery perfusion and less time for adequate ventricular filling. Thus, an excessively rapid heart rate may lead to myocardial ischemia and may compromise cardiac output.

Wandering atrial pacemaker

A wandering atrial pacemaker (WAP) (Figure 7-3 and Box 7-1) occurs when the pacemaker site shifts back and

Box 7-1.
Wandering atrial pacemaker: Identifying ECG features

Rhythm:	Regular or irregular
Rate:	Usually normal (60 to 100 beats/minute) but may be slow (< than 60 beats/minute)
P waves:	Vary in size, shape, and direction across rhythm strip; one P wave precedes each QRS complex
PR interval:	Usually normal duration, but may be abnormal depending on changing pacemaker location
QRS complex:	Normal (0.10 second or less)

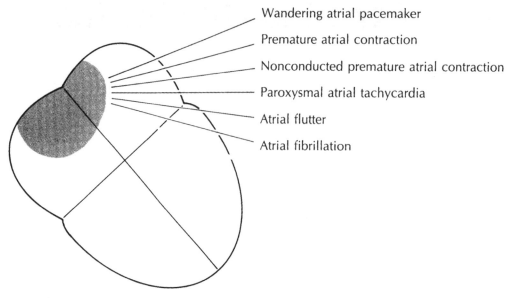

Wandering atrial pacemaker

Premature atrial contraction

Nonconducted premature atrial contraction

Paroxysmal atrial tachycardia

Atrial flutter

Atrial fibrillation

Figure 7-1.   Atrial arrhythmias.

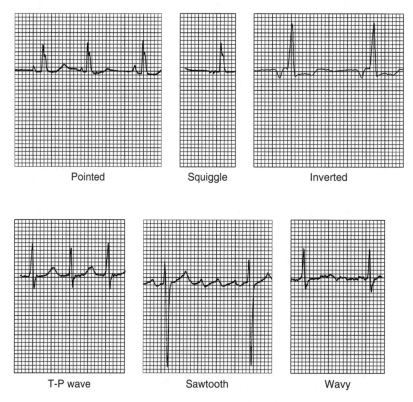

Pointed	Squiggle	Inverted

T-P wave	Sawtooth	Wavy

Figure 7-2.   Atrial P waves.

forth between the sinus node and ectopic atrial sites. The P wave morphology will vary across the rhythm strip as the pacemaker "wanders" between the multiple sites. The ectopic P wave may appear as a small, pointed, and upright waveform; a small squiggle that is barely visible; or it may be inverted if the impulse originates from a site in the lower atrium near the AV junction. Generally, at least

three different P-wave morphologies should be identified before making the diagnosis of WAP.

The heart rate is usually normal, but may be slow. The rhythm may be regular or irregular (each impulse travels through the atria via a slightly different route). The PR interval is usually normal, but may be abnormal because of the different sites of impulse formation. The

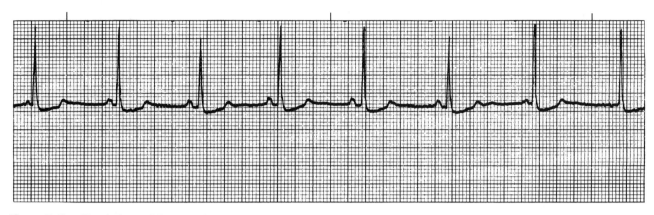

Figure 7-3.   Wandering atrial pacemaker.
Rhythm: Irregular
Rate: 60 beats/minute
P waves: Vary in size, shape, across rhythm strip
PR interval: 0.10 to 0.14 second
QRS complex: 0.04 to 0.08 second.

QRS complex is normal in duration. The distinguishing feature of this rhythm is the changing P-wave morphology across the rhythm strip.

WAP may be a normal phenomenon seen as a result of increased vagal effect on the sinoatrial (SA) node, slowing the sinus rate and allowing other pacemaker sites an opportunity to compete for control of the heart rate. It can also occur due to enhanced automaticity of atrial pacemaker cells that usurp pacemaker control from the SA node. WAP is commonly seen in patients with chronic obstructive pulmonary disease.

WAP usually isn't clinically significant, and treatment is not indicated. If the heart rate is slow, medications should be reviewed and discontinued if possible. If the heart rate is slow and the patient is symptomatic, treatment of the rhythm is the same as for symptomatic sinus bradycardia.

When WAP is associated with a heart rate greater than 100 beats per minute, the rhythm is called *multifocal atrial tachycardia* (MAT) (Figure 7-4). MAT is a relatively infrequent arrhythmia and is most commonly observed in patients with severe chronic obstructive pulmonary disease.

Premature atrial contraction

A premature atrial contraction (PAC) (Figures 7-5 through 7-12 and Box 7-2) is an early beat originating from an

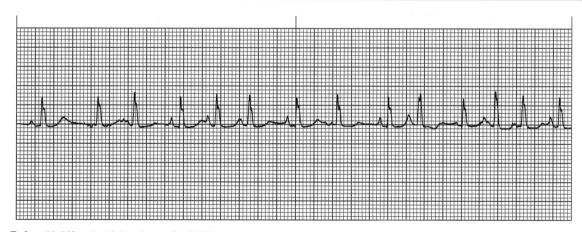

Figure 7-4.   Multifocal atrial tachycardia (MAT).
Rhythm: Irregular
Rate: 140 beats/minute
P waves: Vary in size, shape, and direction across rhythm strip
PR interval: 0.10 to 0.14 second
QRS complex: 0.04 to 0.08 second.

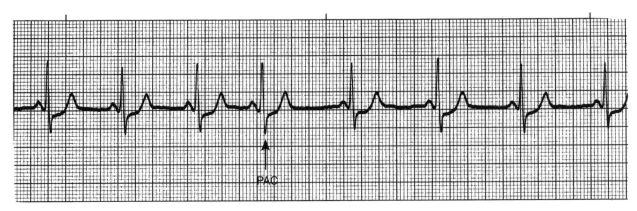

Figure 7-5.   Normal sinus rhythm with premature atrial contraction (PAC).

Rhythm: Basic rhythm regular; irregular with PAC

Rate: Basic rhythm rate 72 beats/minute; rate slows to 60 beats/minute following PAC (Temporary rate suppression is common
               following a pause in the basic rhythm; after several cardiac cycles the rate usually returns to the basic rhythm rate.)

P waves: Sinus P waves with basic rhythm; P wave associated with PAC is premature and closely resembles that of the sinus P waves
               in the underlying rhythm, indicating the ectopic atrial pacemaker site is close to the SA node

PR interval: 0.12 second (basic rhythm and PAC)

QRS complex: 0.08 second (basic rhythm and PAC).

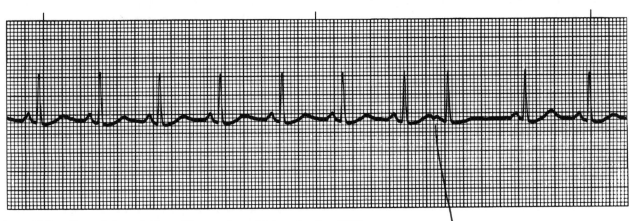

Figure 7-6.   Normal sinus rhythm with premature atrial contraction (PAC).

Rhythm: Basic rhythm regular; irregular with PAC

Rate: Basic rhythm rate 88 beats/minute

P waves: Sinus P waves with basic rhythm; premature, inverted P wave with PAC

PR interval: 0.14 to 0.16 second (basic rhythm); 0.14 second (PAC)

QRS complex: 0.04 to 0.06 second (basic rhythm); 0.06 second (PAC).

Box 7-2.
Premature atrial contraction (PAC): Identifying ECG features

Rhythm:	Underlying rhythm usually regular; irregular with PACs
Rate:	That of underlying rhythm
P waves:	P wave associated with PAC is premature and abnormal in size, shape, and direction (commonly appears small, upright, and pointed; may be inverted); abnormal P wave commonly found hidden in preceding T wave, distorting the T-wave contour
PR interval:	Usually normal; not measurable if hidden in T wave
QRS complex:	Premature; normal duration (0.10 second or less)

ectopic site in the atrium, which interrupts the regularity of the basic rhythm (usually a sinus rhythm). The premature beat occurs in addition to the basic underlying rhythm. PACs may originate from a single ectopic pacemaker site or from multiple sites in the atria. The early beat is characterized by a premature, abnormal P wave and a premature QRS complex that's identical or similar to the QRS complex of the normally conducted beats, and is followed by a pause.

P-wave morphology differs from sinus beats and varies depending on the origin of the impulse in the atria. If the ectopic focus is in the vicinity of the SA node, the P wave may closely resemble the sinus P wave (Figure 7-5). Its sole distinguishing feature may be its prematurity. As a rule,

[handwritten top margin: P wave in T wave makes it higher]
[handwritten left margin: 80 PR QRS]

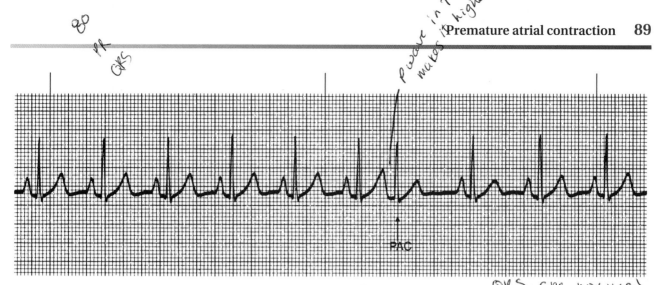

Figure 7-7. **Normal sinus rhythm with premature atrial contraction (PAC).**

Rhythm: Basic rhythm regular; irregular with PAC

Rate: Basic rhythm rate 84 beats/minute

P waves: Sinus P waves with basic rhythm; premature, abnormal P wave with PAC (The P wave of the PAC is hidden in the preceding T wave, distorting the T-wave contour. [T wave is taller and more pointed.])

PR interval: 0.12 to 0.14 second (basic rhythm); not measurable with PAC

QRS complex: 0.06 to 0.08 second (basic rhythm); 0.06 second (PAC).

[handwritten right margin: QRS are normal so ventricles are ok✓ coming from premature atrial contraction]

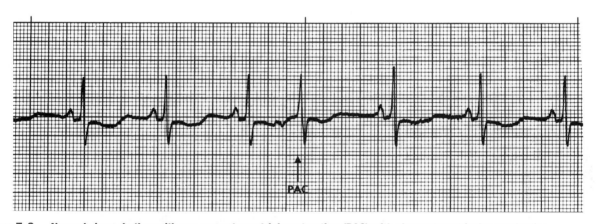

Figure 7-8. **Normal sinus rhythm with one premature atrial contraction (PAC) with aberrant ventricular conduction.**

Rhythm: Basic rhythm regular; irregular with PAC

Rate: Basic rhythm rate 68 beats/minute

P waves: Sinus in basic rhythm; premature, abnormal P wave with PAC

PR interval: 0.16 to 0.18 second (basic rhythm); 0.24 second (PAC)

QRS complex: 0.08 second (basic rhythm); 0.12 second (PAC).

however, the P wave is different from the sinus P waves. In lead II (a positive lead), it's generally upright and pointed (Figure 7-9), or it may be inverted (Figure 7-6) if the pacemaker site is near the AV junction. If the premature beat occurs very early, the abnormal P wave can be found hidden in the preceding T wave, causing a distortion of the T-wave contour (Figure 7-7).

The PR intervals of the PACs are usually normal, similar to those of the underlying rhythm. Occasionally the PR interval may be prolonged if the PAC is very early and finds the AV junction still partially refractory and unable to conduct at a normal rate. The PR interval will be unmeasurable if the abnormal P wave is obscured in the preceding T wave.

The QRS of the PAC usually resembles that of the underlying rhythm because the impulse is conducted normally through the bundle branches into the ventricles. The ventricles depolarize simultaneously, resulting in a normal duration QRS complex. If the PAC occurs very early, it is possible the bundle branches may not be repolarized sufficiently to conduct the premature electrical impulse normally. If the bundle branches are not sufficiently repolarized, the electrical impulse is conducted down one bundle branch (usually the left because it repolarizes quicker)

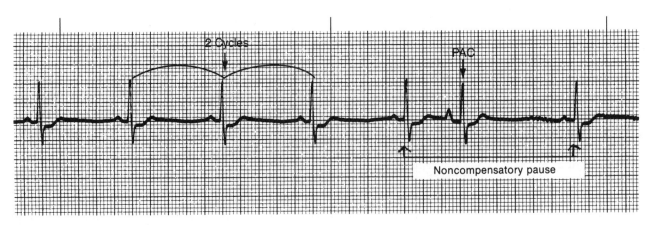

Figure 7-9.   Normal sinus rhythm with premature atrial contraction (PAC).

Rhythm: Basic rhythm regular; irregular with PAC

Rate: Basic rhythm rate 60 beats/minute

P waves: Sinus P waves with basic rhythm; premature, abnormal P wave with PAC

PR interval: 0.12 to 0.16 second (basic rhythm); 0.16 second (PAC)

QRS complex: 0.08 second (basic rhythm and PAC)

Comment: To determine the type of pause after premature beats, measure from the QRS complex before the premature beat to the QRS complex after the premature beat. If the measurement equals two R-R intervals, the pause is compensatory. If the measurement equals less than two R-R intervals, the pause is noncompensatory. ST-segment depression is present.

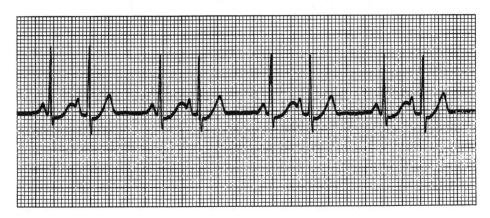

Figure 7-10.   Bigeminal premature atrial contractions.

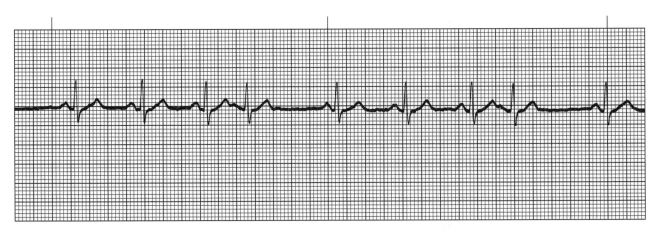

Figure 7-11.   Quadrigeminal premature atrial contractions.

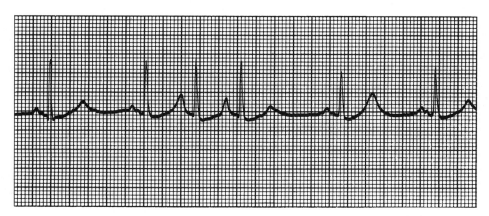

Figure 7-12. Paired premature atrial contractions.

and not conducted down the other. The left ventricle is depolarized first, followed by depolarization of the right ventricle (sequential depolarization). Sequential ventricular depolarization is slower, resulting in a wide QRS complex of 0.12 second or greater. A PAC associated with a wide QRS complex is called a PAC with aberrancy, indicating that conduction through the ventricles is abnormal (aberrant). Figure 7-8 shows a PAC with aberrant ventricular conduction (the QRS is wide) and a long PR interval, indicating conduction through the AV node was also delayed. Aberrantly conducted PACs must be differentiated from a premature ventricular contraction (PVC), especially if the abnormal P wave associated with the PAC is obscured in the preceding T wave. PVCs are discussed in Chapter 9.

The pause associated with the PAC is usually a *noncompensatory pause* (the measurement from the R wave before the premature beat to the R wave after the premature beat is less than two R-R intervals of the underlying regular rhythm) (Figure 7-9). This pause is called an incomplete pause because it doesn't equal two R-R intervals. Less commonly, the PAC may occur with a *compensatory pause* (a pause that is equal to two R-R intervals), but this is usually seen with the PVC. The compensatory pause is called a complete pause because it equals two R-R intervals. To differentiate between a complete pause and an incomplete pause, the underlying rhythm must be regular. Rarely, the PAC may occur with a pause that is longer than compensatory.

PACs may appear as a single beat (Figure 7-9), every other beat (bigeminal PACs, Figure 7-10), every third beat, (trigeminal PACs), every fourth beat (quadrigeminal PACs, Figure 7-11), in pairs (also called couplets, Figure 7-12), or in runs of three or more. Frequent PACs may initiate more serious atrial arrhythmias, such as paroxysmal atrial tachycardia (PAT), atrial flutter, or atrial fibrillation. Three or more beats of PACs in a row at a rate of 140 to 250 beats/minute constitute a run of PAT.

Premature atrial beats are common. They can occur in individuals with a normal heart or in those with heart disease. PACs may be seen with emotional stress (due to an increase in sympathetic tone), or ingestion of certain substances such as alcohol, caffeine, or tobacco. Other causes include hypoxia, electrolyte imbalances, myocardial ischemia or injury, atrial enlargement, congestive heart failure, and the administration of certain drugs, such as epinephrine or nonepinephrine, that increase sympathetic tone. PACs may also occur without apparent cause.

Infrequent PACs require no treatment. Frequent PACs are treated by correcting the underlying cause: reducing stress; reducing or eliminating the consumption of alcohol, caffeine, or tobacco; administering oxygen; correcting electrolyte imbalances; treating congestive heart failure, or discontinuing certain drugs. If needed, frequent PACs may be treated with beta blockers, calcium channel blockers, or antianxiety medications. Runs of PACs may require amiodarone to prevent more serious atrial arrhythmias from developing.

Occasionally, an ectopic atrial beat will occur late instead of early. This beat is called an *atrial escape beat* (Figure 7-13). Atrial escape beats usually occur during a pause in the underlying rhythm when the sinus node fails to initiate an impulse (sinus arrest) or when conduction of the sinus impulse is blocked for any reason (sinus exit block, nonconducted PAC, or Mobitz I second-degree AV block). The pause in the rhythm allows an ectopic pacemaker site in the atria to assume control of the heartbeat. The morphologic characteristics of the late beat will be the same as the PAC. Escape beats act as an electrical backup to maintain the heart rate and require no treatment.

Nonconducted PAC

A nonconducted PAC (Figures 7-14 through 7-16 and Box 7-3) results when an ectopic atrial focus occurs so early that it finds the AV node refractory and the impulse isn't conducted to the ventricles. This results in a premature, abnormal P wave not accompanied by a QRS complex, but followed by a pause (Figure 7-14).

Like the conducted PAC, the P wave associated with the nonconducted PAC will be premature and abnormal in size, shape, or direction. The P wave is commonly found hidden

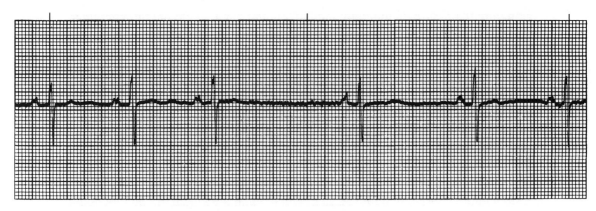

Figure 7-13. Normal sinus rhythm with sinus arrest and atrial escape beat.
Rhythm: Basic rhythm regular; irregular during pause
Rate: Basic rhythm rate 63 beats/minute; rate slows to 58 beats/minute after pause due to temporary rate supression (common
                 following pauses in the basic rhythm)
P waves: Sinus P waves; P waves are notched in basic rhythm which could be due to left atrial enlargement; peaked P wave with
                 escape beat
PR interval: 0.18 to 0.20 second (basic rhythm and escape beat)
QRS complex: 0.08 second (basic rhythm); 0.06 second (escape beat).

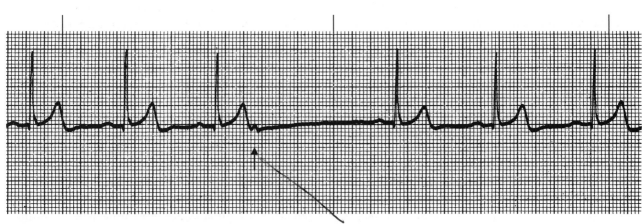

Figure 7-14. Normal sinus rhythm with nonconducted premature atrial contraction (PAC).
Rhythm: Basic rhythm regular; irregular with nonconducted PAC
Rate: Basic rate 60 beats/minute; rate slows following nonconducted PAC (Rate suppression can occur following a pause in the
                 basic rhythm; after several cycles, the rate will return to the basic rhythm rate.)
P waves: Sinus P waves with basic rhythm; premature, abnormal P wave with nonconducted PAC
PR interval: 0.20 second
QRS complex: 0.06 to 0.08 second
Comment: A U wave is present.

Box 7-3.

Nonconducted PACs: Identifying ECG features

Rhythm:	Underlying rhythm usually regular; irregular with nonconducted PACs
Rate:	That of underlying rhythm
P waves:	P wave associated with the nonconducted PAC is premature, and abnormal in size, shape, or direction; often found hidden in preceding T wave, distorting the T wave contour
PR interval:	Absent with nonconducted PAC
QRS complex:	Absent with nonconducted PAC

in the preceding T wave, distorting the T-wave contour (Figure 7-15), and the pause that follows is usually noncompensatory. The nonconducted PAC is the most common cause of unexpected pauses in a regular sinus rhythm.

The nonconducted PAC can be confused with sinus arrest or block (especially if the P wave of the PAC occurs early enough to be hidden in the preceding T wave). All three produce a sudden pause in the rhythm without QRS complexes. To differentiate between these rhythms, one must examine and compare T-wave contours (Figure 7-16). The early, abnormal P wave of the nonconducted PAC will distort the preceding T wave. In sinus arrest or sinus block,

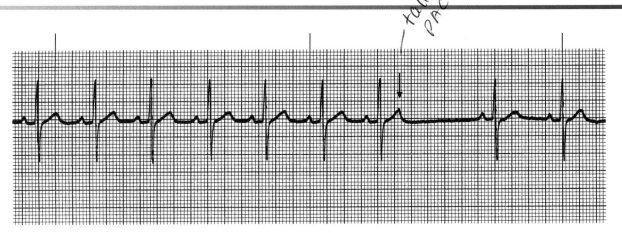

Figure 7-15. Sinus rhythm with nonconducted premature atrial contraction (PAC).

Rhythm: Basic rhythm regular; irregular with nonconducted PACs
Rate: Basic rhythm rate 88 beats/minute
P waves: Sinus P waves with basic rhythm; P wave of nonconducted PAC is premature, abnormal, and hidden in the preceding T wave
                 (T wave is taller and more pointed than those of underlying rhythm.)
PR interval: 0.16 to 0.18 second (basic rhythm); not present with nonconducted PAC
QRS complex: 0.06 to 0.08 second (basic rhythm); not present with nonconducted PAC.

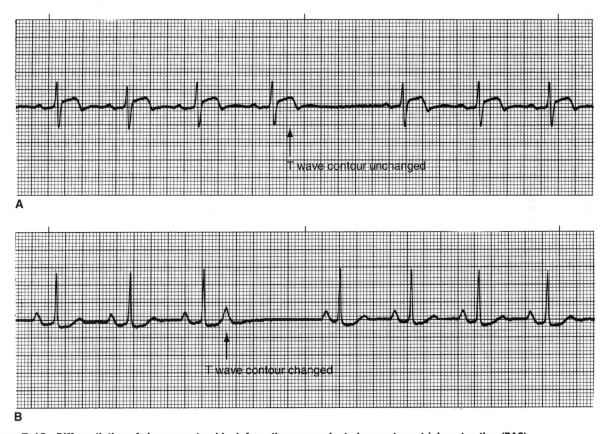

A

B

Figure 7-16. Differentiation of sinus arrest or block from the nonconducted premature atrial contraction (PAC).

A Sinus arrest or block
1. Sudden pause in the basic rhythm
2. No P wave present
3. T-wave contour occurring during pause remains unchanged

B Nonconducted PAC
1. Sudden pause in the basic rhythm
2. Abnormal, premature P wave present and often found hidden in T wave
3. T-wave contour occurring during pause will be different from the contours of the basic rhythm.

no P wave is produced and the T-wave contour remains unchanged.

Nonconducted PACs have the same significance as conducted PACs and may be treated in the same manner.

Paroxysmal atrial tachycardia

Paroxysmal atrial tachycardia (PAT) (Figures 7-17 and 7-18 and Box 7-4) originates in an ectopic pacemaker site in the atria producing a rapid, regular atrial rhythm between 140 and 250 beats per minute. Atrial tachycardia

Box 7-4.
Atrial tachycardia: Identifying ECG features

Rhythm:	Regular
Rate:	140 to 250 beats/minute
P waves:	Abnormal (commonly pointed); usually hidden in preceding T wave, making T wave and P wave appear as one wave deflection (T-P wave); one P wave to each QRS complex unless AV block is present
PR interval:	Usually not measurable
QRS complex:	Normal (0.10 second or less)

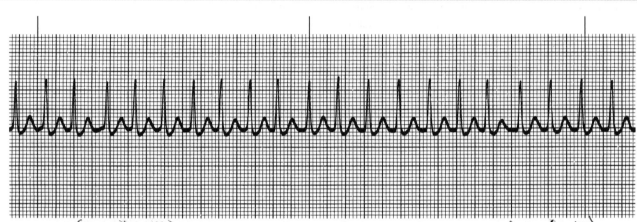

Figure 7-17. Paroxysmal atrial tachycardia.   *(comes & goes) X*   *Supraventricular tachycardia (SVT)*

Rhythm:	Regular
Rate:	188 beats/minute
P waves:	Hidden *- in T waves*
PR interval:	Not measurable
QRS complex:	0.06 to 0.08 second.

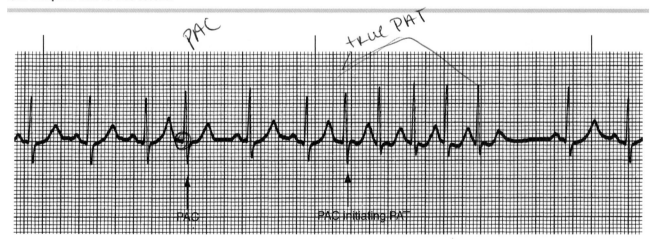

PAC   *true PAT*

PAC   *PAC initiating PAT*

Figure 7-18. Normal sinus rhythm with premature atrial contraction (PAC) and burst of paroxysmal atrial tachycardia (PAT).

Rhythm:	Basic rhythm regular; irregular with PAC and burst of PAT
Rate:	Basic rhythm rate 94 beats/minute; PAT rate 167 beats/minute
P waves:	Sinus P waves with basic rhythm; premature, pointed P waves with PAC and PAT (P waves are superimposed on preceding T waves.)
PR interval:	0.16 second
QRS complex:	0.08 second
Comment:	A run of three or more consecutive PACs is considered PAT.

is often precipitated by a PAC and commonly starts and stops abruptly, occurring in bursts or paroxysms (thus the name paroxysmal atrial tachycardia). By definition, three or more consecutive PACs (at a rate of 140 to 250 beats/minute) is considered to be atrial tachycardia (Figure 7-18). This rhythm may be due to enhanced automaticity of atrial pacemaker cells, resulting in rapid firing of an ectopic atrial focus, or to an atrial reentry circuit in which an impulse travels rapidly and repeatedly around a circular pathway in the atria.

The P waves associated with atrial tachycardia are abnormal (commonly pointed), but may be difficult to identify because they're usually hidden in the preceding T wave (the T wave and P wave appear as one deflection called the T–P wave). One P wave precedes each QRS complex, unless AV block is present. The PR interval is usually not measurable. The duration of the QRS complex is normal. Atrial tachycardia is characterized by regular, narrow QRS complexes, occurring at a rate of 140 to 250 beats per minute, and separated by the T–P wave.

Atrial tachycardia may occur in people with healthy hearts as well as those with diseased hearts. Atrial tachycardia has been associated with ingestion of substances such as caffeine, alcohol, or tobacco; anxiety; hyperthyroidism; use of drugs such as albuterol or theophylline; mitral valve disease; chronic obstructive pulmonary disease; and digitalis toxicity.

During an episode of atrial tachycardia, many individuals can feel the *palpitations* (rapid heart rate), and this is a source of anxiety. When the ventricular rate is rapid, the ventricles are unable to fill completely during diastole, resulting in a significant reduction in cardiac output. In addition, a rapid heart rate increases myocardial oxygen requirements and cardiac workload. Treatment of atrial tachycardia is directed toward controlling the ventricular rate and converting the rhythm.

Priorities of treatment depend on the patient's tolerance of the rhythm. *Cardioversion* (synchronized electrical shock) is the initial treatment of choice in patients whose condition is unstable (patient is symptomatic with low blood pressure; cool, clammy skin; complains of chest pain or dyspnea; and exhibits signs of heart failure). If the patient's condition is stable, sedation alone may terminate the rhythm or slow the rate. If sedation is unsuccessful, vagal maneuvers may terminate some episodes of PAT. Vagal maneuvers work by slowing the heart rate through increasing parasympathetic tone. Vagal maneuvers include coughing, bearing down (the *Valsalva maneuver*), squatting, breath-holding, carotid sinus pressure, stimulation of the gag reflex, and immersion of the face in ice water. If vagal maneuvers fail, administer a 6-mg bolus of adenosine IV rapidly over 1 to 2 seconds, followed by a rapid 10-mL flush of saline. If the initial dose is ineffective after 2 minutes, administer a 12-mg bolus of adenosine IV rapidly over 1 to 2 seconds, followed by a rapid 10-mL flush of saline. If the second

dose is ineffective after 2 minutes, repeat a 12-mg dose of adenosine in the same manner.

If the patient doesn't respond to vagal maneuvers or to the administration of three doses of adenosine, attempt rate control using a calcium channel blocker (such as diltiazem) or a beta blocker. These drugs act primarily on nodal tissue, either to slow the ventricular response by blocking conduction through the AV node or to terminate the reentry mechanism that depends on conduction through the AV node. In the setting of significantly impaired left ventricular (LV) function (clinical evidence of congestive heart failure or moderately to severely reduced LV ejection fraction), caution should be exercised in administering drugs with negative inotropic effects. These include beta blockers and calcium channel blockers, with the exception of diltiazem (a calcium channel blocker that exhibits less depression of contractility when compared with similar drugs).

When AV nodal agents are unsuccessful, cardioversion should be used to terminate the rhythm. Once the rhythm is terminated, antiarrhythmics may be effective in controlling the rhythm. Radiofrequency catheter ablation of the ectopic focus or reentry circuit is successful in many cases.

Atrial flutter

Atrial flutter (Figures 7-19 through 7-22 and Box 7-5) originates in an ectopic pacemaker site in the atria typically depolarizing at a rate between 250 and 400 beats per minute (the average rate is around 300 beats per minute). The atrial muscles respond to this rapid stimulation by producing waveforms that resemble the teeth of a saw. The sawtooth waveforms are called flutter waves (F waves). The typical atrial flutter wave consists of an initial negative component followed by a positive component producing V-shaped waveforms with a sawtooth appearance. The flutter waves affect the whole baseline to such a degree that there is no isoelectric line between the F waves, and the T wave is partially or completely obscured by the flutter waves. Atrial flutter is primarily recognized by this sawtooth baseline. The PR interval is not measurable. The QRS complexes are normal.

Box 7-5.
Atrial flutter: Identifying ECG features

Rhythm:	Regular or irregular (depends on AV conduction ratios)
Rate:	Atrial rate: 250 to 400 beats/minute Ventricular rate: Varies with number of impulses conducted through AV node (will be less than the atrial rate)
P waves:	Sawtooth deflections called flutter waves (F waves) affecting entire baseline
PR interval:	Not measurable
QRS complex:	Normal (0.10 second or less)

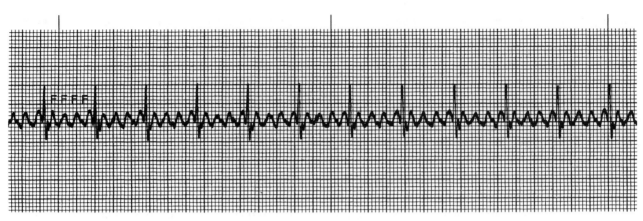

Figure 7-19. Atrial flutter with 4:1 AV conduction.
Rhythm: Regular
Rate: Atrial: 428 beats/minute
               Ventricular: 107 beats/minute
               Note: If the ventricular rate is regular, multiply the number of flutter waves before each QRS × the ventricular rate to deter-
               mine atrial rate.
P waves: Four flutter waves before each QRS (marked as F waves above)
PR interval: Not measurable
QRS complex: 0.06 to 0.08 second.

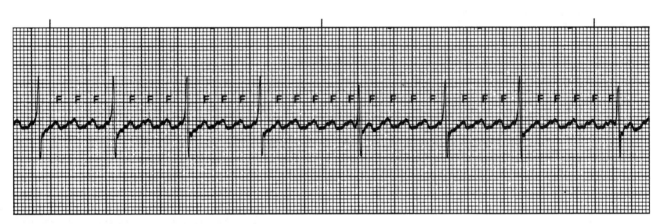

Figure 7-20. Atrial flutter with variable AV conduction.
Rhythm: Irregular
Rate: Atrial: 250 beats/minute
               Ventricular: 60 beats/minute
               Note: If the ventricular rate is irregular, count the number of flutter waves in a 6-second strip and multiply × 10 to obtain
               atrial rate.
P waves: Flutter waves before each QRS (varying ratios)
PR interval: Not measurable
QRS complex: 0.08 second.

While the atria can tolerate the extremely high heart rate reasonably well, the lower chambers (ventricles) cannot. Fortunately, the AV node is present to slow down and diminish the number of impulses that pass through to the ventricles. The AV node conducts the impulses in various ratios. For example, the AV node might allow every second impulse to travel through the AV junction to the ventricles, resulting in a 2:1 AV conduction ratio (a 2:1 conduction ratio indicates that for every two flutter waves,

only one is followed by a QRS complex). Even ratios (2:1, 4:1) are more common than odd ratios (3:1, 5:1). If the conduction ratio remains constant (2:1), the ventricular rhythm will be regular, and the rhythm is described as atrial flutter with 2:1 conduction. If the conduction ratio varies (from 4:1 to 2:1 to 6:1), the ventricular rhythm will be irregular, and the rhythm is described as atrial flutter with variable AV conduction. Conduction ratios are shown in Figures 7-19 and 7-20. In atrial flutter, the ventricular

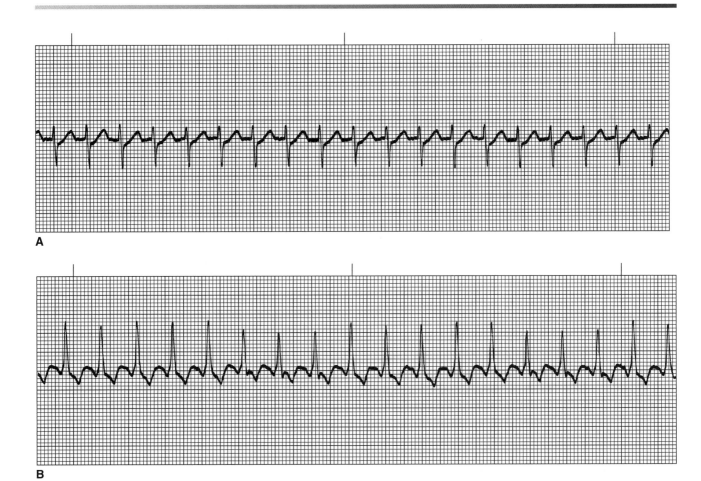

Figure 7-21. **Comparison of atrial flutter with 2:1 AV conduction and paroxysmal atrial tachycardia (PAT).**
Example A. The rhythm shows PAT. This strip shows the T-P wave (the T and P waves appear as one deflection). An isoelectric line is present after the T–P wave.
Example B. The rhythm shows atrial flutter with 2:1 AV conduction. This strip shows two flutter (sawtooth) waves before each QRS complex. There is no isoelectric line.

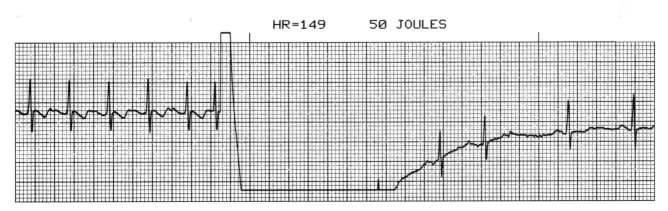

Figure 7-22. Cardioversion of atrial flutter with 2:1 atrioventricular conduction to normal sinus rhythm using 50 joules electrical energy.

rate is slower than the atrial rate, with the rate depending on the number of impulses conducted through the AV node to the ventricles.

Because atrial flutter usually occurs at a rate of 300 beats per minute and the AV node usually blocks at least half of these impulses, a ventricular rate of 150 beats per minute is common (a 2:1 AV conduction ratio). Atrial flutter with 2:1 AV conduction may be difficult to differentiate from atrial tachycardia, especially if the heart rate in both rhythms is 150 beats per minute. These two arrhythmias can be differentiated by closely examining the baseline. In atrial tachycardia, an isoelectric line can usually be seen, whereas in atrial flutter the isoelectric line is absent. A comparison of atrial flutter with 2:1 AV conduction and PAT is shown in Figure 7- 21.

Atrial flutter is rarely seen in people with a normal heart. This arrhythmia most often occurs in patients with mitral or tricuspid valve disease. Atrial flutter is common after cardiac surgery. It may also occur in ischemic heart disease, pulmonary embolism, and in alcohol intoxication.

Like PAT, the ventricular rate in atrial flutter may be rapid, increasing myocardial oxygen requirements and cardiac workload and decreasing cardiac output. In addition, the atria do not contract strongly enough to empty all the blood from the atrial chambers into the ventricles. This results in a loss of the atrial kick, which further decreases cardiac output. Over time some blood in the atria may stagnate and *mural thrombi* (clots in the atrial chambers) may form. Pieces of the clot may break off, leading to a risk of systemic or pulmonary emboli.

Priorities of treatment include controlling the ventricular rate, assessing anticoagulation needs, and restoring sinus rhythm. As with PAT, controlling the ventricular rate should be attempted first using a calcium channel blocker, such as diltiazem, or a beta blocker, using caution in those patients with impaired left ventricular function. Before attempting conversion of the rhythm, it's essential to know the approximate onset of the arrhythmia. If atrial flutter has been present for less than 48 hours, it's safe to convert the rhythm with cardioversion or amiodarone. If atrial flutter has been present for more than 48 hours (or the onset is unknown), pulmonary or systemic embolization

with conversion to sinus rhythm is a risk unless the patient has been adequately anticoagulated. In this situation, attempts to convert the rhythm with cardioversion or an antiarrhythmic should be delayed until the patient is adequately anticoagulated.

One method of anticoagulation involves placing the patient on an oral anticoagulant at home for several weeks, then admitting the patient to the hospital for a transesophageal echocardiogram (TEE). If the TEE is negative for atrial clots, the patient can safely have the rhythm electrically cardioverted. The patient is then discharged home on an oral anticoagulant for several more weeks. Some physicians prefer a quicker approach, using IV heparin or subcutaneous enoxaparin (Lovenox) or dalteparin (Fragmin) in a hospital setting. If the TEE is negative for mural thrombi, cardioversion may be attempted within 24 hours. The patient is discharged home on an oral anticoagulant for several weeks.

Unstable atrial flutter should be treated immediately with cardioversion, regardless of the duration of the arrhythmia. Figure 7-22 is an example of atrial flutter converting to sinus rhythm after cardioversion

Antiarrhythmics are useful in maintaining sinus rhythm after conversion. Radiofrequency catheter ablation of the flutter reentry circuit is becoming the treatment of choice for chronic or recurrent atrial flutter.

Atrial fibrillation

Atrial fibrillation (Figures 7-23 through 7-26 and Box 7-6) is a rapid and highly irregular heart rhythm caused by chaotic electrical impulses that arise from an ectopic site in the atria, depolarizing at a rate greater than

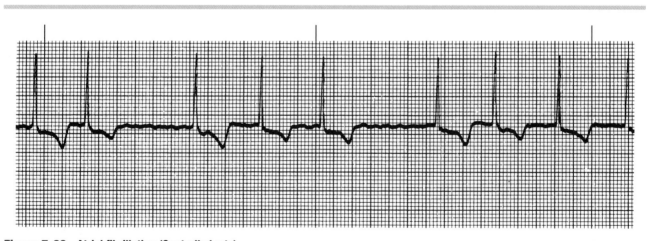

Figure 7-23. Atrial fibrillation (Controlled rate).

Rhythm:	Irregular
Rate:	Ventricular rate 70 beats/minute
P waves:	Fibrillatory waves present
PR interval:	Not measurable
QRS complex:	0.04 to 0.06 second
Comment:	ST-segment depression and T-wave inversion are present.

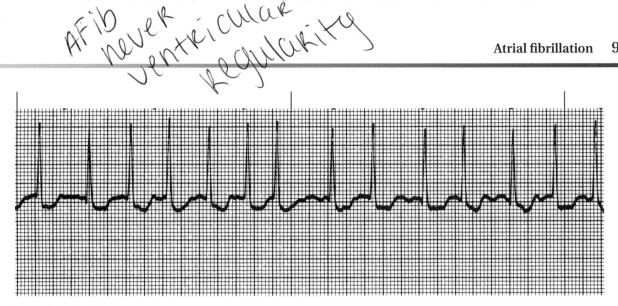

Figure 7-24. Atrial fibrillation (Uncontrolled rate).

Rhythm:	Irregular
Rate:	Ventricular rate 130 beats/minute
P waves:	Fibrillatory waves present
PR interval:	Not measurable
QRS complex:	0.06 to 0.08 second
Comment:	ST-segment depression is present.

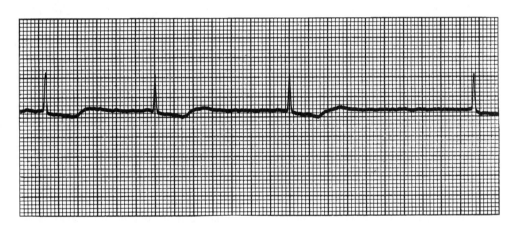

Figure 7-25. Atrial fibrillation with f waves so small they appear to be almost a flat line between QRS complexes.

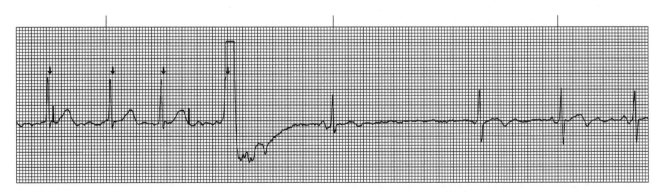

Figure 7-26. Cardioversion of atrial fibrillation to sinus rhythm; junctional escape beat (discussed in Chapter 8) follows the initial sinus beat.

Box 7-6.
Atrial fibrillation: Identifying ECG features

Rhythm: Grossly irregular (unless the ventricular rate is very rapid, in which case the rhythm becomes more regular)

Rate: Atrial rate: 400 beats/minute or more; not measurable on surface ECG
Ventricular rate: Varies with number of impulses conducted through AV node to the ventricles (will be less than the atrial rate)

P waves: Irregular wave deflections called fibrillatory waves (f waves) affecting entire baseline

PR interval: Not measurable

QRS complex: Normal (0.10 second or less)

400 beats per minute. The mechanism of this rhythm is most likely multiple reentry circuits in the atria. These impulses are so rapid that they cause the atria to quiver instead of contract regularly, producing irregular, wavy deflections. These wave deflections are called *fibrillatory waves* (f waves). If the waves are large, they're described as *coarse fibrillatory waves* and if small they're called *fine fibrillatory waves*. Sometimes the f waves are so small they appear to be almost a flat line between the QRS complexes (Figure 7-25). As in atrial flutter, the wavy deflections seen in atrial fibrillation affect the whole baseline. Flutter waves are sometimes seen mixed with the fibrillatory waves. This mixed rhythm is commonly called atrial fib-flutter, meaning the basic rhythm is atrial fibrillation with some flutter waves present. In atrial fib, an actual atrial rate is not measurable. The PR interval is also not measurable. The QRS duration is normal. Because the atrial impulses occur very irregularly, the ventricular response will be irregular also.

As in atrial flutter, the AV node blocks most of the impulses from entering the ventricles, thus protecting the ventricles from excessive rates. The ventricular rate is slower than the atrial rate and depends on the number of impulses conducted through the AV node to the ventricles. When the ventricular rate is less than 100 beats per minute, the rhythm is called controlled atrial fibrillation. When the ventricular rate is greater than 100 beats per minute, the rhythm is called uncontrolled atrial fibrillation or atrial fibrillation with a rapid ventricular response. Atrial fibrillation is primarily recognized by the wavy baseline and the grossly irregular ventricular rhythm (Figure 7-23). If the ventricular rate is very rapid, the ventricular rhythm becomes somewhat more regular (Figure 7-24).

Atrial fibrillation is the most common rhythm seen next to sinus rhythm. Atrial fibrillation can occur in healthy individuals or in those with heart disease. In healthy individuals, the rhythm is usually temporary and may be associated with emotional stress or excessive alcohol consumption ("holiday heart syndrome"). In many patients this type of atrial fibrillation spontaneously reverts to sinus rhythm or is easily converted with drug therapy alone. Other conditions commonly associated with atrial fibrillation include coronary artery disease, hypertension, valvular heart disease, congestive heart failure, and pulmonary disease. It is also common after cardiac surgery.

The clinical consequences of atrial fibrillation are similar to those of atrial flutter. The ventricular rate may be rapid, increasing myocardial oxygen demands and cardiac workload and decreasing cardiac output. Because the atria quiver rather than contract effectively, the atrial kick is lost, which can further reduce cardiac output. Decreased cardiac output is especially marked in patients with underlying cardiac impairment and in the elderly, who appear to be more dependent on atrial contraction for filling of the ventricles. The noncontracting atria cause blood to pool in the atrial chambers, increasing the potential for thrombus formation. Dislodgment of atrial clots may lead to pulmonary or systemic embolization.

Treatment of atrial fibrillation includes controlling the heart rate, providing anticoagulation as a prophylaxis for thromboembolism, and returning the atria to a sinus rhythm. The treatment protocols for atrial fibrillation are the same as those for atrial flutter. Rate control should be achieved first, using a calcium channel blocker, such as diltiazem, or a beta blocker. Use caution in those patients with impaired left ventricular function. If the rhythm is less than 48 hours old, cardioversion or an antiarrhythmic, such as amiodarone, can be used in an attempt to restore the rhythm to a sinus rhythm. If atrial fibrillation has been present for more than 48 hours, the patient must be adequately anticoagulated (refer to anticoagulation protocols for atrial flutter) before attempts are made to restore sinus rhythm using cardioversion or an antiarrhythmic. Unstable atrial fibrillation should be cardioverted immediately, regardless of the duration of the arrhythmia. Patients with chronic atrial fibrillation (present for months or years) may not convert to sinus rhythm with any therapy. Treatment of these patients should be directed at controlling the ventricular rate and providing anticoagulation. An option to medication therapy is radiofrequency catheter ablation, which has been associated with a high success rate.

Cardioversion of atrial fibrillation to a sinus rhythm is shown in Figure 7-26. A summary of the identifying ECG features of atrial arrhythmias can be found in Table 7-1.

Table 7-1.
Atrial arrhythmias: Summary of identifying ECG features

Name	Rhythm	Rate (beats/minute)	P waves (lead II)	PR interval	QRS complex
Wandering atrial pacemaker	Regular or irregular	Normal (60–100) or slow (<60)	Vary in size, shape, and direction; one P wave precedes each QRS complex	Usually normal duration, but may be abnormal depending on changing pacemaker location	Normal (0.10 second or less)
Premature atrial pacemaker	Basic rhythm usually regular; irregular with premature atrial contraction (PAC)	That of basic rhythm	P wave associated with PAC is premature and abnormal in size, shape, or direction (commonly small, upright, and pointed; may be inverted); commonly found hidden in preceding T wave, distorting T-wave contour	Usually normal, but may be abnormal; not measurable if hidden in preceding T wave	Premature; normal duration (0.10 second or less)
Nonconducted premature atrial contraction	Basic rhythm usually regular; irregular with nonconducted PAC	That of basic rhythm	Premature P wave that is abnormal in size, shape, or direction; commonly found in preceding T wave, distorting T-wave contour	Absent with nonconducted PAC	Absent with nonconducted PAC
Paroxysmal atrial tachycardia (PAT)	Regular	140–250	Abnormal P wave (commonly pointed); usually hidden in preceding T wave so that T and P wave appear as one wave deflection (T-P wave); one P wave to each QRS complex unless AV block is present	Usually not measurable	Normal (0.10 second or less)
Atrial flutter	Regular or irregular (depends on atrioventricular [AV] conduction ratios)	Atrial: 250–400 Ventricular: varies with number of impulses conducted through AV node (will be less than atrial rate)	Sawtooth deflections affecting entire baseline	Not measurable	Normal (0.10 second or less)
Atrial fibrillation	Grossly irregular (unless ventricular rate is rapid, in which case rhythm becomes more regular)	Atrial: 400 or more (can't be counted) Ventricular: varies with number of impulses conducted through AV node (will be less than atrial rate; controlled if rate < 100, uncontrolled if > 100)	Wavy deflections affecting entire baseline	Not measurable	Normal (0.10 second or less)

Rhythm strip practice: Atrial arrhythmias

Analyze the following rhythm strips by following the five basic steps:

- Determine *rhythm regularity.*
- Calculate *heart rate.* (This usually refers to the ventricular rate but, if the atrial rate differs, you need to calculate both.)
- Identify and examine *P waves.*

- Measure the *PR interval.*
- Measure the *QRS complex.*

Interpret the rhythm by comparing this data with the ECG characteristics for each rhythm. All rhythm strips are lead II, a positive lead, unless otherwise noted. Check your answers with the answer key in the appendix.

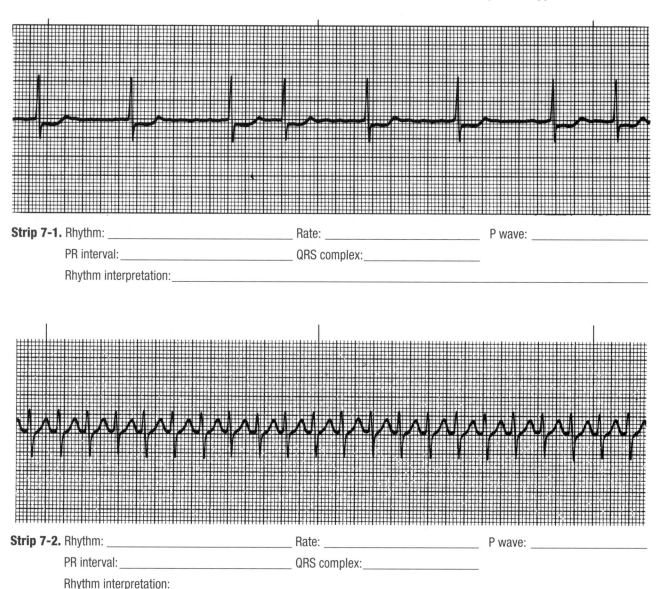

Strip 7-1. Rhythm: _____ Rate: _____ P wave: _____

PR interval: _____ QRS complex: _____

Rhythm interpretation: _____

Strip 7-2. Rhythm: _____ Rate: _____ P wave: _____

PR interval: _____ QRS complex: _____

Rhythm interpretation: _____

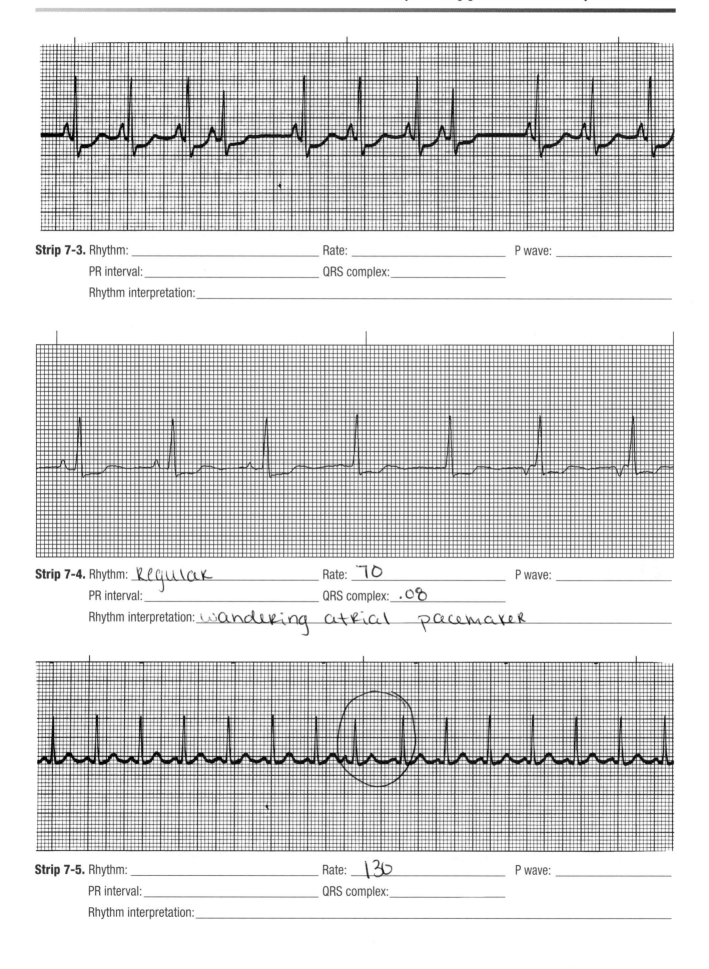

Strip 7-3. Rhythm: _____ Rate: _____ P wave: _____

PR interval: _____ QRS complex: _____

Rhythm interpretation: _____

Strip 7-4. Rhythm: _Regular_____ Rate: _70_____ P wave: _____

PR interval: _____ QRS complex: _.08_____

Rhythm interpretation: _wandering atrial pacemaker_____

Strip 7-5. Rhythm: _____ Rate: _130_____ P wave: _____

PR interval: _____ QRS complex: _____

Rhythm interpretation: _____

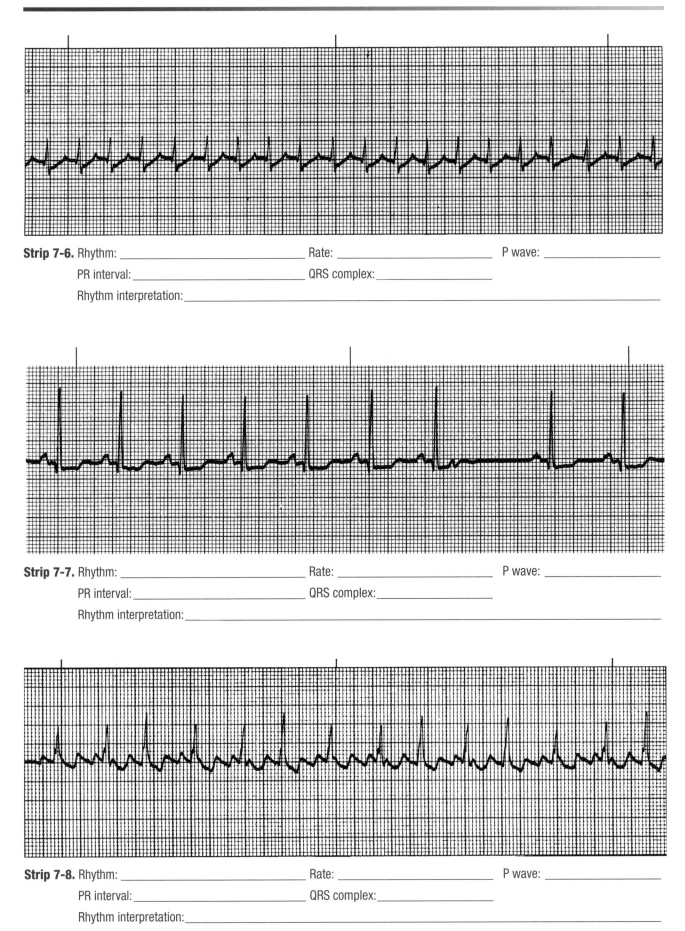

Strip 7-6. Rhythm: _____ Rate: _____ P wave: _____

PR interval: _____ QRS complex: _____

Rhythm interpretation: _____

Strip 7-7. Rhythm: _____ Rate: _____ P wave: _____

PR interval: _____ QRS complex: _____

Rhythm interpretation: _____

Strip 7-8. Rhythm: _____ Rate: _____ P wave: _____

PR interval: _____ QRS complex: _____

Rhythm interpretation: _____

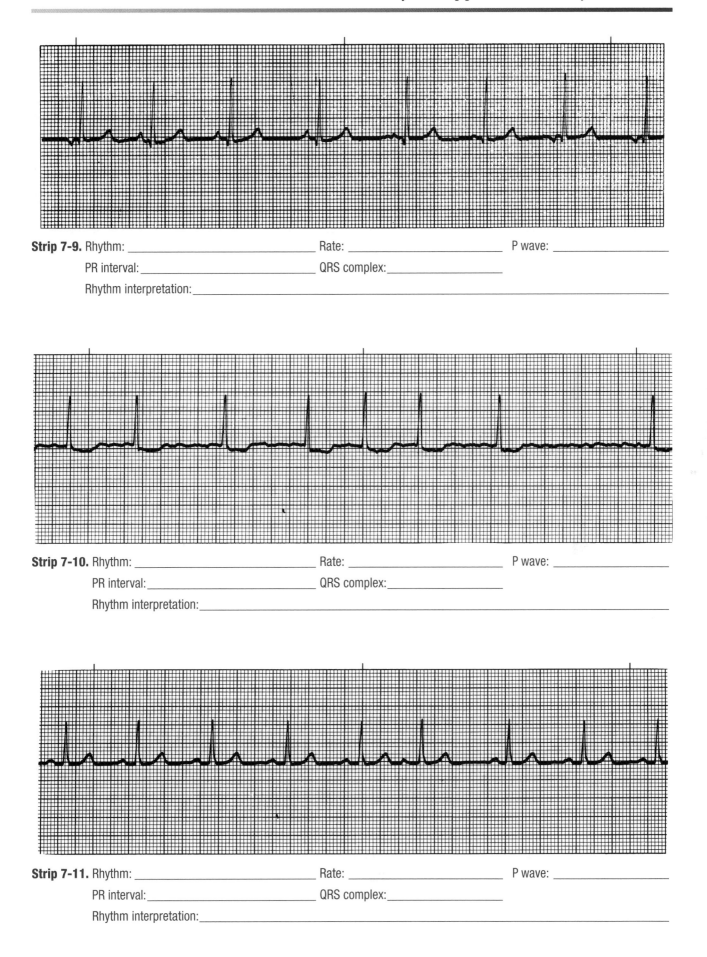

Strip 7-9. Rhythm: _____ Rate: _____ P wave: _____

PR interval: _____ QRS complex: _____

Rhythm interpretation: _____

Strip 7-10. Rhythm: _____ Rate: _____ P wave: _____

PR interval: _____ QRS complex: _____

Rhythm interpretation: _____

Strip 7-11. Rhythm: _____ Rate: _____ P wave: _____

PR interval: _____ QRS complex: _____

Rhythm interpretation: _____

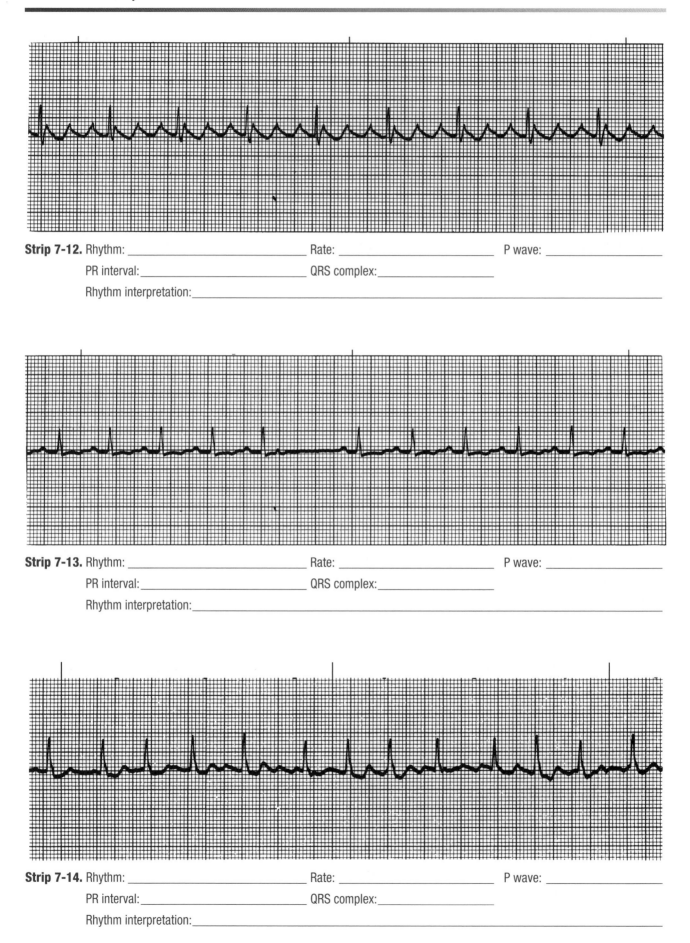

Strip 7-12. Rhythm: _____ Rate: _____ P wave: _____

PR interval: _____ QRS complex: _____

Rhythm interpretation: _____

Strip 7-13. Rhythm: _____ Rate: _____ P wave: _____

PR interval: _____ QRS complex: _____

Rhythm interpretation: _____

Strip 7-14. Rhythm: _____ Rate: _____ P wave: _____

PR interval: _____ QRS complex: _____

Rhythm interpretation: _____

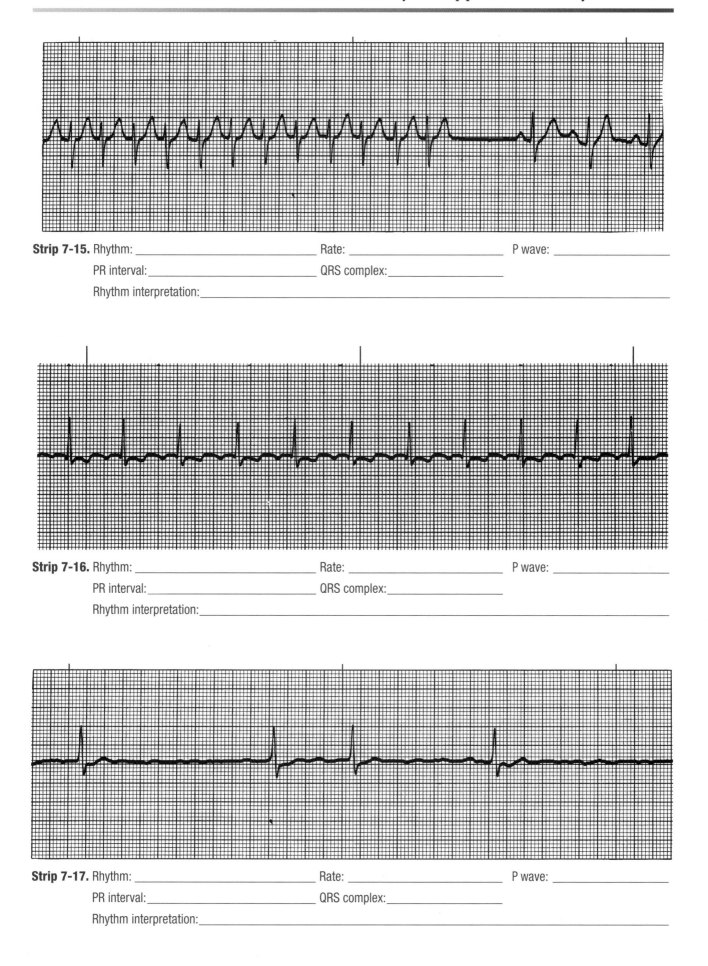

Strip 7-15. Rhythm: _____ Rate: _____ P wave: _____

PR interval:_____ QRS complex:_____

Rhythm interpretation:_____

Strip 7-16. Rhythm: _____ Rate: _____ P wave: _____

PR interval:_____ QRS complex:_____

Rhythm interpretation:_____

Strip 7-17. Rhythm: _____ Rate: _____ P wave: _____

PR interval:_____ QRS complex:_____

Rhythm interpretation:_____

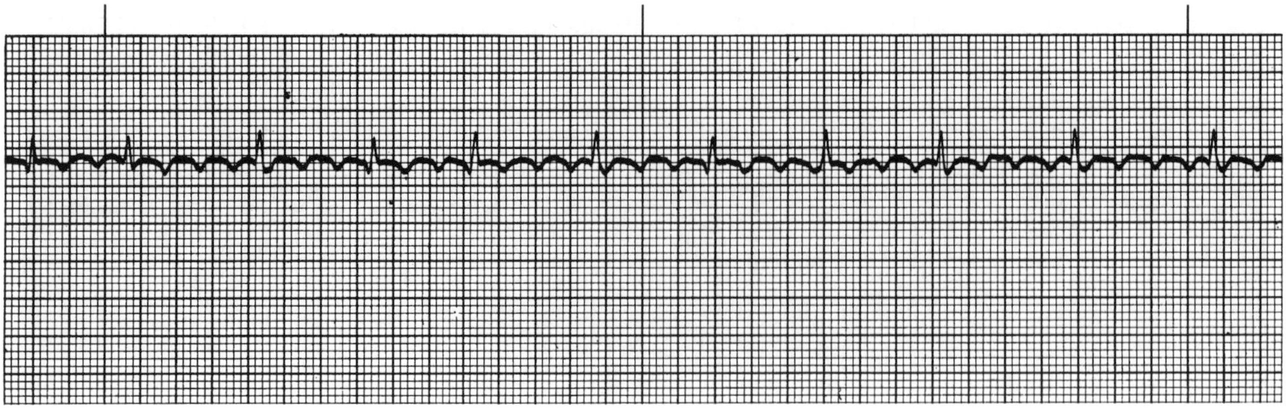

Strip 7-18. Rhythm: _____ Rate: _____ P wave: _____

PR interval:_____ QRS complex:_____

Rhythm interpretation:_____

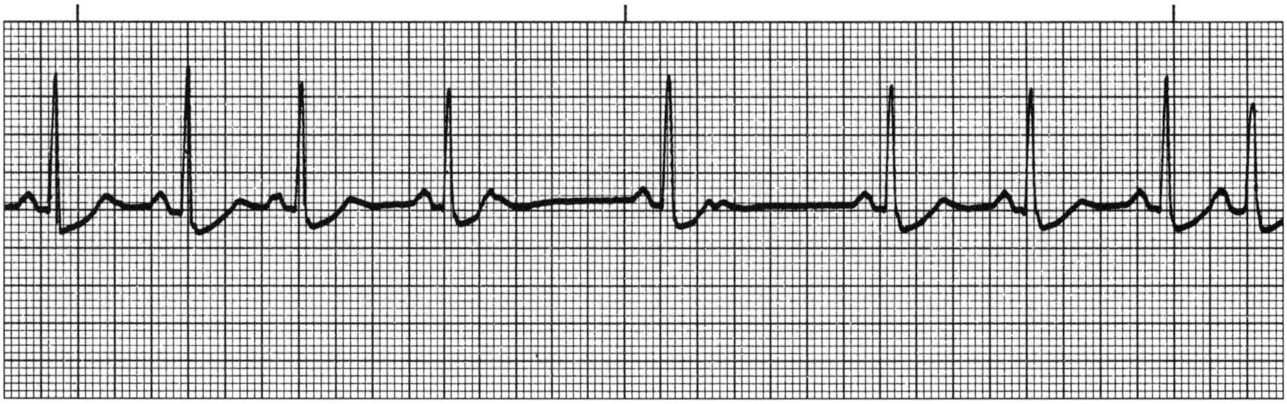

Strip 7-19. Rhythm: _____ Rate: _____ P wave: _____

PR interval:_____ QRS complex:_____

Rhythm interpretation:_____

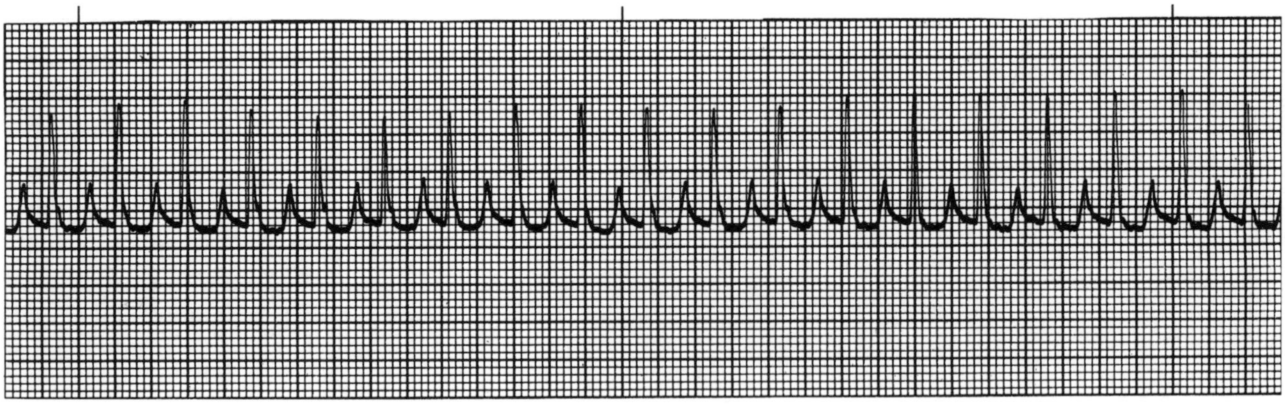

Strip 7-20. Rhythm: _____ Rate: _____ P wave: _____

PR interval:_____ QRS complex:_____

Rhythm interpretation:_____

PAC

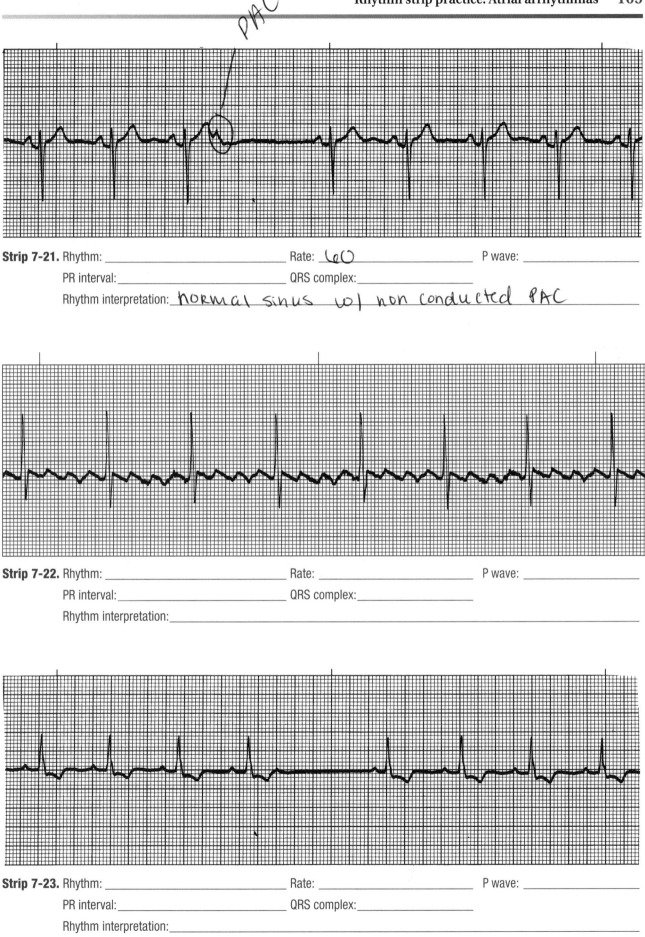

Strip 7-21. Rhythm: _____ Rate: 60 _____ P wave: _____

PR interval: _____ QRS complex: _____

Rhythm interpretation: normal sinus w/ non conducted PAC _____

Strip 7-22. Rhythm: _____ Rate: _____ P wave: _____

PR interval: _____ QRS complex: _____

Rhythm interpretation: _____

Strip 7-23. Rhythm: _____ Rate: _____ P wave: _____

PR interval: _____ QRS complex: _____

Rhythm interpretation: _____

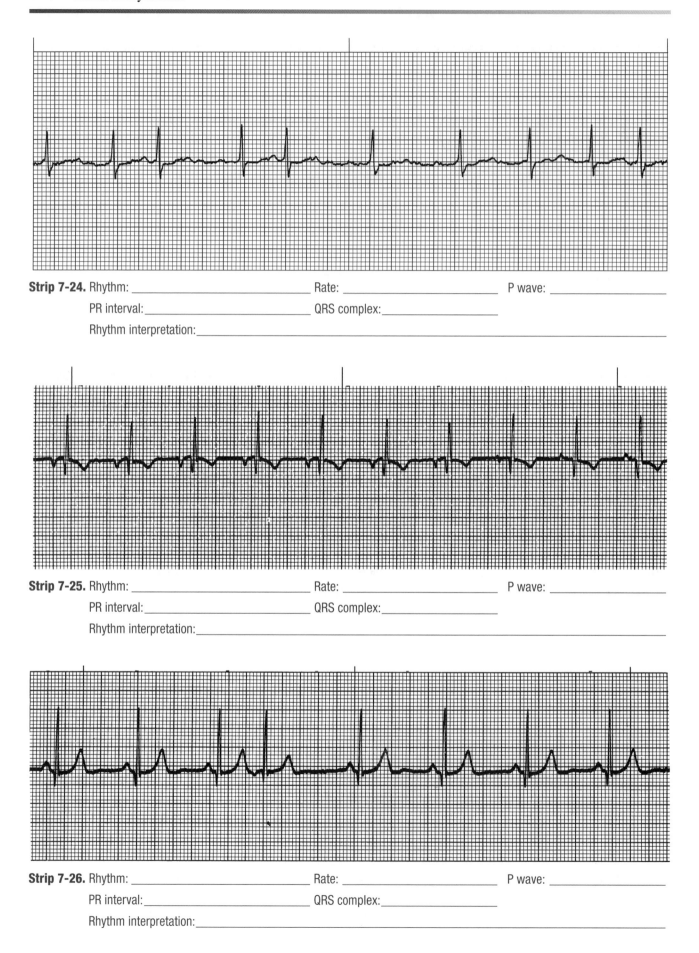

Strip 7-24. Rhythm: _____ Rate: _____ P wave: _____

PR interval: _____ QRS complex: _____

Rhythm interpretation: _____

Strip 7-25. Rhythm: _____ Rate: _____ P wave: _____

PR interval: _____ QRS complex: _____

Rhythm interpretation: _____

Strip 7-26. Rhythm: _____ Rate: _____ P wave: _____

PR interval: _____ QRS complex: _____

Rhythm interpretation: _____

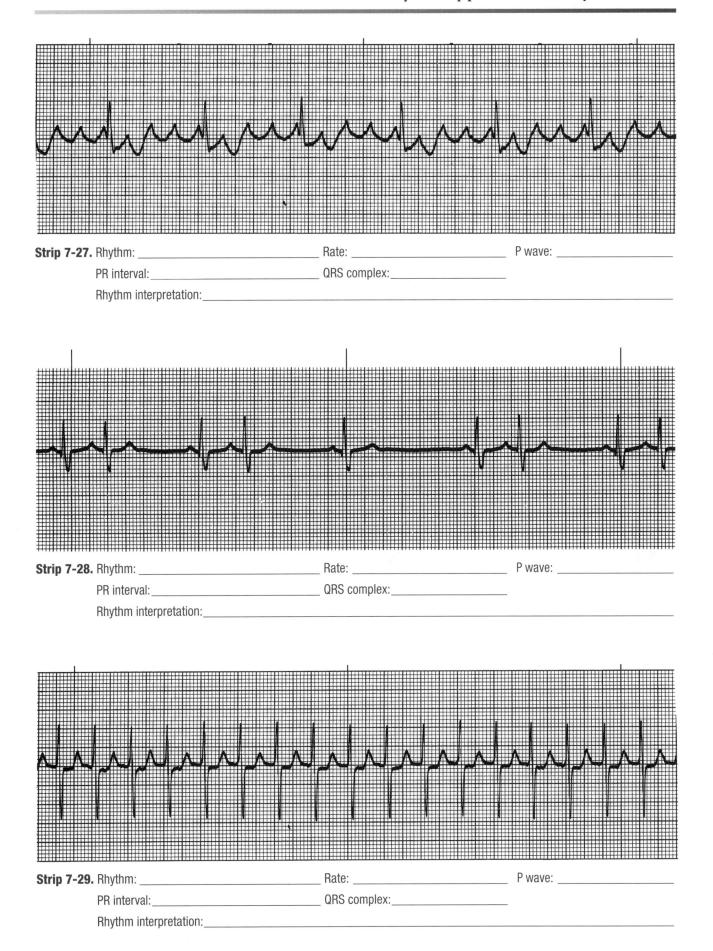

Strip 7-27. Rhythm: _____ Rate: _____ P wave: _____

PR interval:_____ QRS complex:_____

Rhythm interpretation:_____

Strip 7-28. Rhythm: _____ Rate: _____ P wave: _____

PR interval:_____ QRS complex:_____

Rhythm interpretation:_____

Strip 7-29. Rhythm: _____ Rate: _____ P wave: _____

PR interval:_____ QRS complex:_____

Rhythm interpretation:_____

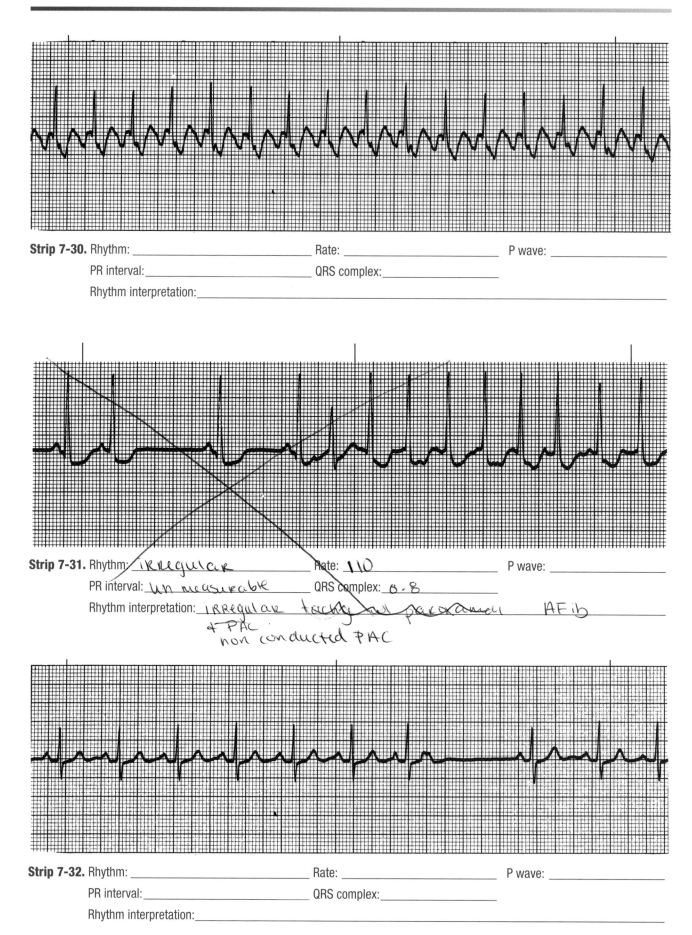

Strip 7-30. Rhythm: _____ Rate: _____ P wave: _____

PR interval: _____ QRS complex: _____

Rhythm interpretation: _____

Strip 7-31. Rhythm: _irregular_____ Rate: _110_____ P wave: _____

PR interval: _un measurable_____ QRS complex: _0.8_____

Rhythm interpretation: _irregular tachy and paroxusmal AFib_____
+ PAC
non conducted PAC

Strip 7-32. Rhythm: _____ Rate: _____ P wave: _____

PR interval: _____ QRS complex: _____

Rhythm interpretation: _____

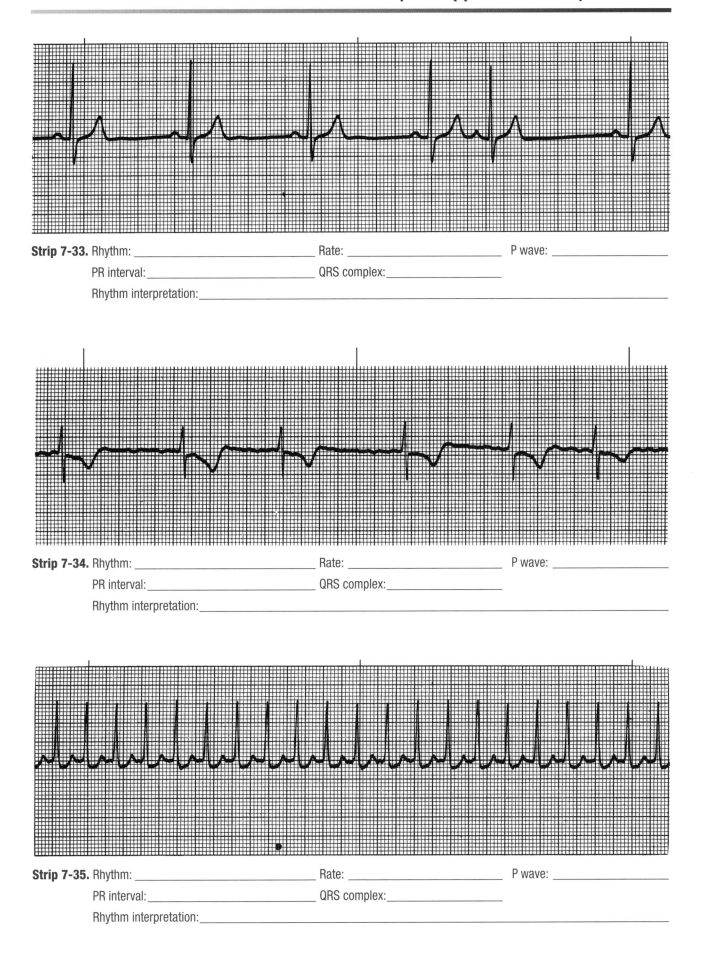

Strip 7-33. Rhythm: _____ Rate: _____ P wave: _____

PR interval: _____ QRS complex: _____

Rhythm interpretation: _____

Strip 7-34. Rhythm: _____ Rate: _____ P wave: _____

PR interval: _____ QRS complex: _____

Rhythm interpretation: _____

Strip 7-35. Rhythm: _____ Rate: _____ P wave: _____

PR interval: _____ QRS complex: _____

Rhythm interpretation: _____

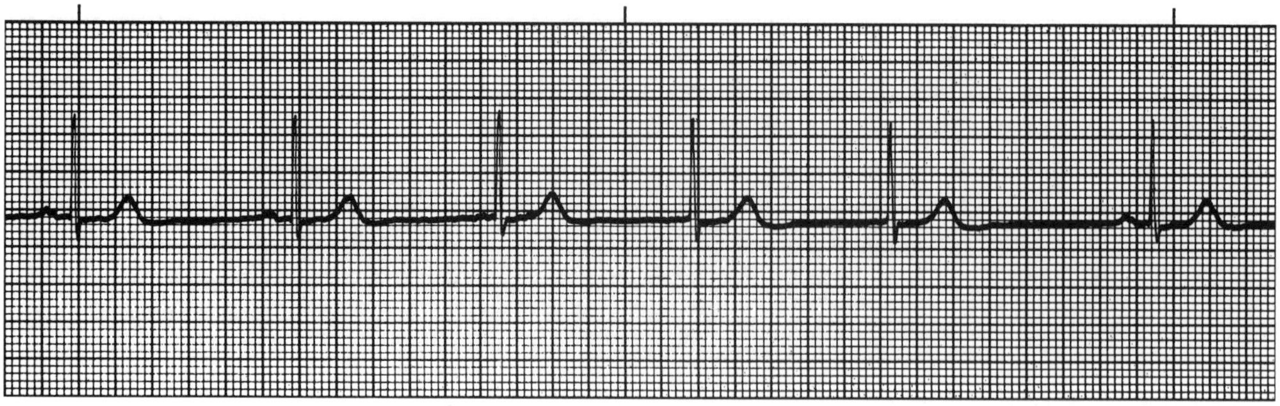

Strip 7-36. Rhythm: _____ Rate: _____ P wave: _____

PR interval:_____ QRS complex:_____

Rhythm interpretation:_____

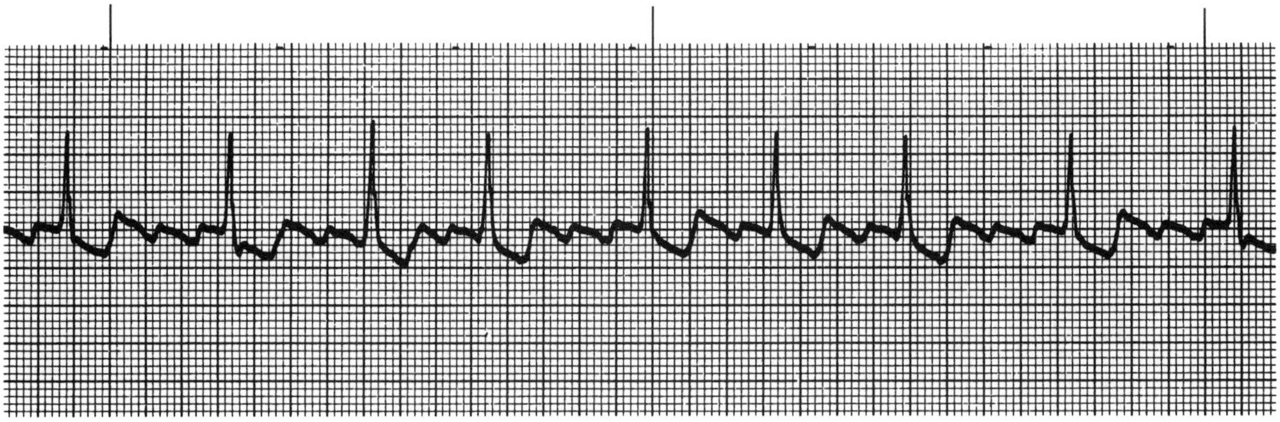

Strip 7-37. Rhythm: _____ Rate: _____ P wave: _____

PR interval:_____ QRS complex:_____

Rhythm interpretation:_____

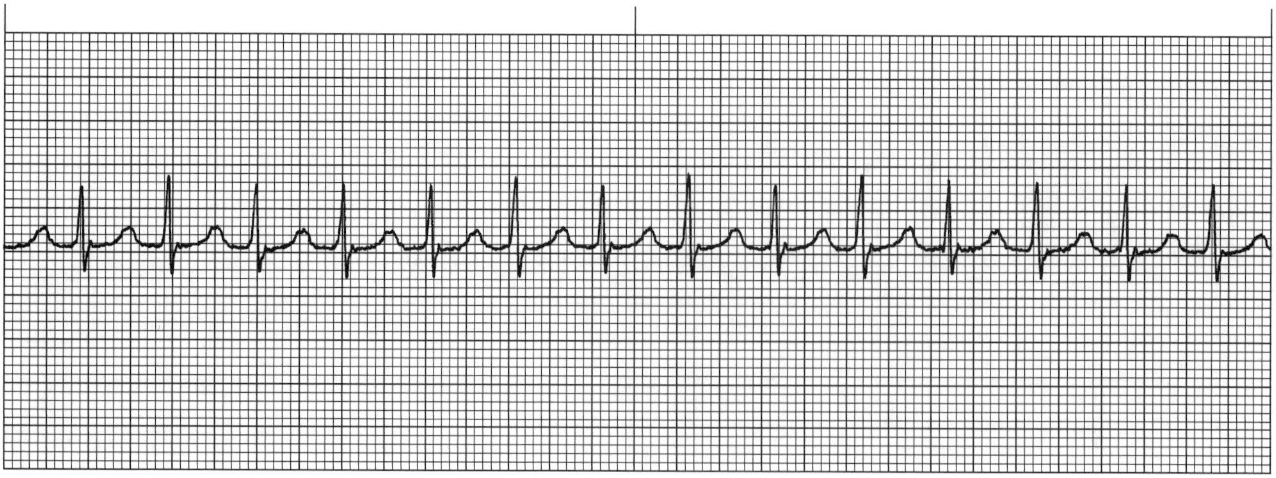

Strip 7-38. Rhythm: _____ Rate: _____ P wave: _____

PR interval:_____ QRS complex:_____

Rhythm interpretation:_____

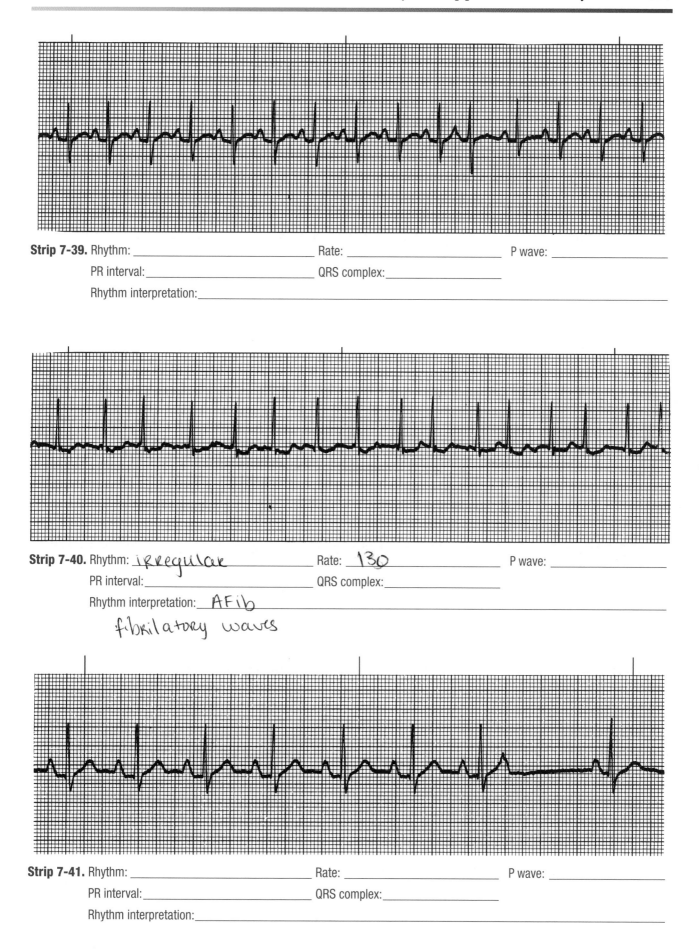

Strip 7-39. Rhythm: _____ Rate: _____ P wave: _____

PR interval: _____ QRS complex: _____

Rhythm interpretation: _____

Strip 7-40. Rhythm: _irregular_____ Rate: _130_____ P wave: _____

PR interval: _____ QRS complex: _____

Rhythm interpretation: _AFib_____

fibrilatory waves

Strip 7-41. Rhythm: _____ Rate: _____ P wave: _____

PR interval: _____ QRS complex: _____

Rhythm interpretation: _____

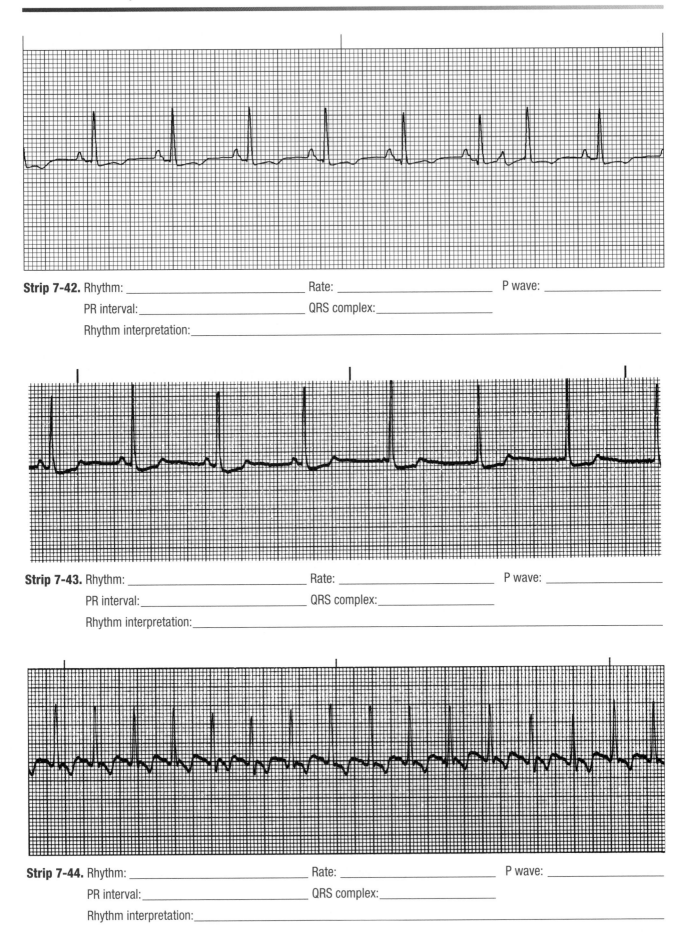

Strip 7-42. Rhythm: _____ Rate: _____ P wave: _____

PR interval: _____ QRS complex: _____

Rhythm interpretation: _____

Strip 7-43. Rhythm: _____ Rate: _____ P wave: _____

PR interval: _____ QRS complex: _____

Rhythm interpretation: _____

Strip 7-44. Rhythm: _____ Rate: _____ P wave: _____

PR interval: _____ QRS complex: _____

Rhythm interpretation: _____

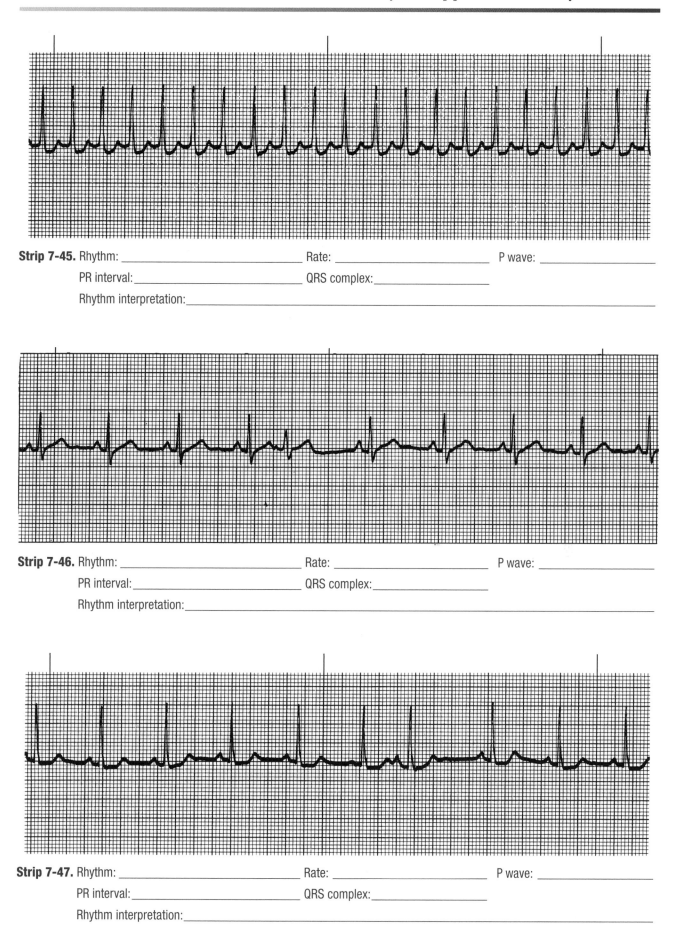

Strip 7-45. Rhythm: _____ Rate: _____ P wave: _____

PR interval:_____ QRS complex:_____

Rhythm interpretation:_____

Strip 7-46. Rhythm: _____ Rate: _____ P wave: _____

PR interval:_____ QRS complex:_____

Rhythm interpretation:_____

Strip 7-47. Rhythm: _____ Rate: _____ P wave: _____

PR interval:_____ QRS complex:_____

Rhythm interpretation:_____

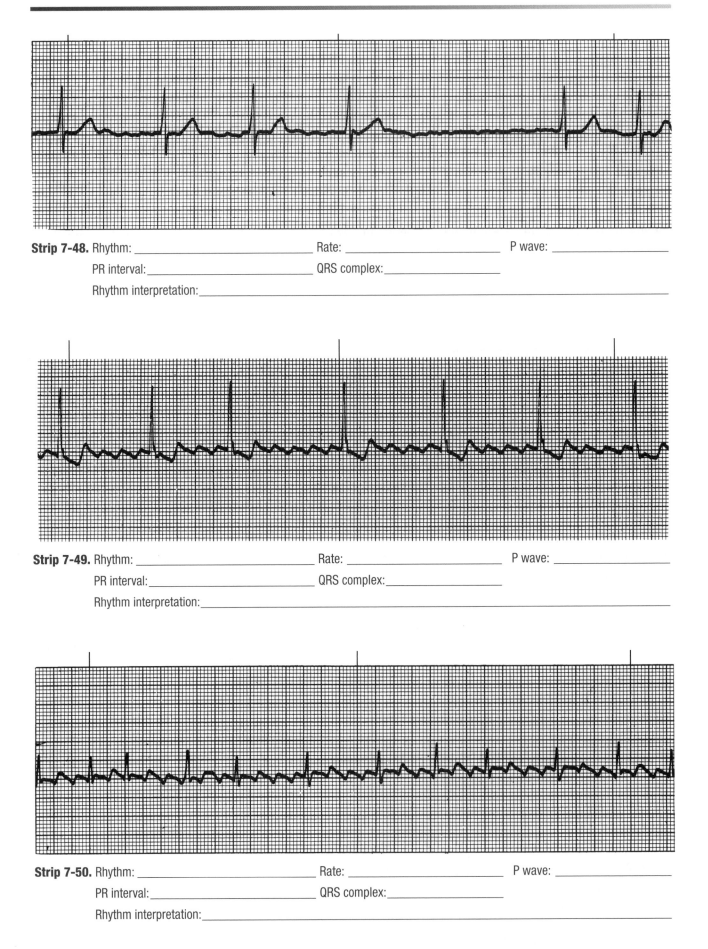

Strip 7-48. Rhythm: _____ Rate: _____ P wave: _____

PR interval: _____ QRS complex: _____

Rhythm interpretation: _____

Strip 7-49. Rhythm: _____ Rate: _____ P wave: _____

PR interval: _____ QRS complex: _____

Rhythm interpretation: _____

Strip 7-50. Rhythm: _____ Rate: _____ P wave: _____

PR interval: _____ QRS complex: _____

Rhythm interpretation: _____

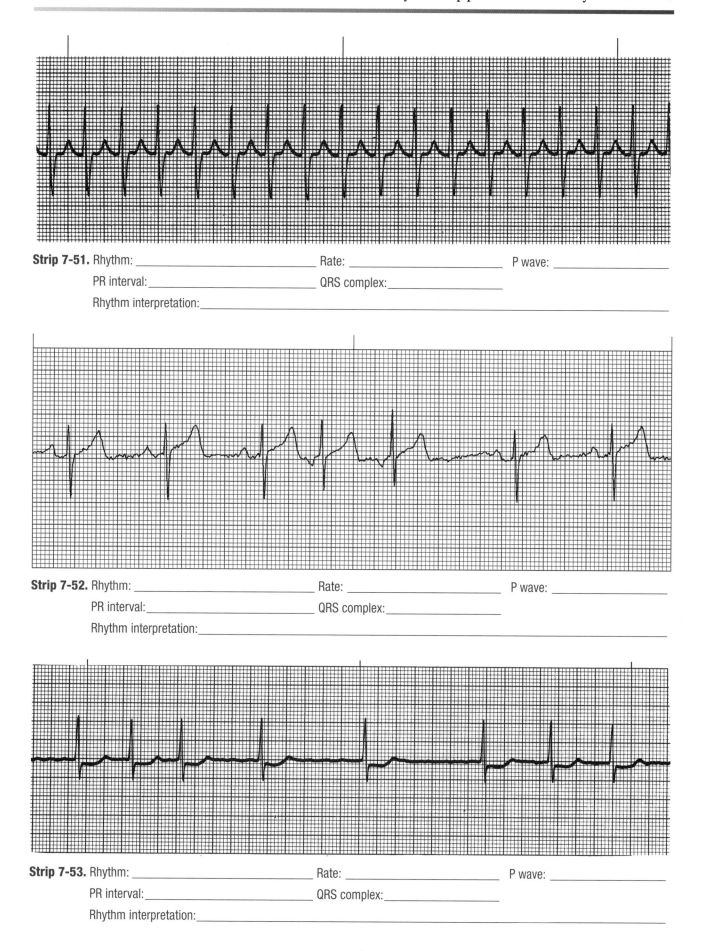

Strip 7-51. Rhythm: _____ Rate: _____ P wave: _____

PR interval:_____ QRS complex:_____

Rhythm interpretation:_____

Strip 7-52. Rhythm: _____ Rate: _____ P wave: _____

PR interval:_____ QRS complex:_____

Rhythm interpretation:_____

Strip 7-53. Rhythm: _____ Rate: _____ P wave: _____

PR interval:_____ QRS complex:_____

Rhythm interpretation:_____

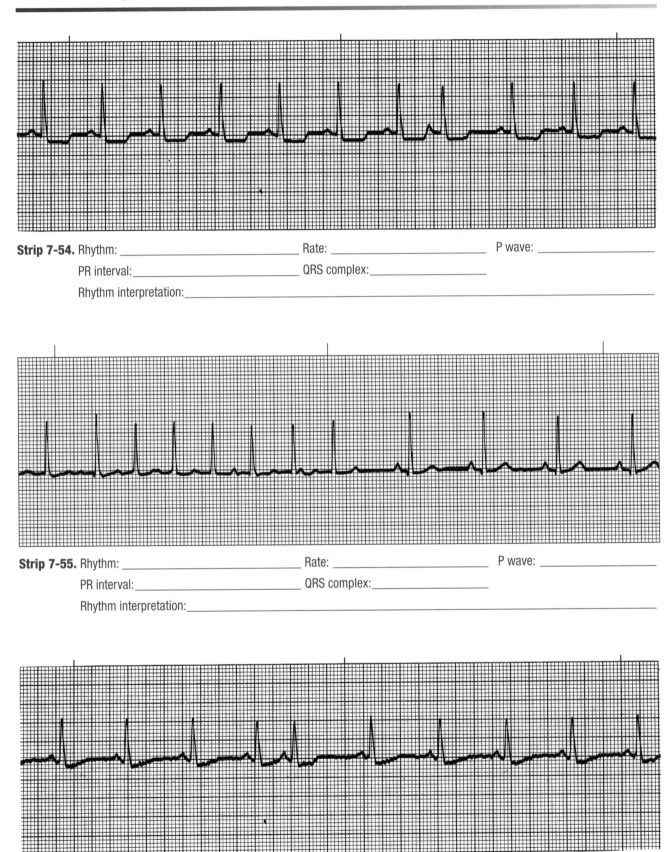

Strip 7-54. Rhythm: _____ Rate: _____ P wave: _____

PR interval: _____ QRS complex: _____

Rhythm interpretation: _____

Strip 7-55. Rhythm: _____ Rate: _____ P wave: _____

PR interval: _____ QRS complex: _____

Rhythm interpretation: _____

Strip 7-56. Rhythm: _____ Rate: _____ P wave: _____

PR interval: _____ QRS complex: _____

Rhythm interpretation: _____

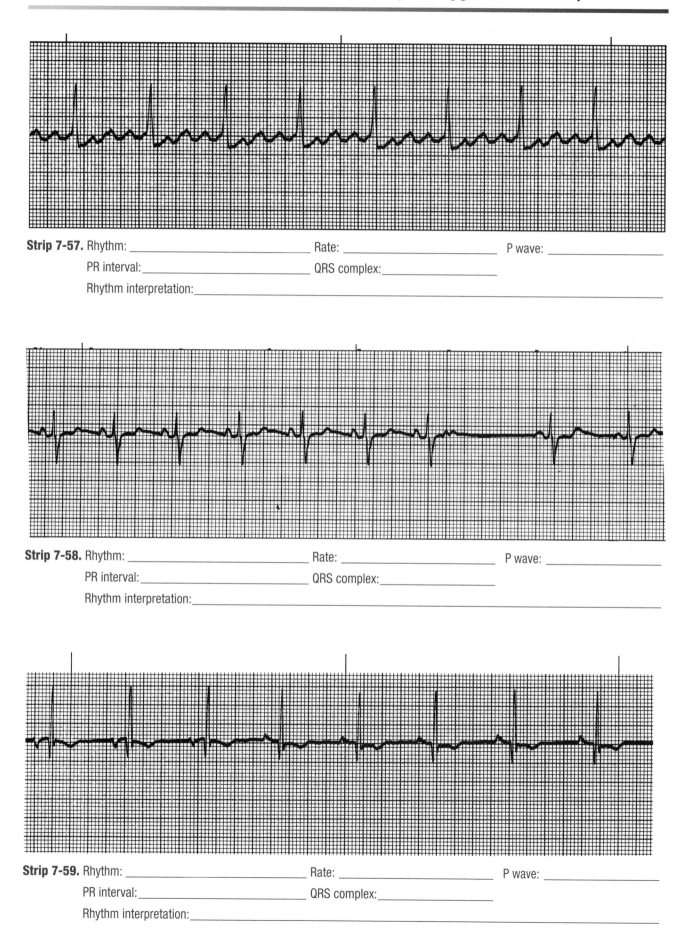

Strip 7-57. Rhythm: _____ Rate: _____ P wave: _____

PR interval: _____ QRS complex: _____

Rhythm interpretation: _____

Strip 7-58. Rhythm: _____ Rate: _____ P wave: _____

PR interval: _____ QRS complex: _____

Rhythm interpretation: _____

Strip 7-59. Rhythm: _____ Rate: _____ P wave: _____

PR interval: _____ QRS complex: _____

Rhythm interpretation: _____

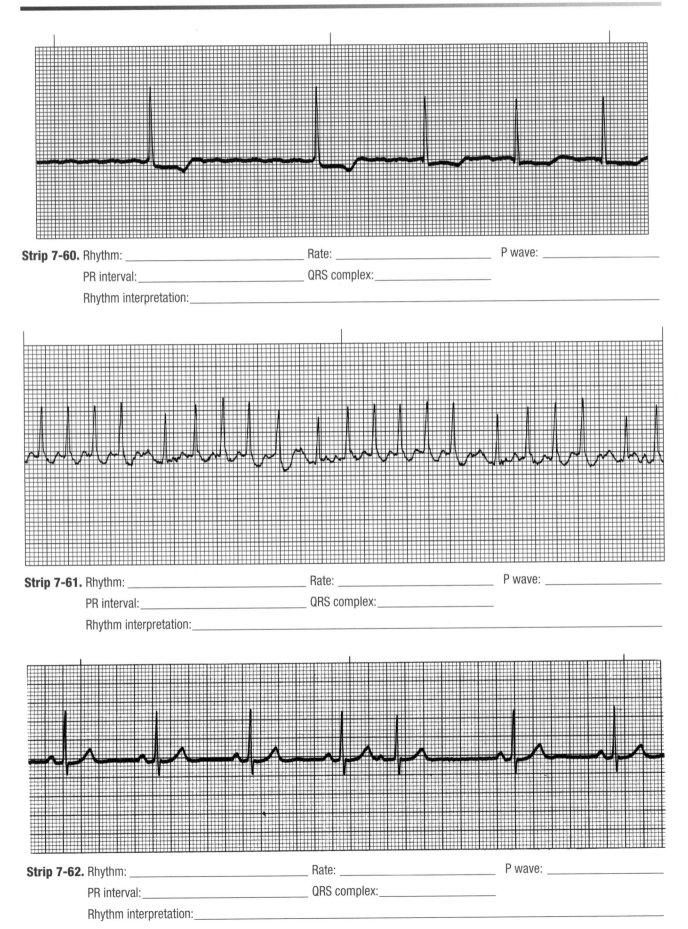

Strip 7-60. Rhythm: _____ Rate: _____ P wave: _____

PR interval: _____ QRS complex: _____

Rhythm interpretation: _____

Strip 7-61. Rhythm: _____ Rate: _____ P wave: _____

PR interval: _____ QRS complex: _____

Rhythm interpretation: _____

Strip 7-62. Rhythm: _____ Rate: _____ P wave: _____

PR interval: _____ QRS complex: _____

Rhythm interpretation: _____

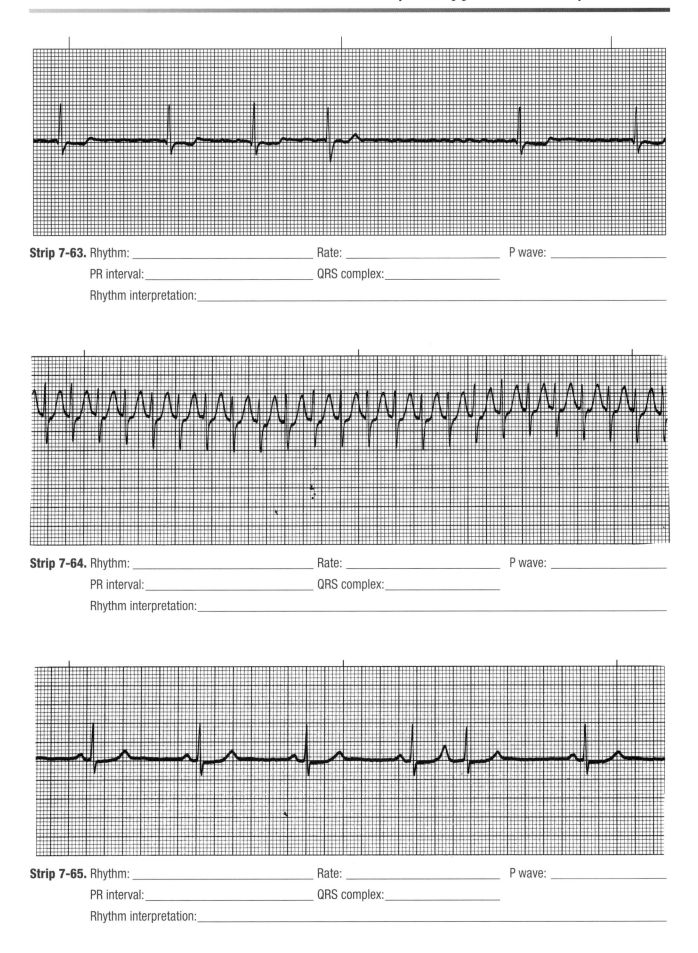

Strip 7-63. Rhythm: _____ Rate: _____ P wave: _____

PR interval: _____ QRS complex: _____

Rhythm interpretation: _____

Strip 7-64. Rhythm: _____ Rate: _____ P wave: _____

PR interval: _____ QRS complex: _____

Rhythm interpretation: _____

Strip 7-65. Rhythm: _____ Rate: _____ P wave: _____

PR interval: _____ QRS complex: _____

Rhythm interpretation: _____

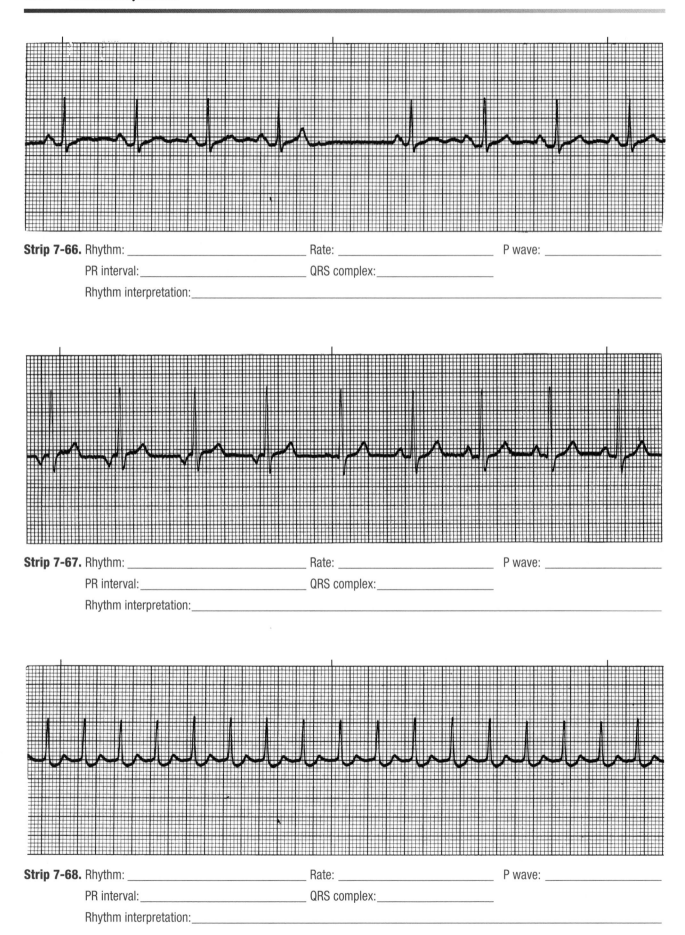

Strip 7-66. Rhythm: _____ Rate: _____ P wave: _____

PR interval: _____ QRS complex: _____

Rhythm interpretation: _____

Strip 7-67. Rhythm: _____ Rate: _____ P wave: _____

PR interval: _____ QRS complex: _____

Rhythm interpretation: _____

Strip 7-68. Rhythm: _____ Rate: _____ P wave: _____

PR interval: _____ QRS complex: _____

Rhythm interpretation: _____

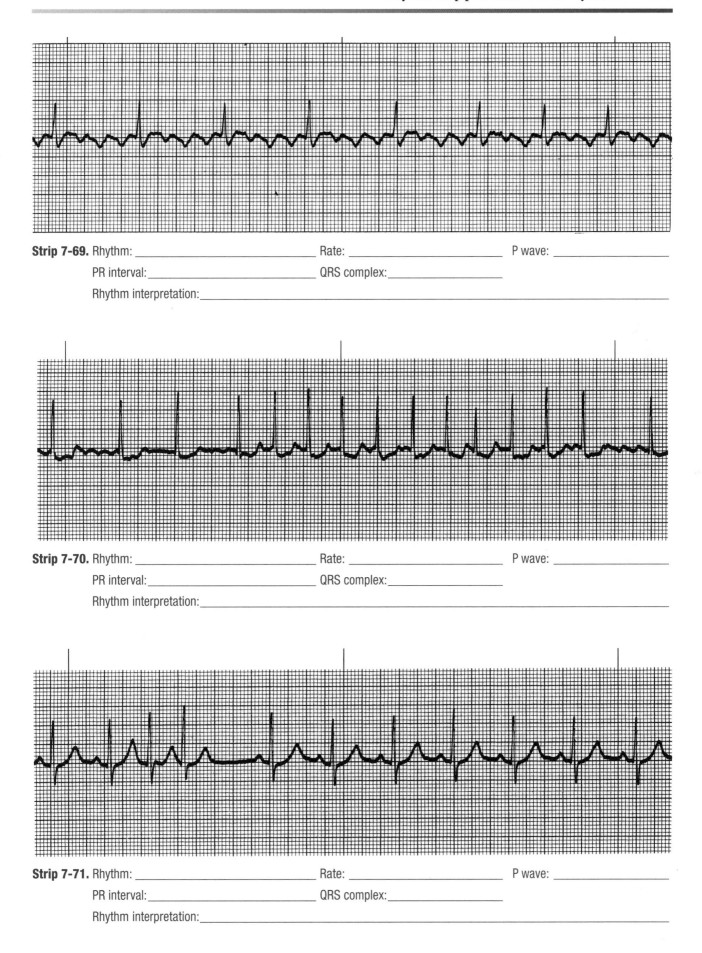

Strip 7-69. Rhythm: _____ Rate: _____ P wave: _____

PR interval: _____ QRS complex: _____

Rhythm interpretation: _____

Strip 7-70. Rhythm: _____ Rate: _____ P wave: _____

PR interval: _____ QRS complex: _____

Rhythm interpretation: _____

Strip 7-71. Rhythm: _____ Rate: _____ P wave: _____

PR interval: _____ QRS complex: _____

Rhythm interpretation: _____

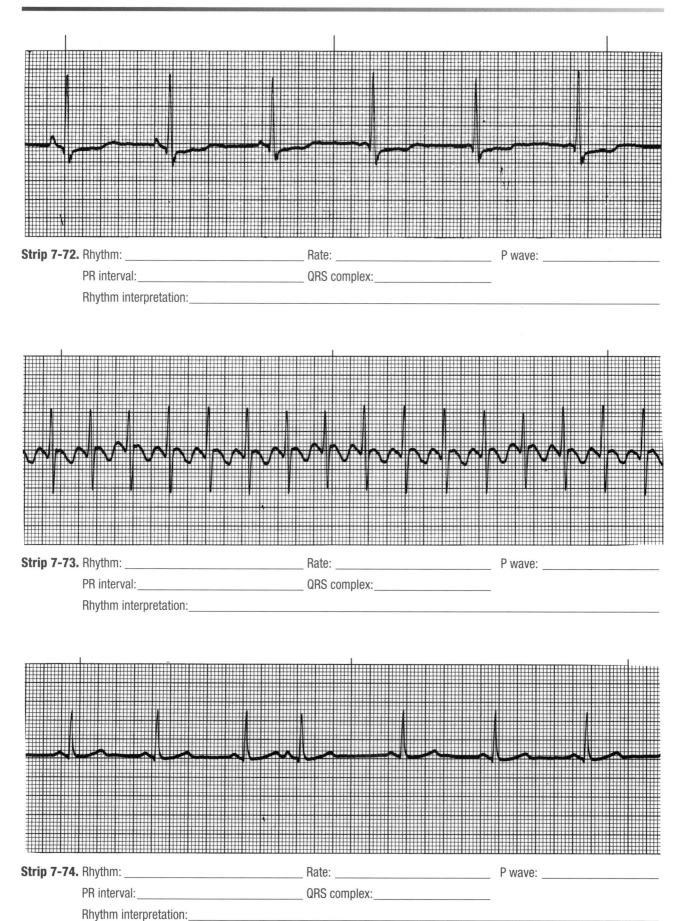

Strip 7-72. Rhythm: _____ Rate: _____ P wave: _____

PR interval:_____ QRS complex:_____

Rhythm interpretation:_____

Strip 7-73. Rhythm: _____ Rate: _____ P wave: _____

PR interval:_____ QRS complex:_____

Rhythm interpretation:_____

Strip 7-74. Rhythm: _____ Rate: _____ P wave: _____

PR interval:_____ QRS complex:_____

Rhythm interpretation:_____

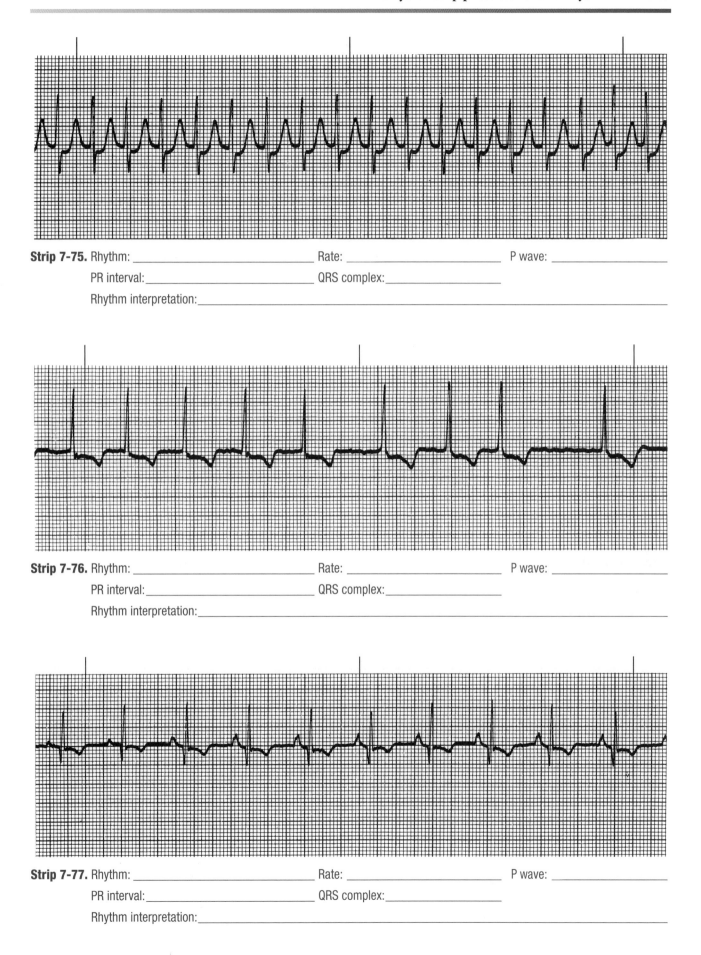

Strip 7-75. Rhythm: _____ Rate: _____ P wave: _____

PR interval:_____ QRS complex:_____

Rhythm interpretation:_____

Strip 7-76. Rhythm: _____ Rate: _____ P wave: _____

PR interval:_____ QRS complex:_____

Rhythm interpretation:_____

Strip 7-77. Rhythm: _____ Rate: _____ P wave: _____

PR interval:_____ QRS complex:_____

Rhythm interpretation:_____

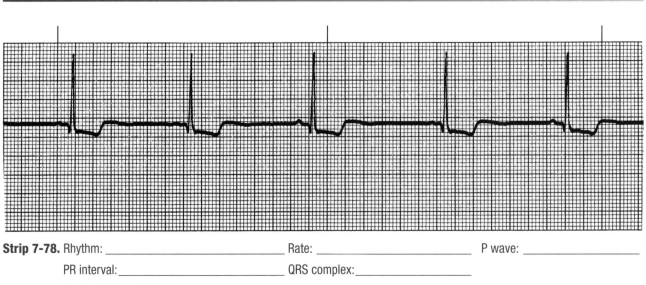

Strip 7-78. Rhythm: _____ Rate: _____ P wave: _____

PR interval:_____ QRS complex:_____

Rhythm interpretation:_____

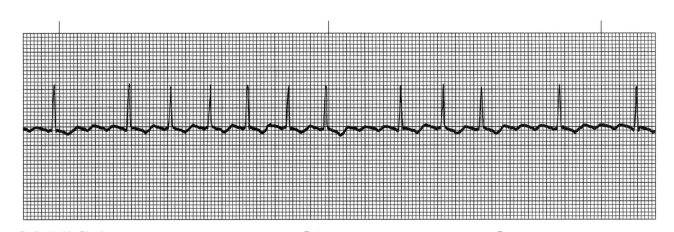

Strip 7-79. Rhythm: _____ Rate: _____ P wave: _____

PR interval:_____ QRS complex:_____

Rhythm interpretation:_____

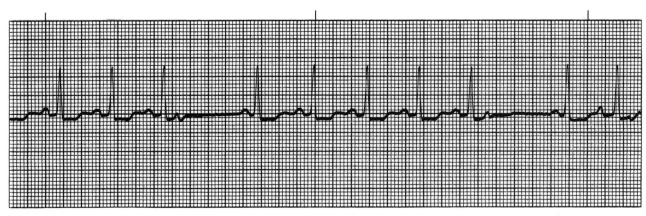

Strip 7-80. Rhythm: _____ Rate: _____ P wave: _____

PR interval:_____ QRS complex:_____

Rhythm interpretation:_____

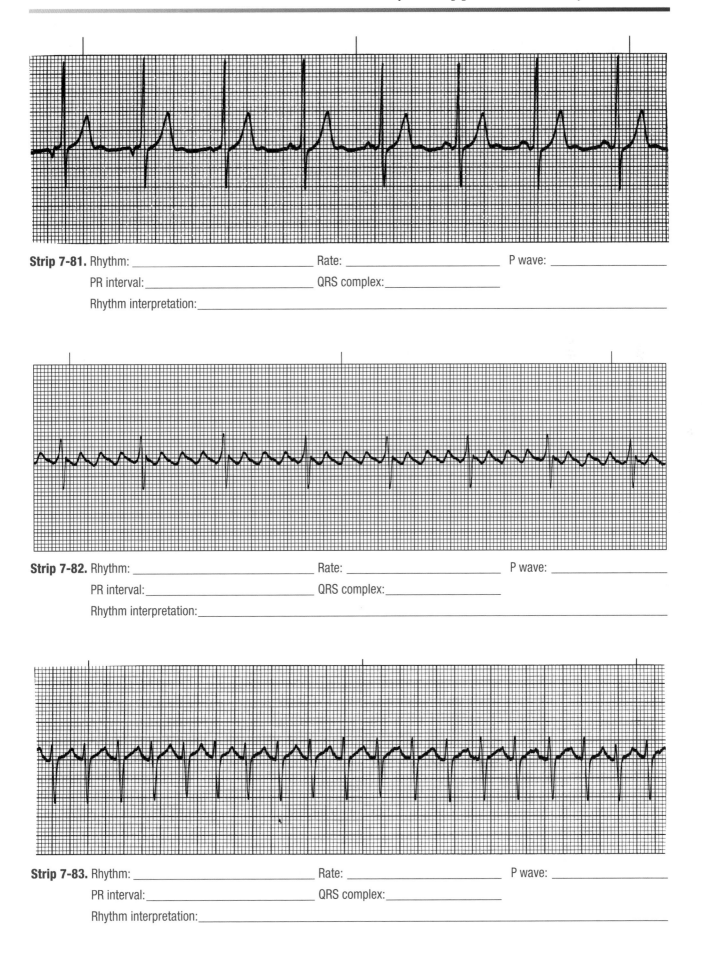

Strip 7-81. Rhythm: _____ Rate: _____ P wave: _____

PR interval: _____ QRS complex: _____

Rhythm interpretation: _____

Strip 7-82. Rhythm: _____ Rate: _____ P wave: _____

PR interval: _____ QRS complex: _____

Rhythm interpretation: _____

Strip 7-83. Rhythm: _____ Rate: _____ P wave: _____

PR interval: _____ QRS complex: _____

Rhythm interpretation: _____

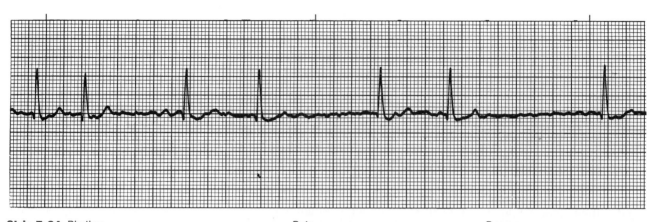

Strip 7-84. Rhythm: _____ Rate: _____ P wave: _____

PR interval:_____ QRS complex:_____

Rhythm interpretation:_____

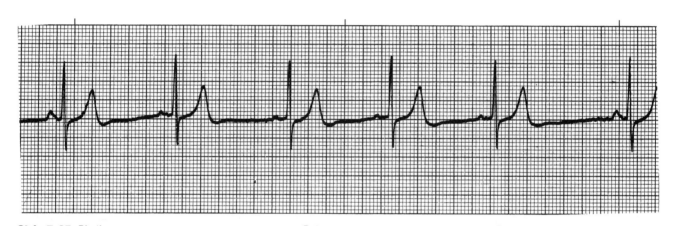

Strip 7-85. Rhythm: _____ Rate: _____ P wave: _____

PR interval:_____ QRS complex:_____

Rhythm interpretation:_____

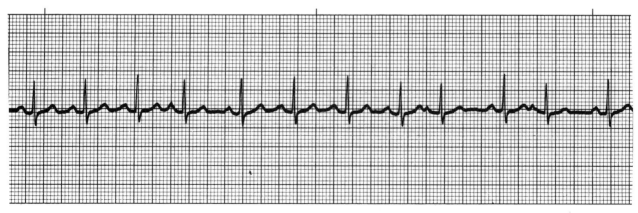

Strip 7-86. Rhythm: _____ Rate: _____ P wave: _____

PR interval:_____ QRS complex:_____

Rhythm interpretation:_____

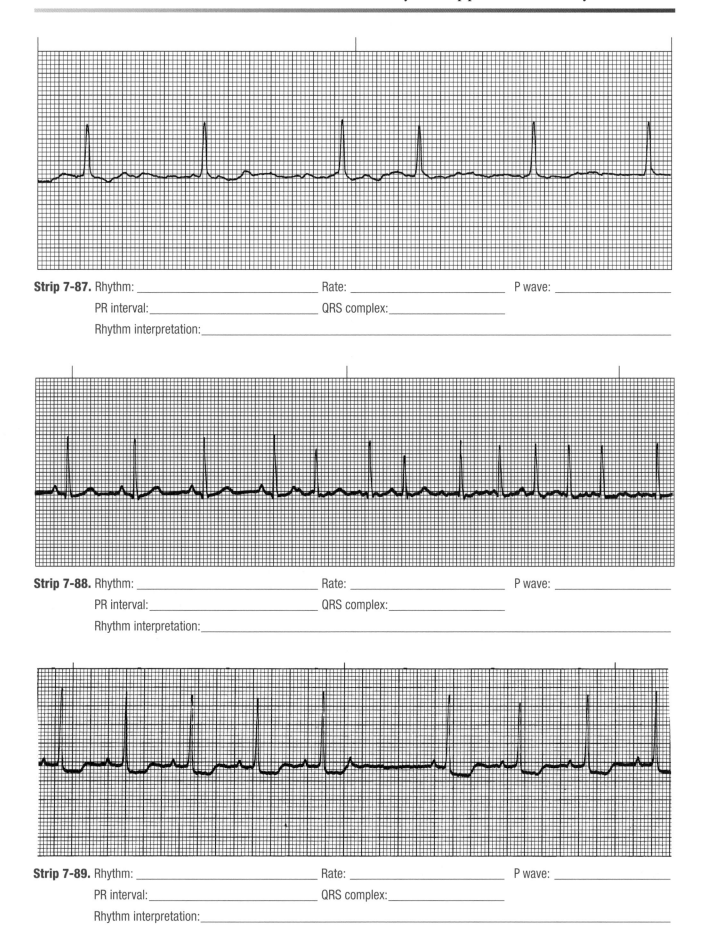

Strip 7-87. Rhythm: _____ Rate: _____ P wave: _____

PR interval:_____ QRS complex:_____

Rhythm interpretation:_____

Strip 7-88. Rhythm: _____ Rate: _____ P wave: _____

PR interval:_____ QRS complex:_____

Rhythm interpretation:_____

Strip 7-89. Rhythm: _____ Rate: _____ P wave: _____

PR interval:_____ QRS complex:_____

Rhythm interpretation:_____

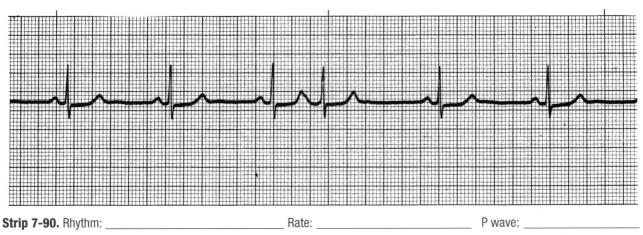

Strip 7-90. Rhythm: _____ Rate: _____ P wave: _____

PR interval: _____ QRS complex: _____

Rhythm interpretation: _____

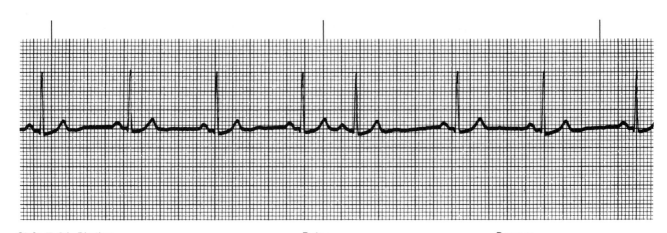

Strip 7-91. Rhythm: _____ Rate: _____ P wave: _____

PR interval: _____ QRS complex: _____

Rhythm interpretation: _____

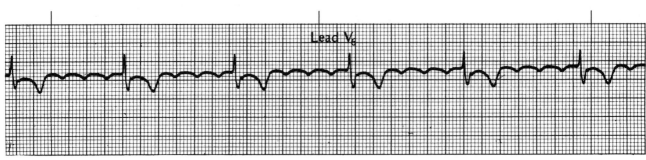

Strip 7-92. Rhythm: _____ Rate: _____ P wave: _____

PR interval: _____ QRS complex: _____

Rhythm interpretation: _____

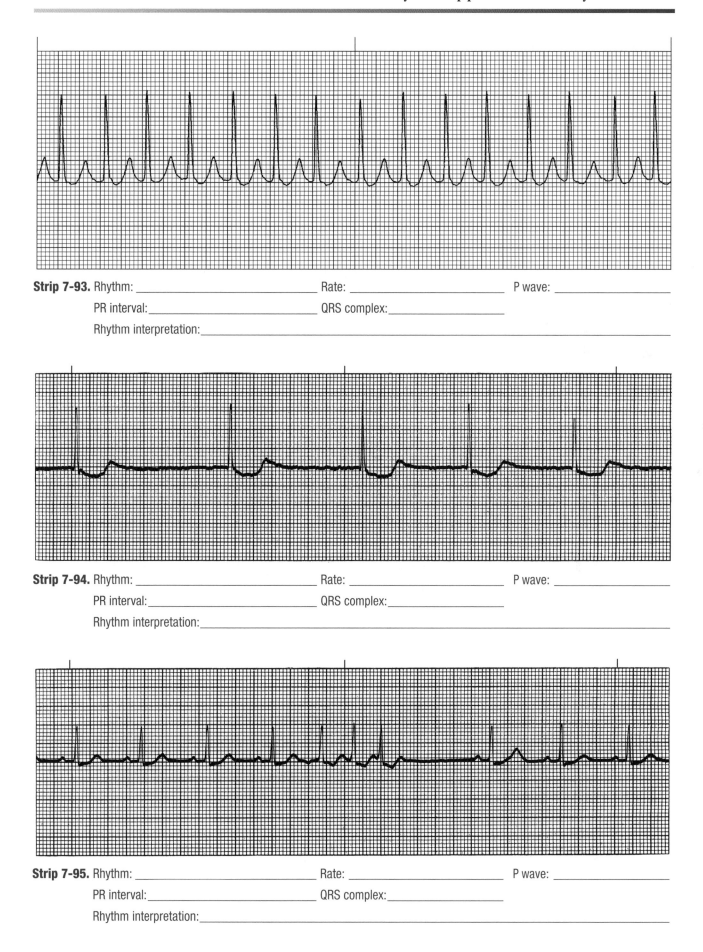

Strip 7-93. Rhythm: _____ Rate: _____ P wave: _____

PR interval: _____ QRS complex: _____

Rhythm interpretation: _____

Strip 7-94. Rhythm: _____ Rate: _____ P wave: _____

PR interval: _____ QRS complex: _____

Rhythm interpretation: _____

Strip 7-95. Rhythm: _____ Rate: _____ P wave: _____

PR interval: _____ QRS complex: _____

Rhythm interpretation: _____

▦ Skillbuilder practice

This section contains mixed *sinus* and *atrial* rhythm strips, allowing the student to practice differentiating between two rhythm groups before progressing to a new group. As before, analyze the rhythm strips using the five-step process. Interepret the rhythm by comparing the data collected with the ECG characteristics for each rhythm. All strips are lead II, a positive lead, unless otherwise noted. Check your answers with the answer key in the appendix.

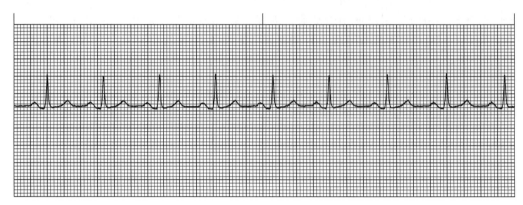

Strip 7-96. Rhythm: _____ Rate: _____ P wave: _____

PR interval: _____ QRS complex: _____

Rhythm interpretation: _____

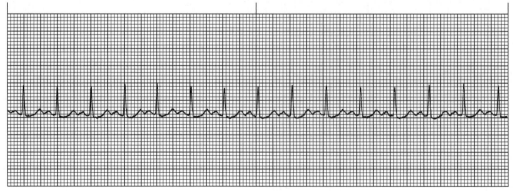

Strip 7-97. Rhythm: _____ Rate: _____ P wave: _____

PR interval: _____ QRS complex: _____

Rhythm interpretation: _____

Strip 7-98. Rhythm: _____ Rate: _____ P wave: _____

PR interval: _____ QRS complex: _____

Rhythm interpretation: _____

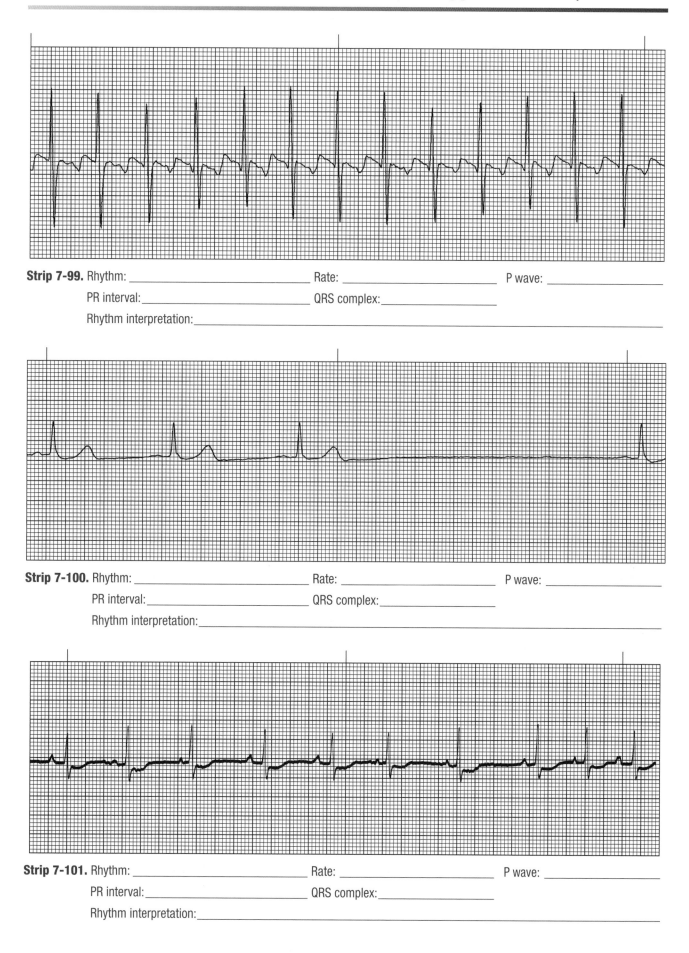

Strip 7-99. Rhythm: _____ Rate: _____ P wave: _____

PR interval: _____ QRS complex: _____

Rhythm interpretation: _____

Strip 7-100. Rhythm: _____ Rate: _____ P wave: _____

PR interval: _____ QRS complex: _____

Rhythm interpretation: _____

Strip 7-101. Rhythm: _____ Rate: _____ P wave: _____

PR interval: _____ QRS complex: _____

Rhythm interpretation: _____

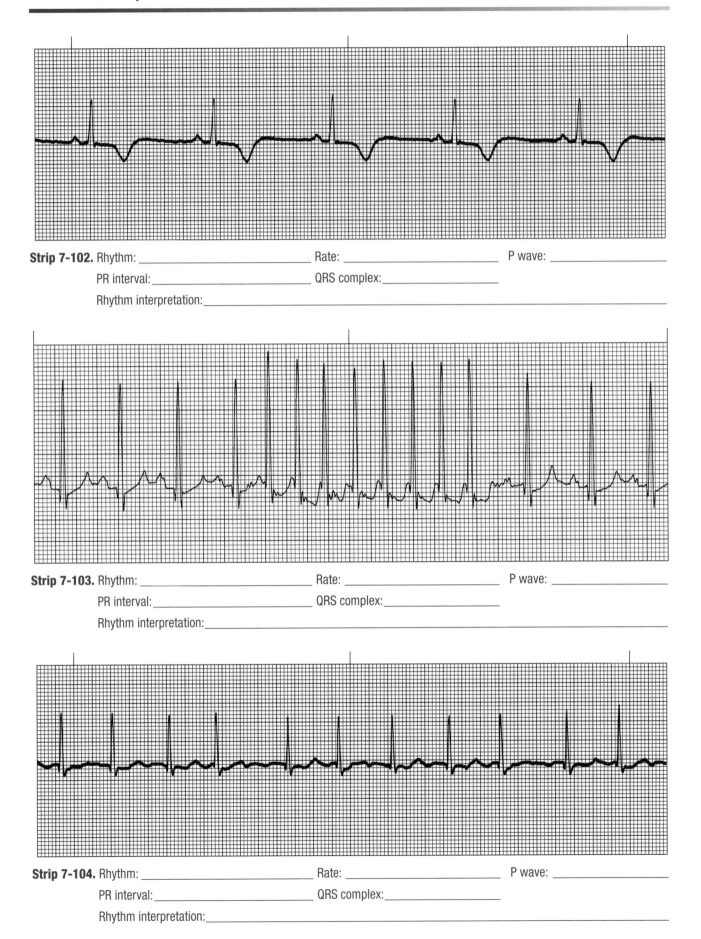

Strip 7-102. Rhythm: _____ Rate: _____ P wave: _____

PR interval: _____ QRS complex: _____

Rhythm interpretation: _____

Strip 7-103. Rhythm: _____ Rate: _____ P wave: _____

PR interval: _____ QRS complex: _____

Rhythm interpretation: _____

Strip 7-104. Rhythm: _____ Rate: _____ P wave: _____

PR interval: _____ QRS complex: _____

Rhythm interpretation: _____

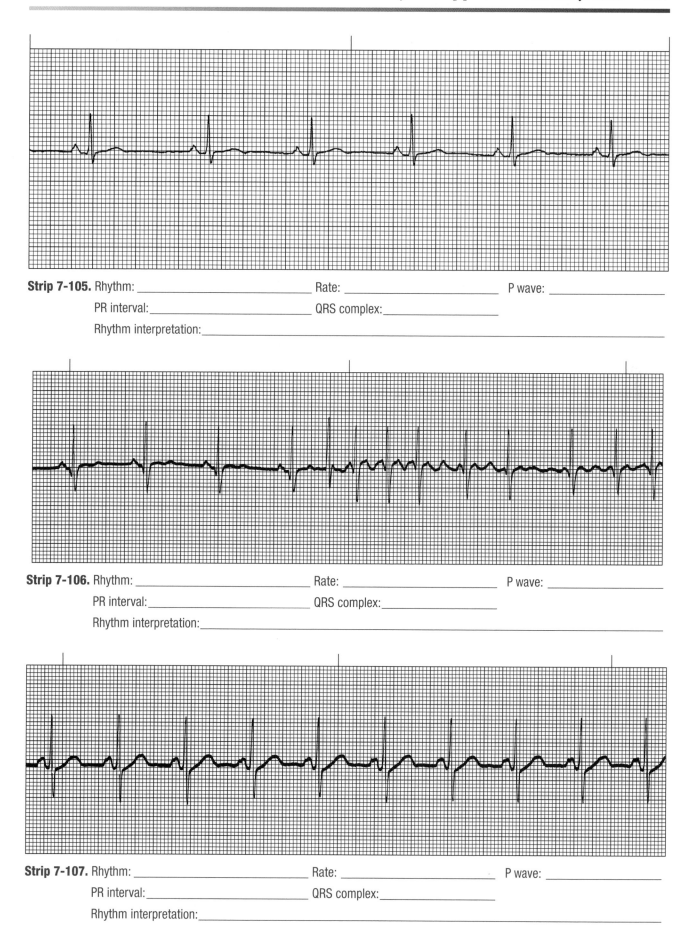

Strip 7-105. Rhythm: _____ Rate: _____ P wave: _____

PR interval:_____ QRS complex:_____

Rhythm interpretation:_____

Strip 7-106. Rhythm: _____ Rate: _____ P wave: _____

PR interval:_____ QRS complex:_____

Rhythm interpretation:_____

Strip 7-107. Rhythm: _____ Rate: _____ P wave: _____

PR interval:_____ QRS complex:_____

Rhythm interpretation:_____

Junctional arrhythmias and AV blocks

Overview

The atrioventricular (AV) node is located in the lower portion of the right atrium. The bundle of His connects the AV node to the two bundle branches. Together, the AV node and the bundle of His are called the AV junction. The AV node doesn't contain pacemaker cells. The main function of the AV node is to slow conduction of the electrical impulse through the AV node to allow the atria to contract and complete filling of the ventricles prior to ventricular contraction. Pacemaker cells nearest the bundle of His in the AV junction are responsible for secondary pacing function. Arrhythmias originating in the AV junction are called junctional rhythms (Figure 8-1).

The inherent firing rate of the junctional pacemaker cells is 40 to 60 beats per minute. A rhythm occurring at this rate is called a *junctional rhythm*. Other rhythms originating in the AV junctional area include premature junctional contraction, accelerated junctional rhythm, and junctional tachycardia.

When the AV junction is functioning as the pacemaker of the heart, the electrical impulse produces a wave of depolarization that spreads backward (*retrograde*) into the atria as well as forward (*antegrade*) into the ventricles. The location of the P wave relative to the QRS complex depends on the speed of antegrade and retrograde conduction:

■ If the electrical impulse from the AV junction depolarizes the atria first and then depolarizes the ventricles, the P wave will be in front of the QRS complex.

■ If the electrical impulse from the AV junction depolarizes the ventricles first and then depolarizes the atria, the P wave will be after the QRS complex.

■ If the electrical impulse from the AV junction depolarizes both the atria and the ventricles simultaneously, the P wave will be hidden in the QRS complex.

Retrograde stimulation of the atria is just opposite the direction of atrial depolarization when normal sinus rhythm is present and produces negative P waves (instead of upright) in lead II (a positive lead). The PR interval is short (0.10 second or less). The ventricles are depolarized normally, resulting in a normal duration QRS complex. Identifying features of junctional rhythms are summarized in Figure 8-2.

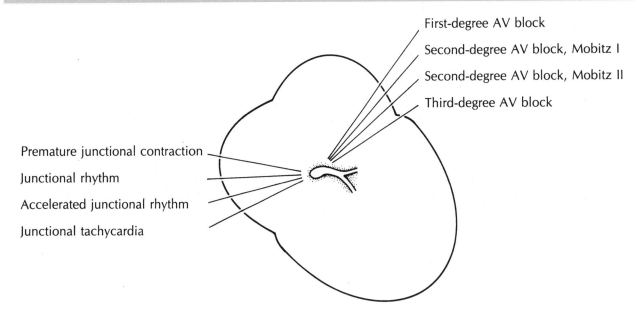

First-degree AV block
Second-degree AV block, Mobitz I
Second-degree AV block, Mobitz II
Third-degree AV block

Premature junctional contraction
Junctional rhythm
Accelerated junctional rhythm
Junctional tachycardia

Figure 8-1. Junctional arrhythmias and AV blocks.

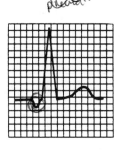 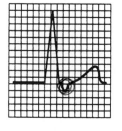 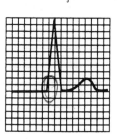

Lead II *pleura...*   Lead II *did...*   Lead II *...rythm*

Figure 8-2. Identifying features of junctional rhythms.

- P waves inverted in lead II.
- P waves will occur in one of three patterns:
  – immediately before the QRS complex
  – immediately after the QRS complex
  – hidden within the QRS complex.
- PR interval will be short (0.10 second or less).
- QRS complex will be normal (0.10 second or less).

P wave before QRS complex   P wave after QRS complex   P wave hidden in QRS complex

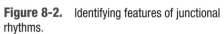

Lead II

Figure 8-3. Premature junctional contractions will appear as a single beat in any of the above three patterns.

Premature junctional contraction

A premature junctional contraction (PJC) (Figures 8-3 through 8-8 and Box 8-1) is an early beat that originates in an ectopic pacemaker site in the AV junction. Like the premature atrial contraction (PAC), the premature junctional beat is characterized by a premature, abnormal P wave and a premature QRS complex that's identical or similar to the QRS complex of the normally conducted beats, and is followed by a pause that is usually noncompensatory. Some differences exist, however, between the two premature beats. Because atrial depolarization occurs in

Box 8-1.
Premature junctional contraction (PJC): Identifying ECG features

Rhythm:	Underlying rhythm usually regular; irregular with PJC
Rate:	That of the underlying rhythm
P waves:	P waves associated with the PJC will be premature, inverted in lead II, and will occur immediately before the QRS complex, immediately after the QRS, or be hidden within the QRS
PR interval:	Short (0.10 second or less)
QRS complex:	Premature; normal duration (0.10 second or less)

a retrograde fashion with the PJC, the P wave associated with the premature beat will be negative in lead II (a positive lead). The inverted P waves will occur immediately before or after the QRS, or will be hidden within the QRS

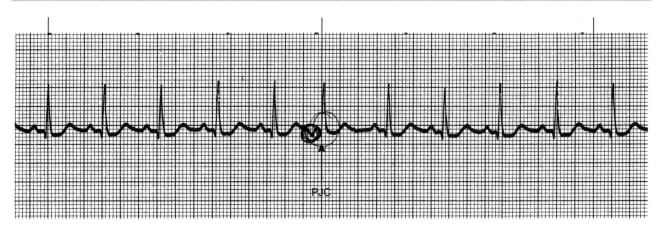

Figure 8-4. Normal sinus rhythm with one premature junctional contraction (PJC).

Rhythm:	Basic rhythm regular; irregular with PJC
Rate:	Basic rhythm rate 94 beats/minute
P waves:	Sinus P waves with basic rhythm; inverted P wave with PJC
PR interval:	0.14 to 0.16 second (basic rhythm); 0.08 second (PJC)
QRS complex:	0.08 second
Comment:	ST-segment depression is present.

atrial fires before ventricle

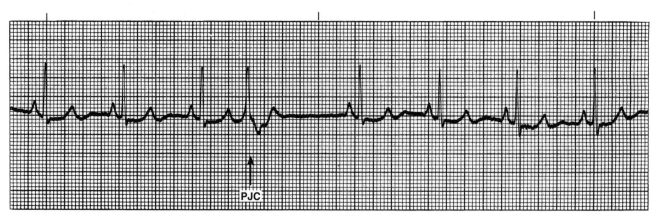

Figure 8-5. **Normal sinus rhythm with one premature junctional contraction (PJC).**

Rhythm:	Basic rhythm regular; irregular with PJC
Rate:	Basic rhythm rate 72 beats/minute
P waves:	Sinus P waves with basic rhythm; inverted P wave after PJC (4th QRS complex)
PR interval:	0.14 to 0.16 second (basic rhythm); 0.06 to 0.08 second (PJC)
QRS complex:	0.06 to 0.08 second (basic rhythm); 0.08 second (PJC)
Comment:	A U wave is present.

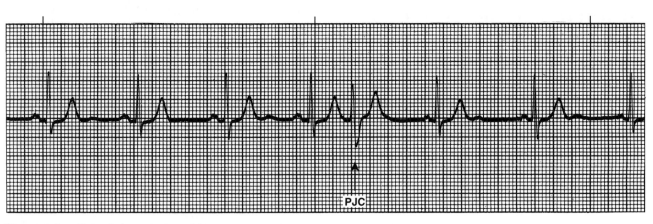

Figure 8-6. **Normal sinus rhythm with one premature junctional contraction (PJC).**

Rhythm:	Basic rhythm regular; irregular with PJC
Rate:	Basic rhythm rate 63 beats/minute; rate slows to 56 beats/minute following PJC due to rate suppression (common following a pause in the basic rhythm)
P waves:	Sinus P waves with basic rhythm; P wave associated with PJC is hidden in the QRS complex
PR interval:	0.16 to 0.18 second (basic rhythm)
QRS complex:	0.06 to 0.08 second (basic rhythm); 0.10 second (PJC)
Comment:	A U wave is present.

complex. The PR interval will be short (0.10 second or less). Figure 8-4 shows a PJC with the P wave before the QRS complex; Figure 8-5 shows a PJC with the P wave after the QRS complex; and in Figure 8-6 the P wave is hidden within the QRS. PJCs are less common than PACs or premature ventricular contractions (PVCs) (discussed in Chapter 9).

Inverted P waves in lead II may also occur with PACs arising from the lower atria, but the associated PR interval is usually normal. If difficulty is encountered in differentiating PJCs from PACs, keep the following in mind: PACs are much more common than PJCs. As a result, narrow complex premature beats are more likely to be PACs. A comparison of ectopic atrial beats and ectopic junctional beats is shown in Figure 8-7. PJCs occur in addition to the underlying rhythm. They occur in the same patterns as PACs: as a single beat; in bigeminal, trigeminal, or quadrigeminal patterns; or in pairs (Figure 8-8). A series of three or more consecutive junctional beats is considered

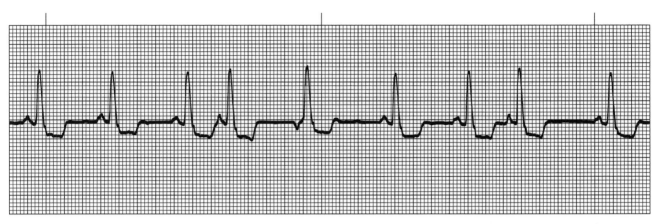

Figure 8-7. Normal sinus rhythm with two premature atrial contractions (PACs) (4th and 8th complexes) and one junctional escape beat (5th complex)

Rhythm:	Regular (basic rhythm); irregular with PACs and junctional escape beat
Rate:	75 beats/minute (basic rhythm)
P waves:	Sinus (basic rhythm); pointed P waves with PACs; inverted P waves with junctional escape beat
PR interval:	0.14 second (basic rhythm); 0.12 second (PACs); 0.08 second (junctional escape beat)
QRS complex:	0.08 to 0.10 second (basic rhythm, PACs, and junctional escape beat).

a rhythm (junctional rhythm, accelerated junctional rhythm, or junctional tachycardia). Differentiation of the rhythm depends on the heart rate.

Like PACs, the premature junctional impulse may (rarely) be conducted to the ventricles abnormally (aberrantly). This results in a wide QRS complex. A PJC associated with a wide QRS complex is called a PJC with aberrancy, indicating that conduction through the ventricles is aberrant. Because of the wide QRS complex, PJCs with aberrancy must be differentiated from PVCs.

Conditions associated with PJCs include ingestion of substances such as caffeine, alcohol, or tobacco; electrolyte imbalances; hypoxia; congestive heart failure; coronary artery disease; and enhanced automaticity of the AV junction caused by digitalis toxicity (the most common cause). PJCs may also occur without apparent cause.

Frequent PJCs are best treated by correcting the underlying cause: decreasing or eliminating the consumption of caffeine, alcohol, or tobacco; correcting electrolyte imbalances; administering oxygen; treating congestive heart failure; and assessing digitalis levels. Frequent PJCs (more than 6/minute) may precede the development of a more serious junctional arrhythmia such as junctional tachycardia.

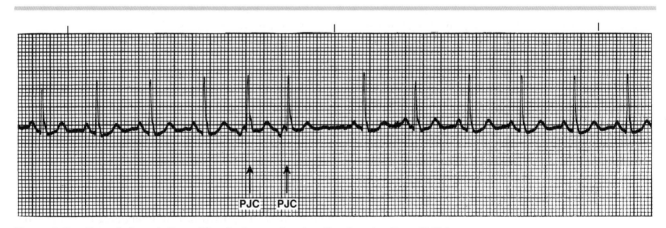

Figure 8-8. Normal sinus rhythm with paired premature junctional contractions (PJCs).

Rhythm:	Basic rhythm regular; irregular following paired PJCs
Rate:	Basic rhythm rate 100 beats/minute
P waves:	Sinus P waves with basic rhythm; inverted P waves with PJCs
PR interval:	0.12 to 0.14 second (basic rhythm); 0.08 second (with PJCs)
QRS complex:	0.06 to 0.08 second (basic rhythm and PJCs).

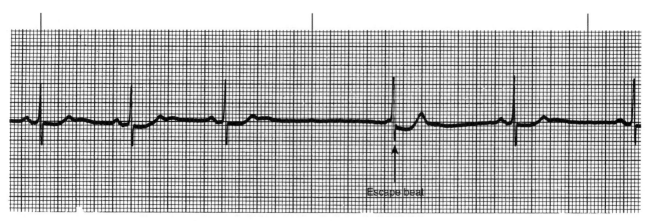

Figure 8-9.   **Normal sinus rhythm with a pause followed by a junctional escape beat.**
Rhythm: Basic rhythm regular; irregular with escape beat
Rate: Basic rhythm 60 beats/minute; rate slows to 45 beats/minute after escape beat (Rate suppression can occur following any pause in the basic rhythm. After several cycles the rate will return to the basic rate.)
P waves: Sinus P waves with basic rhythm; hidden P wave with escape beat
PR interval: 0.16 second
QRS complex: 0.06 second
Comment: ST-segment depression and a U wave are present.

Occasionally, an ectopic junctional beat will occur late instead of early. The late beat usually occurs after a pause in the underlying rhythm in which the dominant pacemaker (usually the sinoatrial [SA] node) fails to initiate an impulse. If the ventricles are not activated by the SA node within a certain amount of time, a focus in the AV junction may "escape" and pace the heart. These are called *junctional escape beats* (Figure 8-9).

Junctional rhythm

Junctional rhythm (Figures 8-10 through 8-13 and Box 8-2) is an arrhythmia originating in the AV junction with a rate between 40 and 60 beats per minute. Junctional rhythm is the normal rhythm of the AV junction. Junctional rhythm can occur under either of the following conditions:

■ The heart rate of the dominant pacemaker (usually the SA node) becomes less than the heart rate of the AV junction.

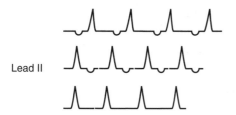

Lead II

Figure 8-10.   Junctional rhythm will appear as a continuous rhythm at a rate of 40 to 60 beats/minute in either of the above three patterns.

Box 8-2.
Junctional rhythm: Identifying ECG features

Rhythm:	Regular
Rate:	40 to 60 beats/minute
P waves:	Inverted in lead II and occurs immediately before the QRS complex, immediately after the QRS complex, or is hidden within the QRS complex
PR interval:	Short (0.10 second or less)
QRS complex:	Normal (0.10 second or less)

■ Electrical impulses from the SA node or atria fail to reach the ventricles because of sinus arrest, sinus exit block, or third-degree AV block.

If the ventricles are not activated by the SA node or atria, a focus in the AV junction can "escape" and pace the heart. For this reason, junctional rhythm is commonly referred to as *junctional escape rhythm.*

Junctional rhythm is regular with a heart rate between 40 and 60 beats per minute. The P waves are inverted in lead II (a positive lead), and will occur immediately before or after the QRS or will be hidden within the QRS complex. The PR interval is short (0.10 second or less). The QRS duration is normal. Junctional rhythm has the same characteristics as accelerated junctional rhythm and junctional tachycardia. This rhythm is differentiated from the other junctional rhythms by the heart rate.

Junctional rhythm may be seen in acute myocardial infarction (MI) (particularly inferior-wall MI), increased parasympathetic tone, disease of the SA node, and hypoxia. It can also occur in patients taking digitalis, calcium channel blockers, or beta blockers.

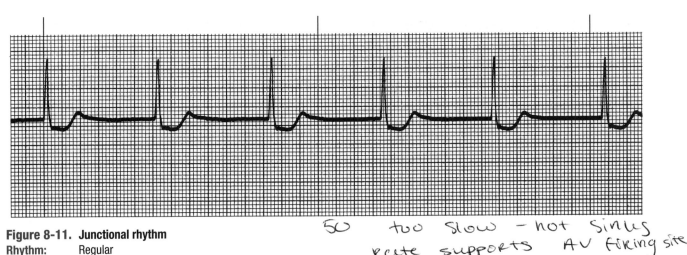

Figure 8-11. Junctional rhythm

Rhythm:	Regular
Rate:	50 beats/minute
P waves:	Hidden in QRS complex
PR interval:	Not measurable
QRS complex:	0.06 to 0.08 second
Comment:	ST-segment depression is present.

[handwritten: 50 too slow - not sinus, rate supports AV firing site]

The slow rate and loss of normal atrial contraction (atrial kick) secondary to retrograde atrial depolarization may cause a decrease in cardiac output. Treatment for symptomatic junctional rhythm includes following the protocols for significant bradycardia (atropine, pacing, dopamine, or epinephrine infusions to increase blood pressure). Treatment should also be directed at identifying and correcting the underlying cause of the rhythm if possible. All medications should be reviewed and discontinued if indicated.

Accelerated junctional rhythm

Accelerated junctional rhythm (Figures 8-14 through 8-16 and Box 8-3) is an arrhythmia originating in the AV junction with a rate between 60 and 100 beats per minute. The term "accelerated" denotes a rhythm that occurs at a rate that exceeds the junctional escape rate of 40 to 60, but isn't fast enough to be junctional tachycardia.

Accelerated junctional rhythm is regular with a heart rate between 60 and 100 beats per minute. The P waves are

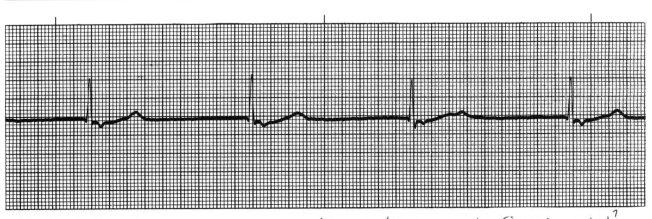

Figure 8-12. Junctional rhythm.

Rhythm:	Regular
Rate:	33 beats/minute
P waves:	Inverted after QRS complex
PR interval:	0.08 to 0.10 second
QRS complex:	0.08 to 0.10 second.

[handwritten: 40 <60 not sinus -AV? Regular, inverted P after QRS]

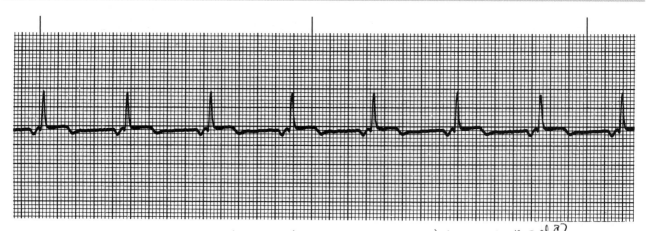

Figure 8-13. Junctional rhythm.

Rhythm:	Regular
Rate:	35 beats/minute
P waves:	Inverted before the QRS
PR interval:	0.06 to 0.08 second
QRS complex:	0.06 to 0.08 second.

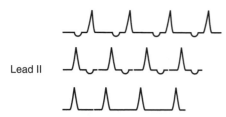

Lead II

Figure 8-14. Accelerated junctional rhythm will appear as a continuous rhythm at a rate of 60 to 100 beats/minute in any of the above three patterns.

Box 8-3.

Accelerated junctional rhythm: Identifying ECG features

Rhythm:	Regular
Rate:	60 to 100 beats/minute
P waves:	Inverted in lead II and occurs immediately before the QRS complex, immediately after the QRS complex, or is hidden within the QRS complex
PR interval:	Short (0.10 second or less)
QRS complex:	Normal (0.10 second or less)

Figure 8-15. Accelerated junctional rhythm.

Rhythm:	Regular
Rate:	65 beats/minute
P waves:	Inverted before each QRS complex
PR interval:	0.08 to 0.10 second
QRS complex:	0.08 second
Comment:	ST-segment elevation and T wave inversion are present.

junctional rhythm w/ HR 70   >60 SA node?
rhythm >60
>60   still AV node   not SA

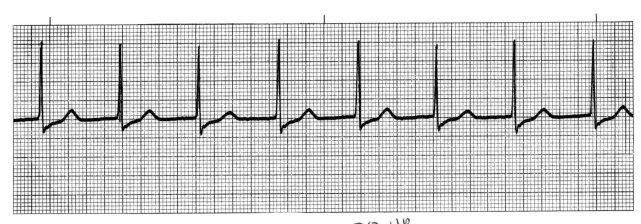

Figure 8-16. Accelerated junctional rhythm.

Rhythm:	Regular
Rate:	68 beats/minute
P waves:	Hidden in QRS complex
PR interval:	Not measurable
QRS complex:	0.06 to 0.08 second.

70 HR
junctional Rhythm
w/ HR ↓ 60

inverted in lead II (a positive lead), and will occur immediately before or after the QRS or will be hidden within the QRS complex. The PR interval is short (0.10 second or less). The QRS duration is normal. Accelerated junctional rhythm has the same characteristics as junctional rhythm and junctional tachycardia. This rhythm is differentiated from the other junctional rhythms by the heart rate. Accelerated junctional rhythm is not a common arrhythmia.

Accelerated junctional rhythm may result from enhanced automaticity of the AV junction caused by digitalis toxicity (the most common cause). Other causes include damage to the AV junction from MI (usually inferior-wall MI), heart failure, and electrolyte imbalances.

Usually the heart rate associated with accelerated junctional rhythm isn't a problem because it corresponds to that of the sinus node (60 to 100 beats per minute). Problems are more likely to occur from the loss of the atrial kick secondary to retrograde depolarization of the atria, resulting in a reduction in cardiac output. Treatment is directed at reversing the consequences of reduced cardiac output, if present, as well as identifying and correcting the underlying cause of the rhythm. All medications should be reviewed and discontinued if indicated.

Paroxysmal junctional tachycardia

Paroxysmal junctional tachycardia (PJT) (Figures 8-17 and 8-18 and Box 8-4) is an arrhythmia originating in the AV junction with a heart rate exceeding 100 beats per minute. Junctional tachycardia commonly starts and stops abruptly (like paroxysmal atrial tachycardia) and is often precipitated by a premature junctional complex. Three or more PJCs in a row at a rate exceeding 100 per minute constitute a run of junctional tachycardia.

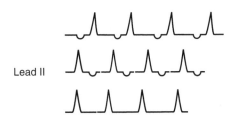

Lead II

Figure 8-17. Paroxysmal junctional tachycardia will appear as a continuous rhythm at a rate exceeding 100 beats/minute in any of the above three patterns.

Junctional tachycardia is regular with a heart rate exceeding 100 beats per minute. The P waves are inverted in lead II (a positive lead), and will occur immediately before or after the QRS or will be hidden within the QRS complex. The PR interval will be short (0.10 second or less). The QRS duration is normal. Junctional tachycardia has the same characteristics as junctional rhythm and accelerated junctional rhythm. This rhythm is differentiated from the other junctional rhythms by the heart rate. Junctional tachycardia is not a common arrhythmia.

Box 8-4.
Paroxysmal junctional tachycardia: Identifying ECG features

Rhythm:	Regular
Rate:	Greater than 100 beats/minute
P waves:	Inverted in lead II and occurs immediately before the QRS complex, immediately after the QRS complex, or is hidden within the QRS complex
PR interval:	Short (0.10 second or less)
QRS complex:	Normal (0.10 second or less)

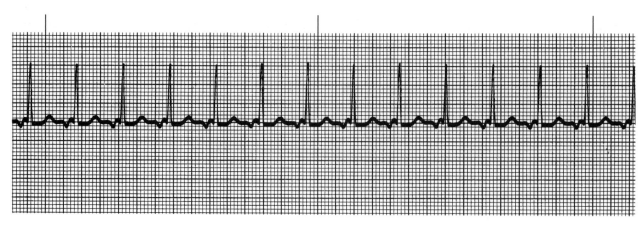

Figure 8-18. Paroxysmal junctional tachycardia.
Rhythm: Regular
Rate: 115 beats/minute
P waves: Inverted before each QRS complex
PR interval: 0.08 second
QRS complex: 0.06 to 0.08 second.

Junctional tachycardia may result from enhanced automaticity of the AV junction caused by digitalis toxicity (the most common cause). Other causes include damage to the AV junction from MI (usually inferior-wall MI) and heart failure.

Junctional tachycardia may lead to a decrease in cardiac output related to the faster heart rate as well as the loss of the atrial kick secondary to retrograde depolarization of the atria. Treatment is directed at reversing the consequences of reduced cardiac output, as well as identifying and correcting the underlying cause of the rhythm. Symptomatic junctional tachycardia may respond to diltiazem, beta blockers (use caution in patients with pulmonary disease or heart failure), or amiodarone.

AV heart blocks

The term *heart block* is used to describe arrhythmias in which there is delayed conduction or failed conduction of impulses through the AV node into the ventricles. Normally the AV node acts as a bridge between the atria and the ventricles. The PR interval is primarily a measure of conduction between the initial stimulation of the atria and the initial stimulation of the ventricles. This measurement is normally 0.12 to 0.20 second.

The site of pathology of the AV blocks may be at the level of the AV node, the bundle of His, or the bundle branches. When located at the level of the AV node or bundle of His, the QRS complexes will be normal duration. The QRS complex will be wide if the site of pathology is located in the bundle branches.

AV blocks are classified into first-degree, second-degree (type I and II), and third-degree. This classification system is based on the degree (type) of block and the location of the block. It is important to remember that the PR interval is the key to identifying the type of block present. The width of the QRS complex and the ventricular rate are keys to differentiating the location of the block (the lower the location of the block in the conduction system, the wider the QRS complex and the slower the ventricular rate).

In first-degree AV block (the mildest form), the electrical impulses are delayed in the AV node longer than normal, but all impulses are conducted to the ventricles. In second-degree AV block (type I and II), some impulses are conducted to the ventricles and some are blocked. The most extreme form of heart block is third-degree AV block, in which no impulses are conducted from the atria to the ventricles. The clinical significance of an AV block depends on the degree of block, the ventricular rate, and patient response.

The ability to accurately diagnose AV blocks depends on a systematic approach. The following steps are suggested:
■ Look for the P wave. Is there one P wave before each QRS or more than one?
■ Measure the regularity of the atrial rhythm (the P-P interval) and the ventricular rhythm (the R-R interval).
■ Measure the PR interval. Is the PR interval consistent or does it vary? *Remember, the PR interval is the key to identifying the type of AV block present.*
■ Look at the QRS complex. Is it narrow or wide?

First-degree AV block

In first-degree AV block (Figure 8-19 and Box 8-5), the sinus impulse is normally conducted to the AV node, where it's delayed longer than usual before being conducted to the ventricles. This delay in the AV node results in a prolonged PR interval (> 0.20 second). This rhythm is reflected on the ECG by a regular rhythm (both atrial

[handwritten: PR interval longer than normal]

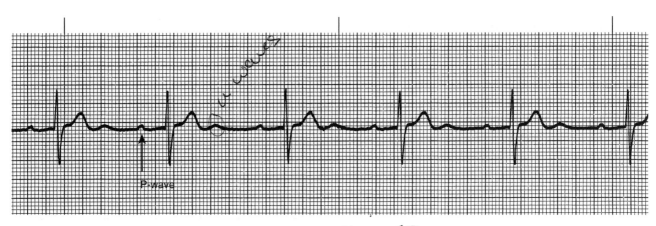

[handwritten annotations on figure: "U waves", "P-wave"]

Figure 8-19. Sinus bradycardia with first-degree AV block. *[handwritten: with U waves 40]*

Rhythm:	Regular
Rate:	48 beats/minute
P waves:	Sinus P waves present; one P wave to each QRS complex
PR interval:	0.28 to 0.32 second (remains constant) *[handwritten: 0.26 rate > .20]*
QRS complex:	0.08 to 0.10 second *[handwritten: .08]*
Note:	A U wave is present.

and ventricular), one P wave preceding each QRS complex, a consistent but prolonged PR interval, and a narrow QRS complex. This conduction disorder is located at the level of the AV node (thus the narrow QRS complex) and isn't a serious form of heart block.

The underlying sinus rhythm is usually identified along with the AV block when interpreting the rhythm (for example, normal sinus rhythm with first-degree AV block).

First-degree AV block may occur from ischemia or injury to the AV node or junction secondary to acute MI (usually inferior-wall MI), increased parasympathetic (vagal) tone, drug effects (beta blockers, calcium channel blockers, digitalis, amiodarone), hyperkalemia, degeneration of the conduction pathways associated with aging, and unknown causes.

First-degree AV block produces no symptoms and requires no treatment. Because first-degree heart block can progress to a higher degree of AV block under certain conditions, the rhythm should continue to be monitored until the block resolves or stabilizes. Drugs causing AV block should be reviewed and discontinued if indicated.

Box 8-5.
First-degree AV block: Identifying ECG features

Rhythm:	Regular
Rate:	That of the underlying sinus rhythm; both atrial and ventricular rates will be the same
P waves:	Sinus; one P wave to each QRS complex
PR interval:	Prolonged (> 0.20 second); remains consistent
QRS complex:	Normal (0.10 second or less)

Second-degree AV block, type I (Mobitz I or Wenckebach)

Second-degree AV block, type I is commonly known as Mobitz I or Wenckebach (for the early 20th century physician who discovered it). This rhythm (Figures 8-20 through 8-23 and Box 8-6) is characterized by a failure of some of the sinus impulses to be conducted to the ventricles. In Mobitz I, the sinus impulse is normally conducted to the AV node, but each successive impulse has increasing difficulty passing through the AV node, until finally an impulse does not pass through (isn't conducted). This rhythm is reflected on the ECG by P waves that occur at regular intervals across the rhythm strip and PR intervals that progressively lengthen from beat to beat until a P wave appears that is not followed by a QRS complex, but instead by a pause. The missing QRS complex (dropped beat) causes

Box 8-6.
Second-degree AV block (Mobitz I): Identifying ECG features

Rhythm:	Regular atrial rhythm; irregular ventricular rhythm
Rate:	Atrial: That of the underlying sinus rhythm Ventricular: Varies depending on number of impulses conducted through AV node (will be less than the atrial rate)
P waves:	Sinus
PR interval:	Varies; progressively lengthens until a P wave isn't conducted (P wave occurs without the QRS complex); a pause follows the dropped QRS complex
QRS complex:	Normal (0.10 second or less)

SU R
7o Atrical

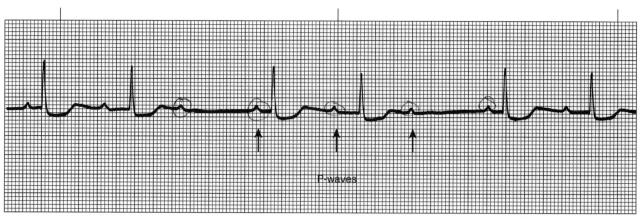

P-waves

Figure 8-20. Second-degree AV block, Mobitz I.

Rhythm:	Regular atrial rhythm; irregular ventricular rhythm
Rate:	Atrial: 72 beats/minute
	Ventricular: 50 beats/minute
P waves:	Sinus P waves present
PR interval:	Progressively lengthens from 0.20 to 0.30 second
QRS complex:	0.06 to 0.08 second
Note:	ST-segment depression is present.

P's are all regular

the ventricular rhythm to be irregular. After each dropped beat the cycle repeats itself. The overall appearance of the rhythm demonstrates group beating (groups of beats separated by pauses) and is a distinguishing characteristic of Mobitz I. Escape beats (atrial, junctional, or ventricular) may occasionally occur during the pause in the ventricular rhythm, and may obscure the diagnosis because they interrupt the group beating pattern (Figure 8-22). The location of the conduction disturbance is at the level of the AV node and therefore the QRS complex will be narrow.

Mobitz I can be confused with the nonconducted PAC (Figure 8-23). Both rhythms have episodes where P waves are not followed by a QRS complex, but instead by a pause. To differentiate between the two rhythms, one must examine the configuration of the P waves and measure the P-P regularity. The nonconducted PAC will have an abnormal P wave and will occur prematurely. In Mobitz I, the P wave is normal and occurs on schedule, not prematurely.

Mobitz I is common following acute inferior-wall MI due to AV node ischemia. Other causes include increased

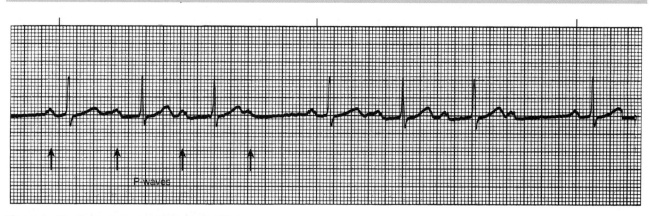

P-waves

Figure 8-21. Second-degree AV block, Mobitz I.

Rhythm:	Regular atrial rhythm; irregular ventricular rhythm
Rate:	Atrial: 75 beats/minute
	Ventricular: 60 beats/minute
P waves:	Sinus P waves present
PR interval:	Progressively lengthens from 0.24 to 0.38 second
QRS complex:	0.08 second
Comment:	Good example of group beating.

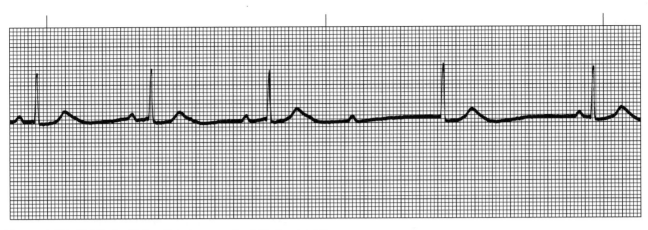

Figure 8-22. Mobitz I with junctional escape beat (during pause).

Rhythm:	Regular (basic rhythm); irregular during pause
Rate:	Atrial (50 beats/minute); ventricular (48 beats/minute)
P waves:	Sinus (basic rhythm); hidden P wave with junctional escape beat
PR interval:	Progressively lengthens from 0.20 to 0.24 second
QRS complex:	0.04 to 0.06 second (basic rhythm and junctional escape beat).

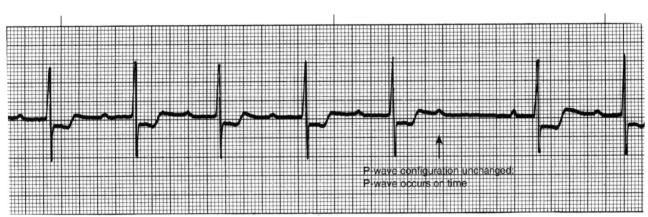

P wave configuration unchanged; P-wave occurs on time

MOBITZ I
- Pause in basic ventricular rhythm
- P-P regularity unchanged (P wave occurs on time)
- P wave configuration same as sinus beats
- PR interval of basic rhythm varies

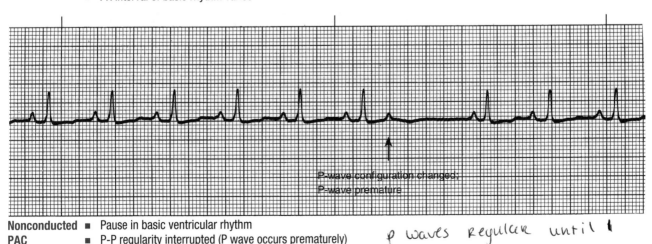

P-wave configuration changes; P-wave premature

Nonconducted PAC
- Pause in basic ventricular rhythm
- P-P regularity interrupted (P wave occurs prematurely)
- P wave configuration different from sinus beats
- PR interval of basic rhythm remains constant

p waves regular until ↑

Figure 8-23.   Differentiation of the nonconducted premature atrial contraction from Mobitz I.

parasympathetic (vagal) tone, effects of medications (digitalis, beta blockers, calcium channel blockers), and hyperkalemia. Mobitz I may also occur as a normal variant in athletes because of physiologic increase in vagal tone. Mobitz I, under certain conditions, may progress to a higher degree of AV block, but generally this is not the case. This type of AV block is usually temporary and resolves spontaneously.

Mobitz I is usually asymptomatic because the ventricular rate remains nearly normal and cardiac output is usually not affected. If the ventricular rate is slow and the patient develops symptoms, protocols for symptomatic bradycardia (atropine, external or transvenous pacing, dopamine or epinephrine infusions to increase blood pressure) should be followed. Conduction usually improves in response to the administration of atropine. Drugs causing AV block should be discontinued if indicated.

Second-degree AV block, type II (Mobitz II)

Mobitz II (Figures 8-24 and 8-25 and Box 8-7), like Mobitz I, is characterized by a failure of some of the sinus impulses to be conducted to the ventricles. There are differences, however, in the location and severity of the conduction disturbance, as well as in the ECG features. In Mobitz II, there's more than one P wave before each QRS complex (usually two or three, but sometimes more) with only one of the impulses being conducted to the ventricles. The rhythm would be described as Mobitz II with 2:1, 3:1, or 4:1 AV conduction. The P waves are identical and occur regularly. In Mobitz II with higher conduction ratios (3:1 or more), the P waves may be hidden in the ST segment

Box 8-7.
Second-degree AV block (Mobitz II): Identifying ECG features

Rhythm:	Atrial: Regular
	Ventricular: Usually regular but may be irregular if AV conduction ratios vary
Rate:	Atrial: That of the underlying sinus rhythm
	Ventricular: Varies depending on number of impulses conducted through AV node (will be less than the atrial rate)
P waves:	Sinus; two or three P waves (sometimes more) before each QRS complex
PR interval:	May be normal or prolonged; remains consistent
QRS complex:	Normal if block located at level of bundle of His; wide if block located in bundle branches

or T wave (Figure 8-25). The PR interval of the conducted beat may be normal or prolonged, but remains consistent. The ventricular rhythm is usually regular unless the AV conduction ratio varies (alternating among 2:1, 3:1, and 4:1). The location of the conduction disturbance is below the AV node in the bundle of His or bundle branches. As a result, the QRS complex may be narrow (if located in the bundle of His) or wide (if located in the bundle branches). The most common location is the bundle branches.

Mobitz II is usually associated with an anterior-wall MI and, unlike Mobitz I, is not the result of increased vagal tone or drug toxicity. Other causes include acute myocarditis and degeneration of the electrical conduction system seen in the elderly.

The patient's response to Mobitz II is usually related to the ventricular rate. If the ventricular rate is within normal

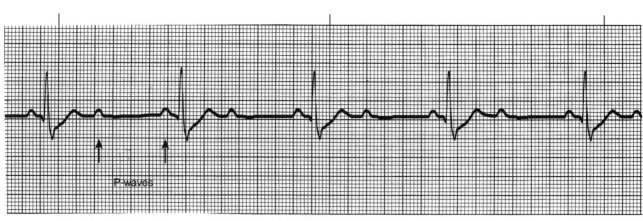

Figure 8-24.   Second-degree AV block, Mobitz II.
Rhythm:	Regular atrial and ventricular rhythm
Rate:	Atrial: 82 beats/minute
	Ventricular: 41 beats/minute
P waves:	Two sinus P waves to each QRS complex
PR interval:	0.16 second (remains constant)
QRS complex:	0.14 second.

40   80
PR interval equal

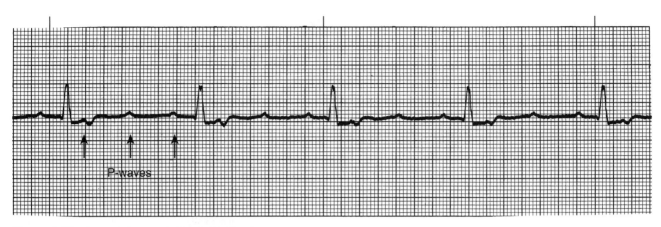

Figure 8-25. Second-degree AV block, Mobitz II.

Rhythm:	Regular atrial and ventricular rhythm
Rate:	Atrial: 123 beats/minute
	Ventricular: 41 beats/minute
P waves:	Three sinus P waves to each QRS complex
PR interval:	0.24 to 0.26 second (remains constant)
QRS complex:	0.12 second.

limits (rare), the patient may be asymptomatic. More commonly, the ventricular rate is extremely slow, cardiac output is decreased, and symptoms are present (hypotension, shortness of breath, heart failure, chest pain, or syncope). The syncopal episodes (called *Stokes-Adams attacks* or Stokes-Adams syncope) are caused by a sudden slowing or stopping of the heartbeat.

Mobitz II is less common but more serious than Mobitz I. Mobitz II has the potential to progress suddenly to third-degree AV block or ventricular standstill (asystole) with little or no warning. Treatment is required immediately for symptomatic Mobitz II and for asymptomatic Mobitz II with wide QRS complexes in the setting of acute anterior-wall MI. An external pacemaker should be applied while preparations are made for insertion of a temporary transvenous pacemaker. Atropine is usually not effective in reversing Mobitz II second-degree AV block and may actually worsen the conduction disturbance. A dopamine infusion may be used to increase blood pressure. Unresolved Mobitz II will require a permanent pacemaker.

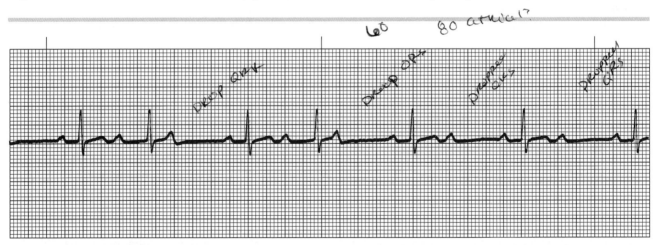

Figure 8-26. Mobitz I. This strip shows a typical Wenckebach pattern during the first part of the strip changing to a 2:1 conduction ratio at the end of the strip. Even though 2:1 conduction is seen (common with Mobitz II), the presence of a Wenckebach pattern confirms the diagnosis of Mobitz I.

Rhythm:	Atrial (regular); ventricular (irregular)
Rate:	Atrial (100 beats/minute); ventricular (60 beats/minute)
P waves:	Sinus
PR interval:	Progressively lengthens from 0.24 to 0.36 second
QRS complex:	0.06 to 0.08 second.

A comment about 2:1 conduction: A 2:1 conduction ratio is common with Mobitz II (two P waves to one QRS complex). A 2:1 conduction ratio may also occasionally occur with Mobitz I. In Mobitz I with 2:1 conduction, every other impulse is not conducted and the ECG shows two P waves to one QRS complex. The only difference on the ECG would be a narrow QRS (seen in Mobitz I) and a wide QRS (seen more commonly, but not exclusively, with Mobitz II). Typically, if Mobitz I with 2:1 conduction is present, an occasional Wenckebach pattern will usually assert itself when a longer rhythm strip is viewed, thus confirming the diagnosis of Mobitz I. Figure 8-26 shows such an example.

The AV block strips with consistent 2:1 AV conduction and a narrow QRS complex have been interpreted in the answer keys as Mobitz II with a notation that clinical correlation may be necessary to determine a definite diagnosis.

Third-degree AV block (complete heart block)

Third-degree AV block (Figures 8-27 and 8-28 and Box 8-8) represents complete absence of conduction between the atria and the ventricles. This rhythm is also called complete heart block. With third-degree heart block, the atria and ventricles beat independently of each other and there's no relationship between atrial activity and ventricular activity (AV dissociation). The atria are usually paced by the sinus node at its inherent rate of 60 to 100 beats per minute and the ventricles are either paced by a pacemaker in the AV junction at a rate of 40 to 60 beats per minute or in the ventricles at a rate of 30 to 40 beats per minute. The P waves have no relationship with the QRS complexes, and will be seen marching across the rhythm strip, hiding inside QRS complexes or in the ST segment or T wave. The

Box 8-8.
Third-degree AV block (complete heart block): Identifying ECG features

Rhythm:	Atrial: Regular
	Ventricular: Regular
Rate:	Atrial: That of the underlying sinus rhythm
	Ventricular: 40 to 60 beats/minute if paced by AV junction; 30 to 40 beats/minute (or less) if paced by ventricles; will be less than the atrial rate
P waves:	Sinus P waves with no constant relationship to the QRS complex; P waves can be found hidden in QRS complexes, ST segments, and T waves
PR interval:	Varies greatly
QRS complex:	Normal if block located at level of AV node or bundle of His; wide if block located at level of bundle branches

"hidden" P waves can be found by measuring the regularity of the atrial rhythm (the P-P interval). The PR intervals are completely variable. Both the atrial rhythm and the ventricular rhythm are usually regular. The width of the QRS complex and the ventricular rate reflect the location of the blockage. If the block is at the level of the AV node or bundle of His, the QRS complex will be narrow and the ventricular rate will be between 40 and 60 beats per minute. If the blockage is in the bundle branches, the QRS complex will be wide and the ventricular rate much slower (40 beats per minute or less). Generally, complete heart block with wide QRS complexes tends to be less stable than complete heart block with narrow QRS complexes.

Complete heart block associated with inferior-wall MI is usually a result of a block at the level of the AV node or bundle of His. The rhythm is usually stable and the

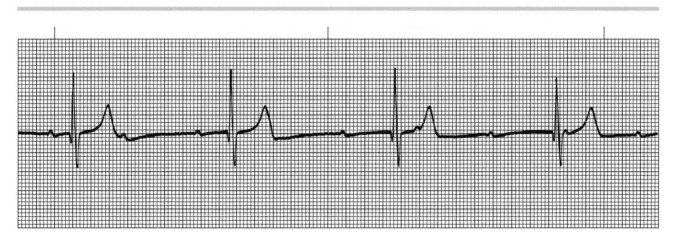

Figure 8-27. Third-degree AV block.

Rhythm:	Regular (atrial); regular (ventricular) off by 2 squares
Rate:	Atrial (75 beats/minute); ventricular (33 to 34 beats/minute)
P waves:	Sinus P waves (have no relationship to QRS complexes; found hidden in QRS complexes, ST segments, and T waves)
PR interval:	Varies greatly (is not consistent)
QRS complex:	0.12 second.

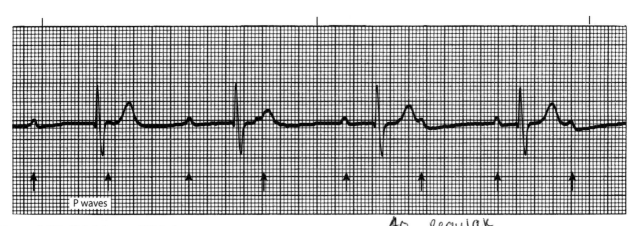

P waves

Figure 8-28. Third-degree AV block.

Rhythm:	Regular atrial and ventricular rhythm
Rate:	Atrial: 72 beats/minute
	Ventricular: 40 beats/minute
P waves:	Sinus P waves present (bear no constant relationship to QRS complexes; found hidden in QRS complexes and T waves)
PR interval:	Varies greatly
QRS complex:	0.12 second.

40 Regular atrial

ventricles are paced by a junctional pacemaker with narrow QRS complexes and a ventricular rate of 40 to 60 beats per minute. Third-degree AV block associated with an inferior-wall MI often resolves on its own. Complete heart block associated with an anterior-wall MI is usually a result of a block within the bundle branches. The rhythm is usually unstable and the ventricles are paced by a ventricular pacemaker with wide QRS complexes and a ventricular rate of 40 beats per minute or less. Third-degree AV block associated with an anterior MI often does not resolve on its own and may require permanent pacing. Complete heart block can also be seen in older patients who have chronic degenerative changes in their conduction system not related to acute MI. It has also been reported with Lyme disease. Complete heart block may occur with digitalis toxicity.

The patient's response to complete heart block is usually related to the ventricular rate. If the ventricular rate is within normal limits, the patient may be relatively asymptomatic with minor symptoms such as weakness, fatigue, dizziness, or exercise intolerance. More commonly, the ventricular rate is extremely slow, cardiac output is decreased, and symptoms are present (hypotension, dyspnea, heart failure, chest pain, or Stokes-Adams syncope).

Regardless of its cause, complete heart block is a serious and potentially life-threatening arrhythmia. Third-degree AV block, like Mobitz II, can quickly progress to ventricular standstill (asystole) with little or no warning. Treatment is required immediately for symptomatic third-degree heart block and for asymptomatic third-degree heart block with wide QRS complexes in the setting of acute anterior-wall MI. An external pacemaker should be applied while preparations are made for insertion of a temporary transvenous

pacemaker. Third-degree AV block with narrow QRS complexes may occasionally respond to atropine. Hypotension should be treated with vasopressors. Unresolved complete heart block will require a permanent pacemaker.

Tips on heart blocks

To distinguish one heart block from another, remember these important tips:

■ Measure the P-P interval. The P-P interval is regular in all the blocks. If you measure the P-P interval, you will be able to track the P waves. This is very important in finding hidden P waves seen in third-degree AV block or Mobitz II with higher conduction ratios (3:1 or more).

■ Measure the R-R interval. First-degree and third-degree AV block have a regular ventricular rhythm. Mobitz I has an irregular ventricular rhythm. The ventricular rhythm in Mobitz II may be regular or irregular, depending on conduction ratios.

■ Measure the PR interval. If the PR interval is consistent, choose between first-degree and Mobitz II AV block. First-degree AV block has one P wave to each QRS while Mobitz II AV block has two or more P waves to each QRS. If the PR interval is not consistent, choose between Mobitz I AV block and third-degree AV block. In Mobitz I the PR interval is not consistent and the ventricular rhythm is irregular. In third-degree AV block the PR interval is not consistent and the ventricular rhythm is regular.

Table 8-1 compares the ECG characteristics of each type of AV block. A summary of the identifying ECG features of junctional rhythms and AV blocks can be found in Table 8-2.

Table 8-1.
AV block comparisons

PR constant *(First-degree)*	PR varies *(Second-degree, Mobitz I)*
PR constant	PR varies
PR prolonged One P wave to each QRS	PR progressively gets longer until a QRS is dropped
Regular atrial rhythm; regular ventricular rhythm	Regular atrial rhythm; irregular ventricular rhythm
(Second-degree, Mobitz II)	*(Third-degree)*
PR constant	PR varies
PR normal or prolonged; two or three P waves (possibly more) to each QRS	P waves have no constant rela- tionship to QRS (found hidden in QRS complexes, ST segments, and T waves)
Regular atrial rhythm; regular ventricular rhythm (unless conduction ratios vary)	Regular atrial rhythm; regular ventricular rhythm

Table 8-2.

Junctional arrhythmias and AV blocks: Summary of identifying ECG features

Name	Rhythm	Rate (beats/minute)	P waves (lead II)	PR interval	QRS complex
Premature junctional contraction (PJC)	Basic rhythm usually regular; irregular with PJC	That of basic rhythm	Premature P wave; inverted in lead II and will occur immediately before the QRS complex or immediately after the QRS, or be hidden within the QRS	0.10 second or less	Premature QRS complex; normal duration (0.10 second or less)
Junctional rhythm	Regular	40 to 60	Inverted in lead II and will occur immediately before the QRS complex or immediately after the QRS, or be hidden within the QRS	Short (0.10 second or less)	Normal (0.10 second or less)
Accelerated junctional rhythm	Regular	60 to 100	Inverted in lead II and will occur immediately before the QRS complex or immediately after the QRS, or be hidden within the QRS	Short (0.10 second or less)	Normal (0.10 second or less)
Junctional tachycardia	Regular	>100	Inverted in lead II and will occur immediately before the QRS complex or immediately after the QRS, or be hidden within the QRS	Short (0.10 second or less)	Normal (0.10 second or less)
First-degree atrioventricular (AV) block	Regular	That of underlying sinus rhythm; both atrial and ventricular rates will be the same	Sinus origin; one P wave to each QRS complex	Prolonged (more than 0.20 second); remains consistent	Normal (0.10 second or less)
Second-degree AV block, Mobitz I	Atrial: regular Ventricular: irregular	Atrial: that of underlying sinus rhythm Ventricular: depends on number of impulses conducted through AV node; will be less than atrial late	Sinus origin	Varies; progressively lengthens until a P wave isn't conducted (P wave occurs without the QRS complex); a pause follows the dropped QRS complex	Normal (0.10 second or less)
Second-degree AV block, Mobitz II	Atrial: regular Ventricular: usually regular, but may be irregular if conduction ratios vary	Atrial: that of underlying sinus rhythm Ventricular: depends on number of impulses conducted through AV node; will be less than atrial late	Sinus origin; two or three P waves (sometimes more) before each QRS complex	Normal or prolonged; remains consistent	Normal if block at level of bundle of His; wide if block in bundle branches
Third-degree AV block	Atrial: regular Ventricular: regular	Atrial: that of underlying sinus rhythm Ventricular: 40 to 60 if paced by AV junction; 30 to 40 (sometimes less) if paced by ventricles; will be less than atrial rate	Sinus P waves with no constant relationship to the QRS complex; P waves found hidden in QRS complexes, ST segments, and T waves	Varies greatly	Normal if block at level of AV node or bundle of His; wide if block in bundle branches

Rhythm strip practice: Junctional arrhythmias and AV blocks

Analyze the following rhythm strips by following the five basic steps:
- Determine *rhythm regularity*.
- Calculate *heart rate*. (This usually refers to the ventricular rate, but if atrial rate differs you need to calculate both.)
- Identify and examine *P waves*.
- Measure *PR interval*.
- Measure *QRS complex*.

Interpret the rhythm by comparing this data with the ECG characteristics for each rhythm. All rhythm strips are lead II, a positive lead, unless otherwise noted. Check your answers with the answer keys in the appendix.

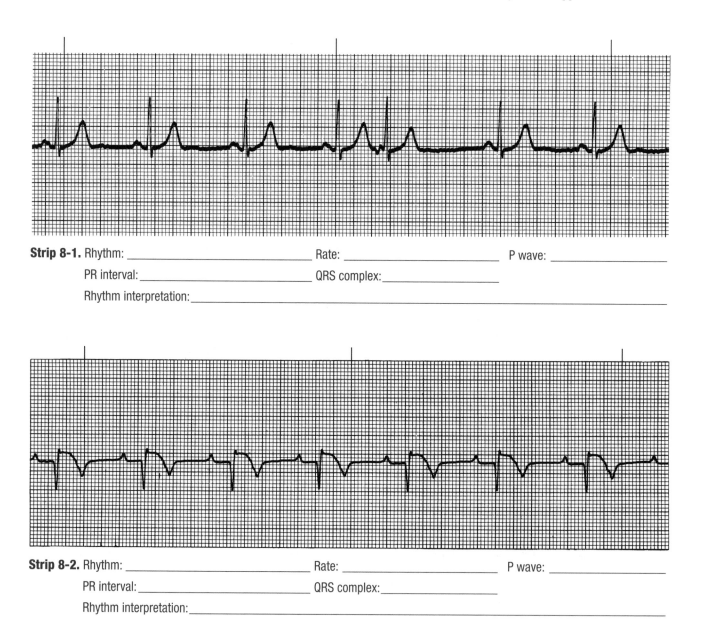

Strip 8-1. Rhythm: _____ Rate: _____ P wave: _____

PR interval: _____ QRS complex: _____

Rhythm interpretation: _____

Strip 8-2. Rhythm: _____ Rate: _____ P wave: _____

PR interval: _____ QRS complex: _____

Rhythm interpretation: _____

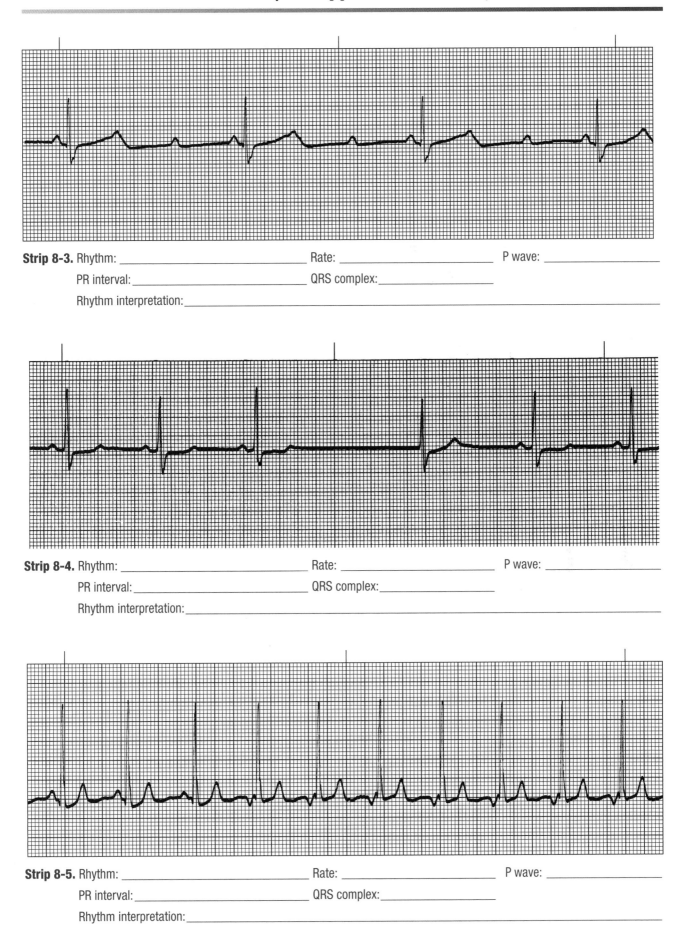

Strip 8-3. Rhythm: _____ Rate: _____ P wave: _____

PR interval: _____ QRS complex: _____

Rhythm interpretation: _____

Strip 8-4. Rhythm: _____ Rate: _____ P wave: _____

PR interval: _____ QRS complex: _____

Rhythm interpretation: _____

Strip 8-5. Rhythm: _____ Rate: _____ P wave: _____

PR interval: _____ QRS complex: _____

Rhythm interpretation: _____

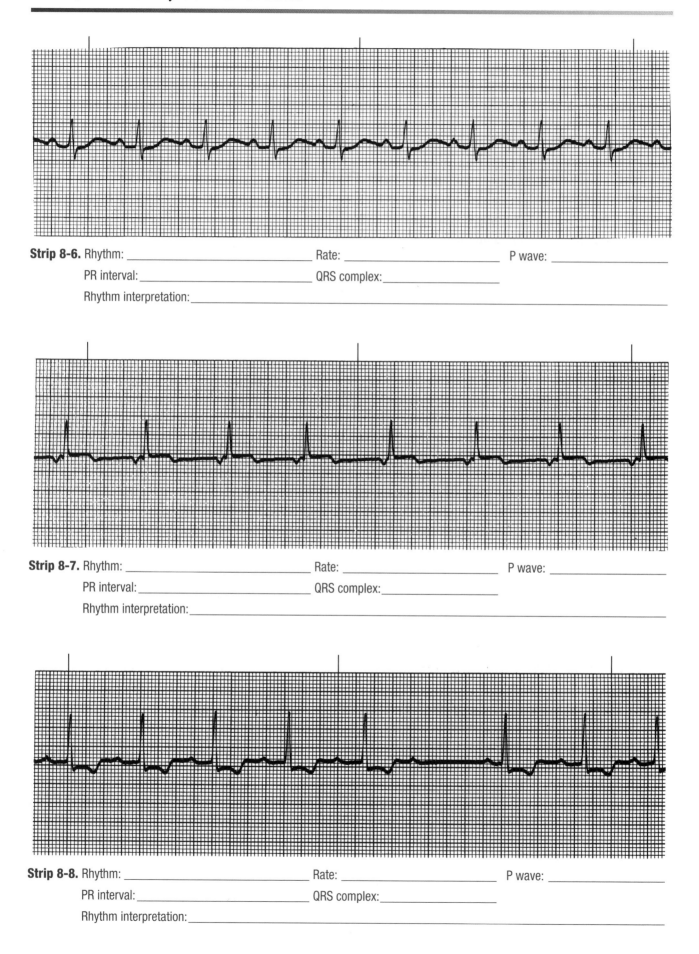

Strip 8-6. Rhythm: _____ Rate: _____ P wave: _____

PR interval: _____ QRS complex: _____

Rhythm interpretation: _____

Strip 8-7. Rhythm: _____ Rate: _____ P wave: _____

PR interval: _____ QRS complex: _____

Rhythm interpretation: _____

Strip 8-8. Rhythm: _____ Rate: _____ P wave: _____

PR interval: _____ QRS complex: _____

Rhythm interpretation: _____

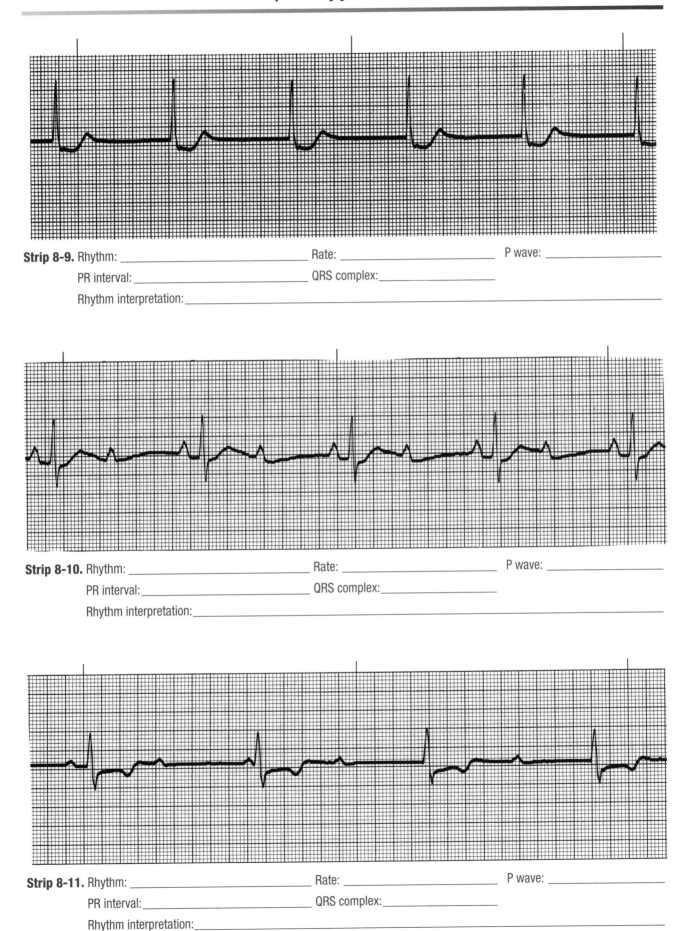

Strip 8-9. Rhythm: _____ Rate: _____ P wave: _____

PR interval: _____ QRS complex: _____

Rhythm interpretation: _____

Strip 8-10. Rhythm: _____ Rate: _____ P wave: _____

PR interval: _____ QRS complex: _____

Rhythm interpretation: _____

Strip 8-11. Rhythm: _____ Rate: _____ P wave: _____

PR interval: _____ QRS complex: _____

Rhythm interpretation: _____

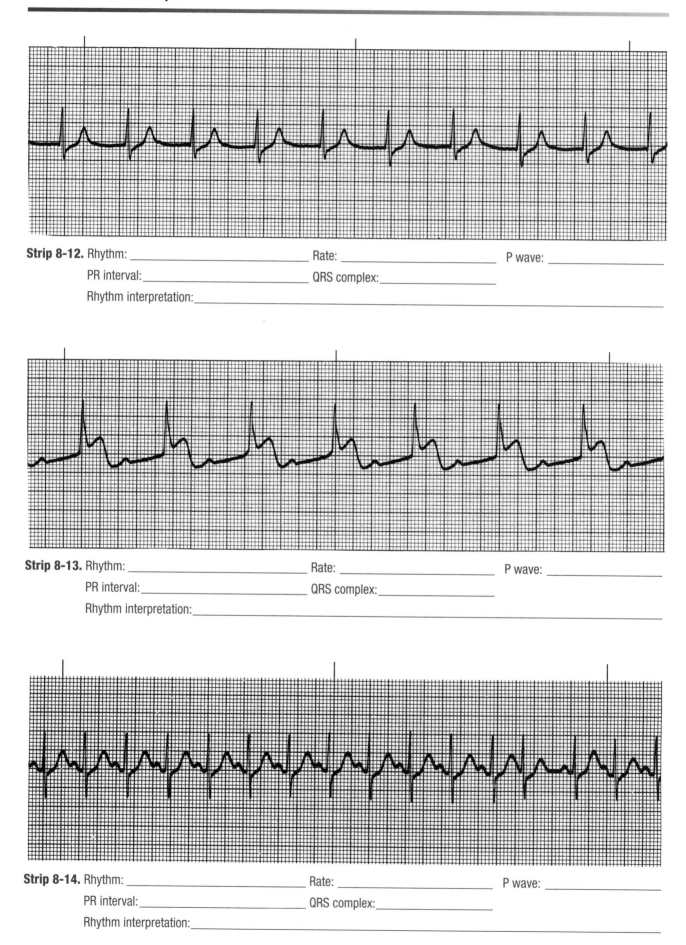

Strip 8-12. Rhythm: _____ Rate: _____ P wave: _____

PR interval:_____ QRS complex:_____

Rhythm interpretation:_____

Strip 8-13. Rhythm: _____ Rate: _____ P wave: _____

PR interval:_____ QRS complex:_____

Rhythm interpretation:_____

Strip 8-14. Rhythm: _____ Rate: _____ P wave: _____

PR interval:_____ QRS complex:_____

Rhythm interpretation:_____

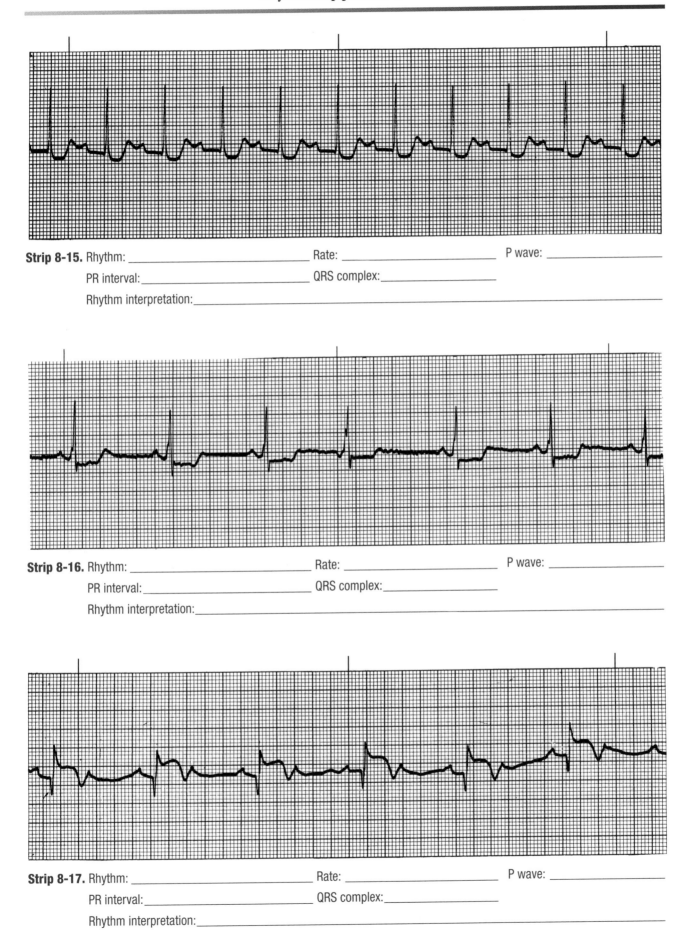

Strip 8-15. Rhythm: _____ Rate: _____ P wave: _____

PR interval: _____ QRS complex: _____

Rhythm interpretation: _____

Strip 8-16. Rhythm: _____ Rate: _____ P wave: _____

PR interval: _____ QRS complex: _____

Rhythm interpretation: _____

Strip 8-17. Rhythm: _____ Rate: _____ P wave: _____

PR interval: _____ QRS complex: _____

Rhythm interpretation: _____

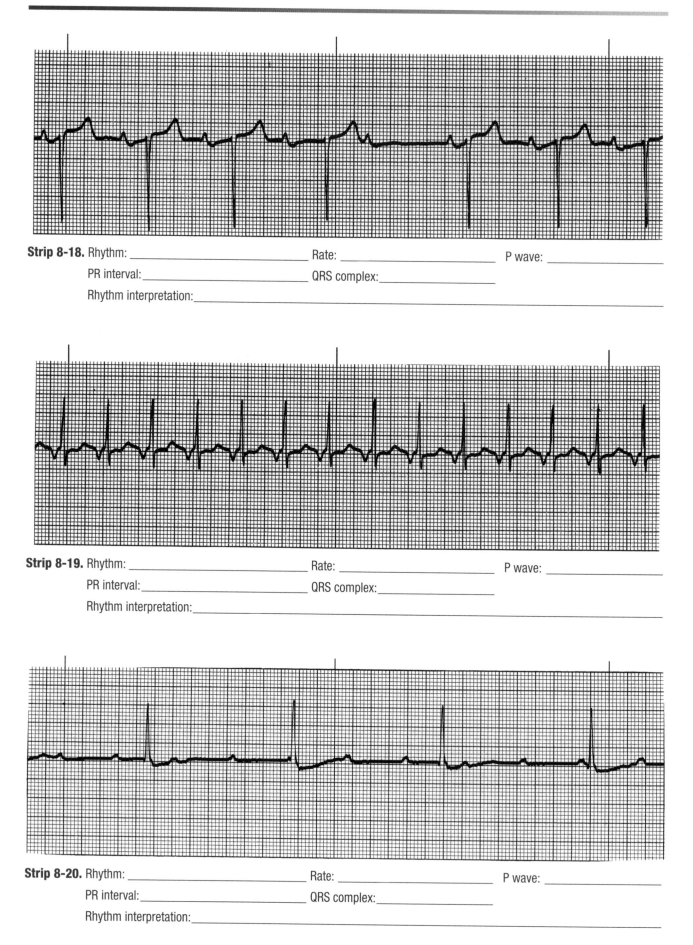

Strip 8-18. Rhythm: _____ Rate: _____ P wave: _____

PR interval: _____ QRS complex: _____

Rhythm interpretation: _____

Strip 8-19. Rhythm: _____ Rate: _____ P wave: _____

PR interval: _____ QRS complex: _____

Rhythm interpretation: _____

Strip 8-20. Rhythm: _____ Rate: _____ P wave: _____

PR interval: _____ QRS complex: _____

Rhythm interpretation: _____

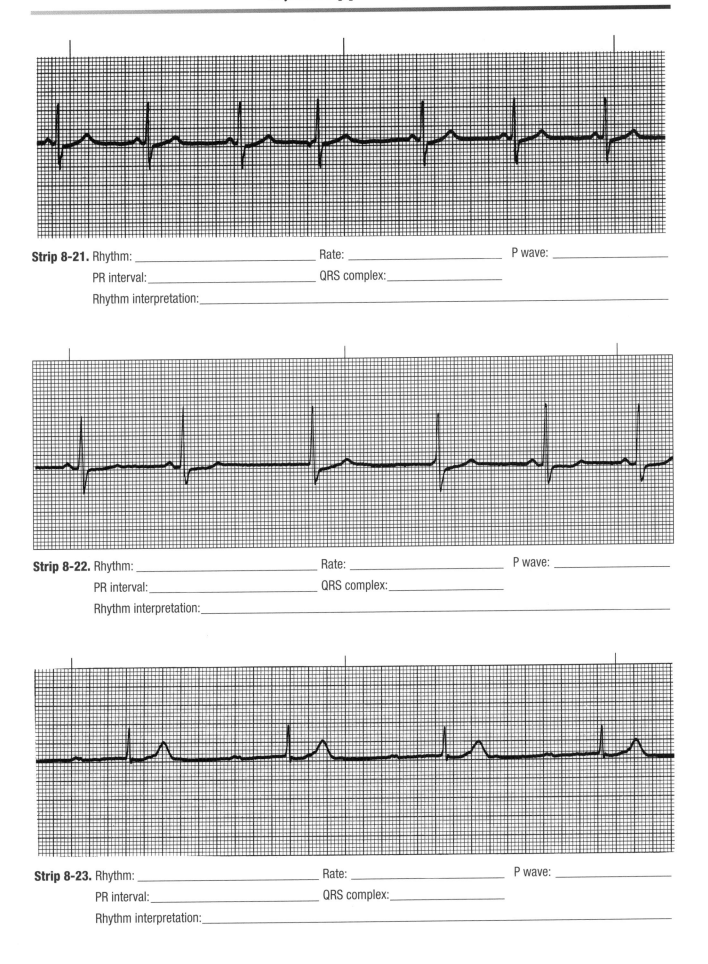

Strip 8-21. Rhythm: _____ Rate: _____ P wave: _____

PR interval: _____ QRS complex: _____

Rhythm interpretation: _____

Strip 8-22. Rhythm: _____ Rate: _____ P wave: _____

PR interval: _____ QRS complex: _____

Rhythm interpretation: _____

Strip 8-23. Rhythm: _____ Rate: _____ P wave: _____

PR interval: _____ QRS complex: _____

Rhythm interpretation: _____

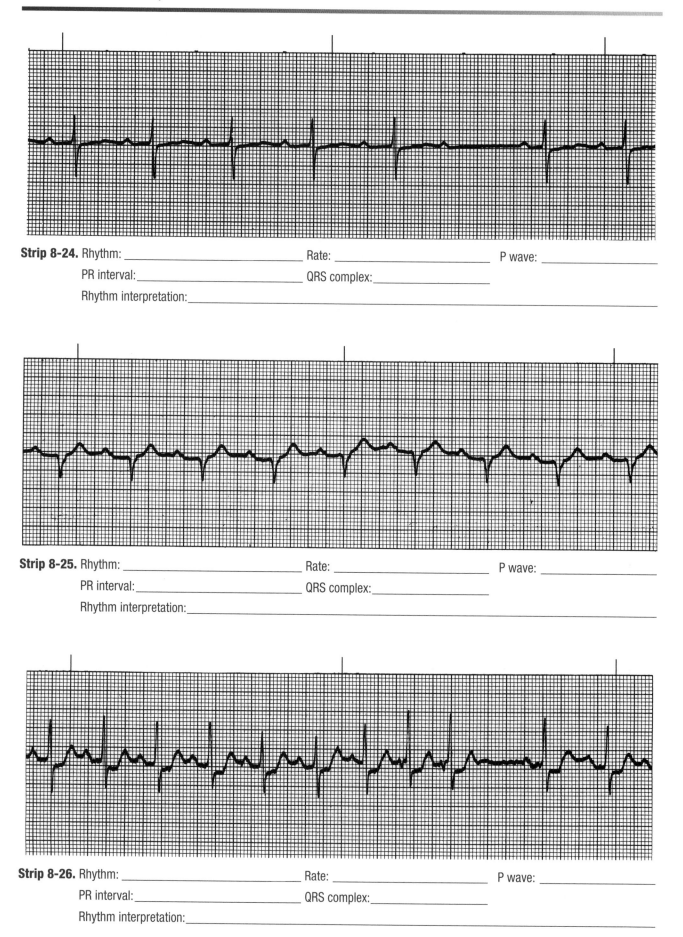

Strip 8-24. Rhythm: _____ Rate: _____ P wave: _____

PR interval: _____ QRS complex: _____

Rhythm interpretation: _____

Strip 8-25. Rhythm: _____ Rate: _____ P wave: _____

PR interval: _____ QRS complex: _____

Rhythm interpretation: _____

Strip 8-26. Rhythm: _____ Rate: _____ P wave: _____

PR interval: _____ QRS complex: _____

Rhythm interpretation: _____

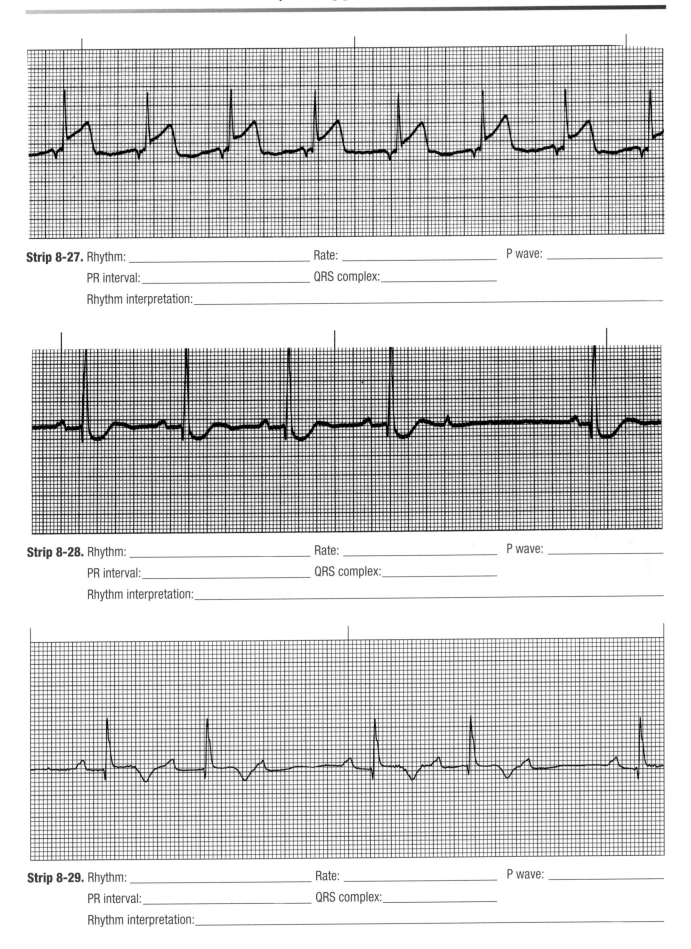

Strip 8-27. Rhythm: _____ Rate: _____ P wave: _____

PR interval: _____ QRS complex: _____

Rhythm interpretation: _____

Strip 8-28. Rhythm: _____ Rate: _____ P wave: _____

PR interval: _____ QRS complex: _____

Rhythm interpretation: _____

Strip 8-29. Rhythm: _____ Rate: _____ P wave: _____

PR interval: _____ QRS complex: _____

Rhythm interpretation: _____

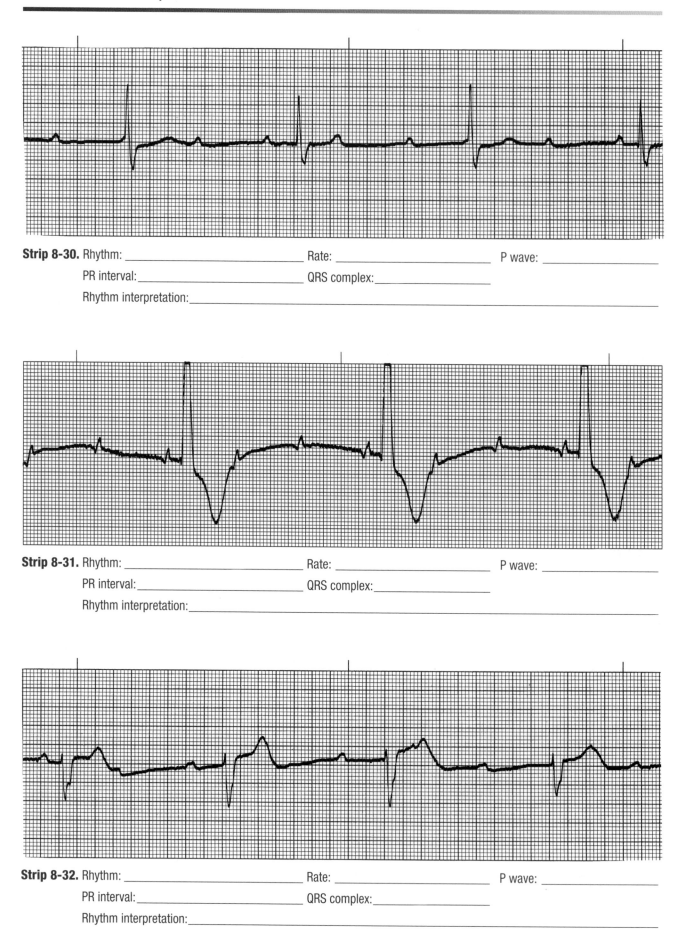

Strip 8-30. Rhythm: _____ Rate: _____ P wave: _____

PR interval: _____ QRS complex: _____

Rhythm interpretation: _____

Strip 8-31. Rhythm: _____ Rate: _____ P wave: _____

PR interval: _____ QRS complex: _____

Rhythm interpretation: _____

Strip 8-32. Rhythm: _____ Rate: _____ P wave: _____

PR interval: _____ QRS complex: _____

Rhythm interpretation: _____

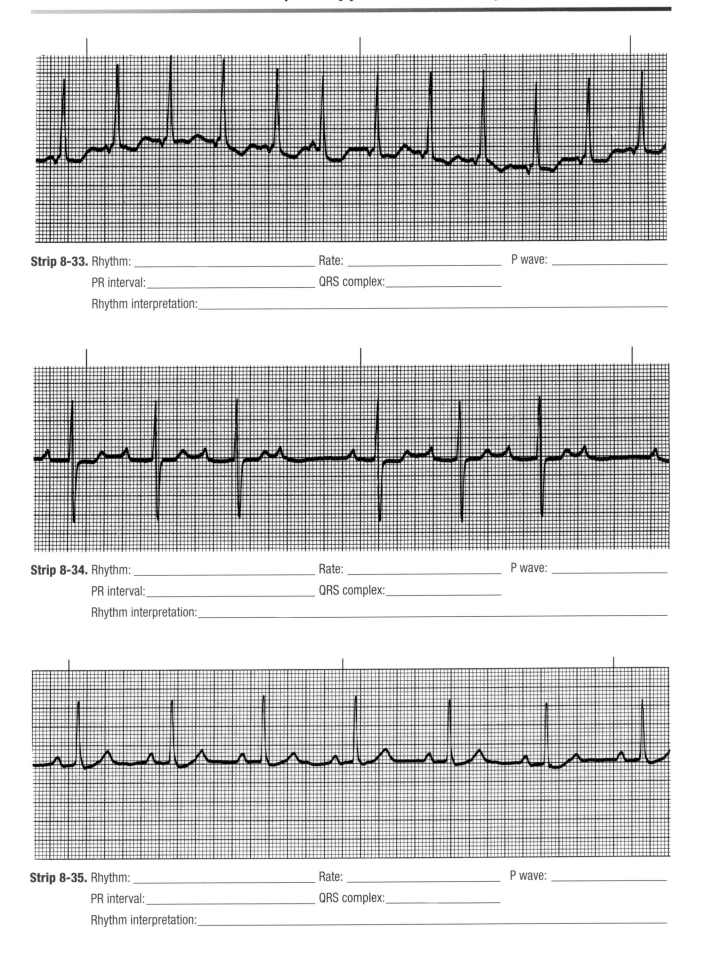

Strip 8-33. Rhythm: _____ Rate: _____ P wave: _____

PR interval: _____ QRS complex: _____

Rhythm interpretation: _____

Strip 8-34. Rhythm: _____ Rate: _____ P wave: _____

PR interval: _____ QRS complex: _____

Rhythm interpretation: _____

Strip 8-35. Rhythm: _____ Rate: _____ P wave: _____

PR interval: _____ QRS complex: _____

Rhythm interpretation: _____

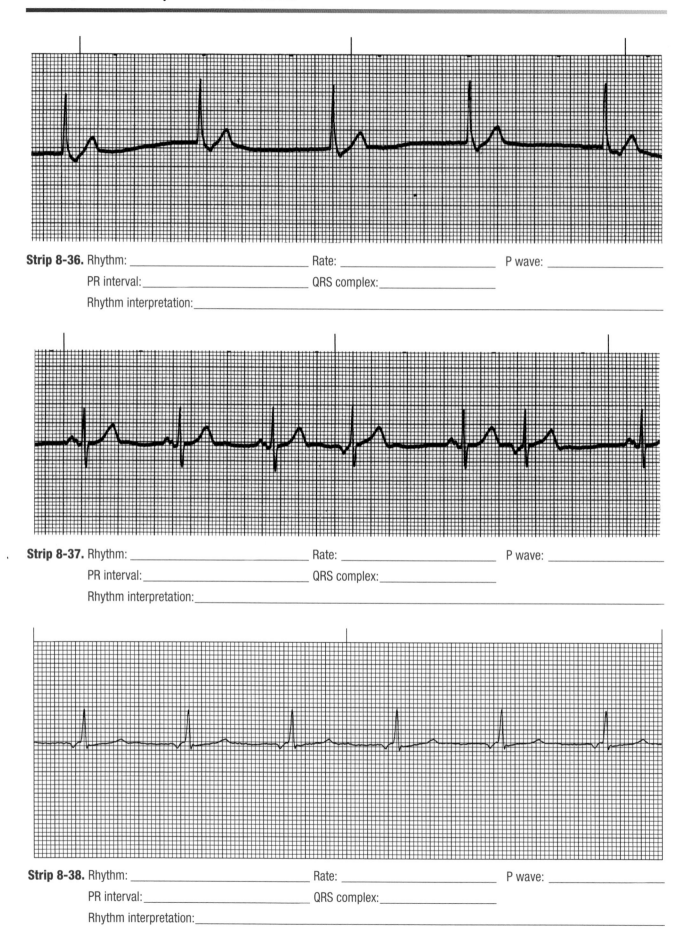

Strip 8-36. Rhythm: _____ Rate: _____ P wave: _____

PR interval: _____ QRS complex: _____

Rhythm interpretation: _____

Strip 8-37. Rhythm: _____ Rate: _____ P wave: _____

PR interval: _____ QRS complex: _____

Rhythm interpretation: _____

Strip 8-38. Rhythm: _____ Rate: _____ P wave: _____

PR interval: _____ QRS complex: _____

Rhythm interpretation: _____

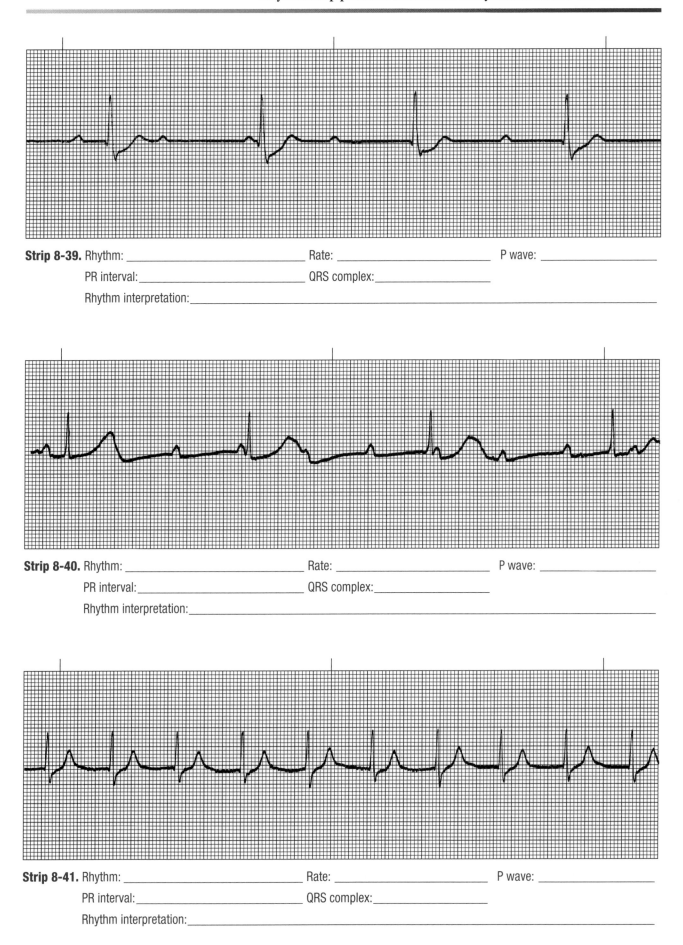

Strip 8-39. Rhythm: _____ Rate: _____ P wave: _____

PR interval: _____ QRS complex: _____

Rhythm interpretation: _____

Strip 8-40. Rhythm: _____ Rate: _____ P wave: _____

PR interval: _____ QRS complex: _____

Rhythm interpretation: _____

Strip 8-41. Rhythm: _____ Rate: _____ P wave: _____

PR interval: _____ QRS complex: _____

Rhythm interpretation: _____

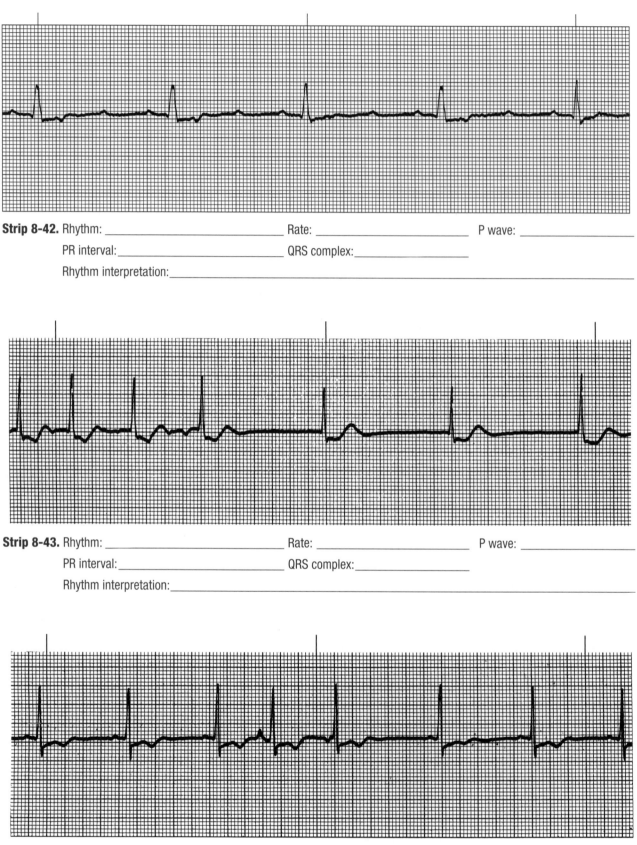

Strip 8-42. Rhythm: _____ Rate: _____ P wave: _____

PR interval: _____ QRS complex: _____

Rhythm interpretation: _____

Strip 8-43. Rhythm: _____ Rate: _____ P wave: _____

PR interval: _____ QRS complex: _____

Rhythm interpretation: _____

Strip 8-44. Rhythm: _____ Rate: _____ P wave: _____

PR interval: _____ QRS complex: _____

Rhythm interpretation: _____

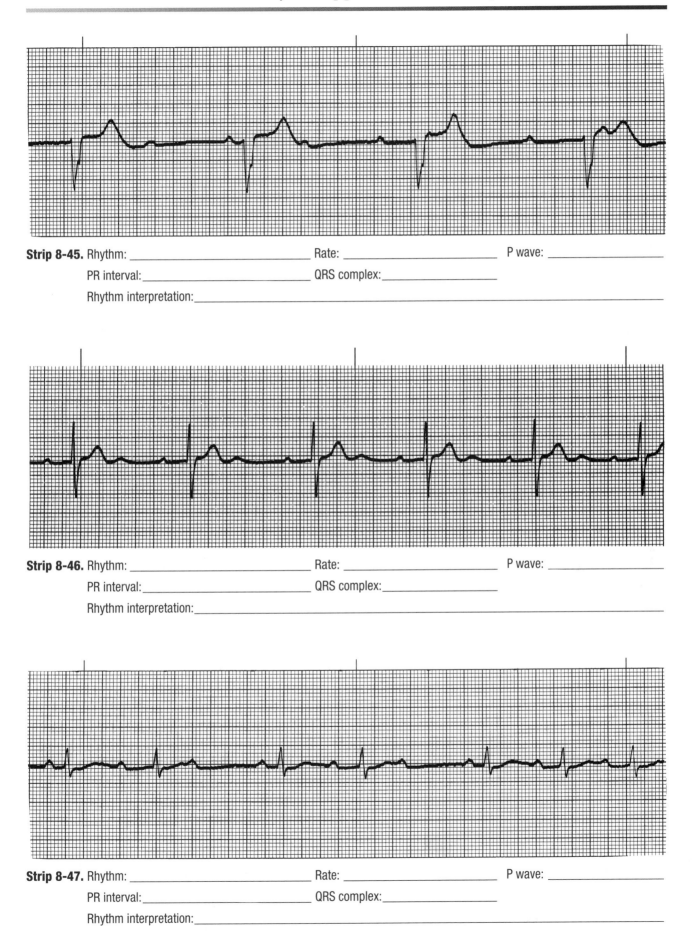

Strip 8-45. Rhythm: _____ Rate: _____ P wave: _____

PR interval: _____ QRS complex: _____

Rhythm interpretation: _____

Strip 8-46. Rhythm: _____ Rate: _____ P wave: _____

PR interval: _____ QRS complex: _____

Rhythm interpretation: _____

Strip 8-47. Rhythm: _____ Rate: _____ P wave: _____

PR interval: _____ QRS complex: _____

Rhythm interpretation: _____

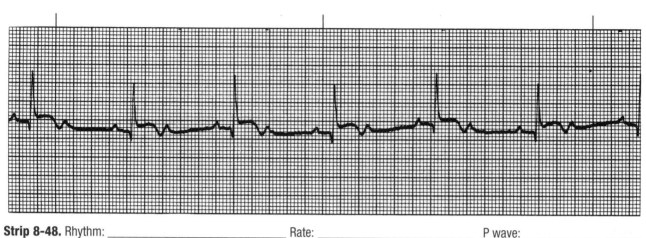

Strip 8-48. Rhythm: _____ Rate: _____ P wave: _____

PR interval:_____ QRS complex:_____

Rhythm interpretation:_____

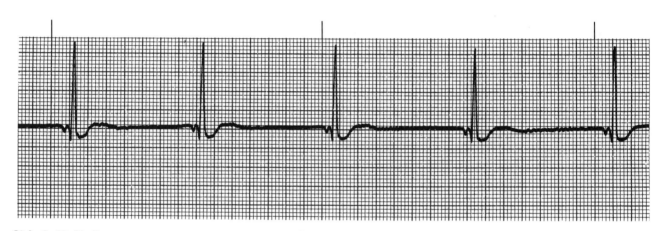

Strip 8-49. Rhythm: _____ Rate: _____ P wave: _____

PR interval:_____ QRS complex:_____

Rhythm interpretation:_____

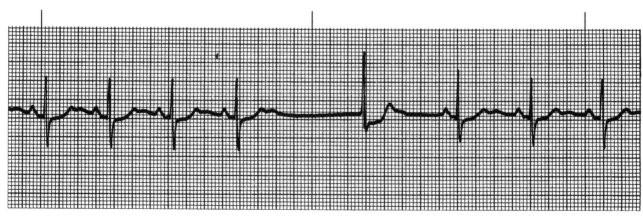

Strip 8-50. Rhythm: _____ Rate: _____ P wave: _____

PR interval:_____ QRS complex:_____

Rhythm interpretation:_____

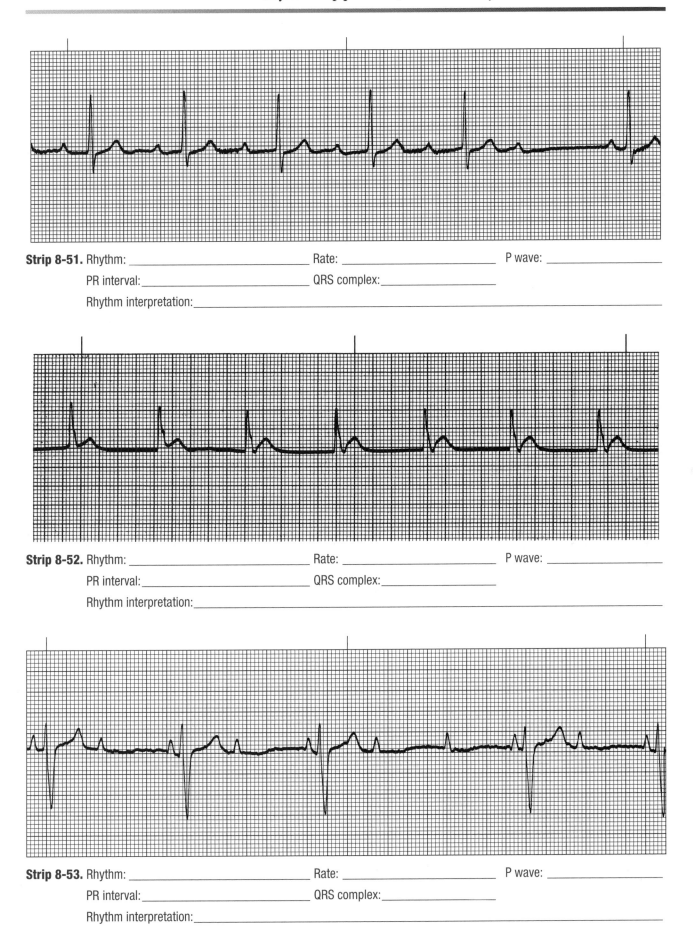

Strip 8-51. Rhythm: _____ Rate: _____ P wave: _____

PR interval: _____ QRS complex: _____

Rhythm interpretation: _____

Strip 8-52. Rhythm: _____ Rate: _____ P wave: _____

PR interval: _____ QRS complex: _____

Rhythm interpretation: _____

Strip 8-53. Rhythm: _____ Rate: _____ P wave: _____

PR interval: _____ QRS complex: _____

Rhythm interpretation: _____

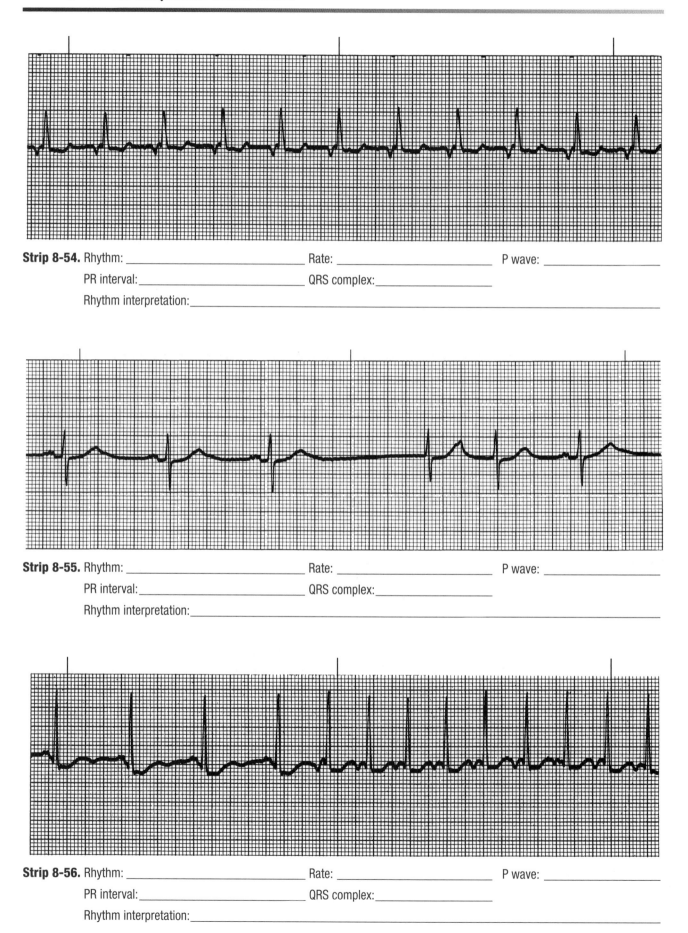

Strip 8-54. Rhythm: _____ Rate: _____ P wave: _____

PR interval:_____ QRS complex:_____

Rhythm interpretation:_____

Strip 8-55. Rhythm: _____ Rate: _____ P wave: _____

PR interval:_____ QRS complex:_____

Rhythm interpretation:_____

Strip 8-56. Rhythm: _____ Rate: _____ P wave: _____

PR interval:_____ QRS complex:_____

Rhythm interpretation:_____

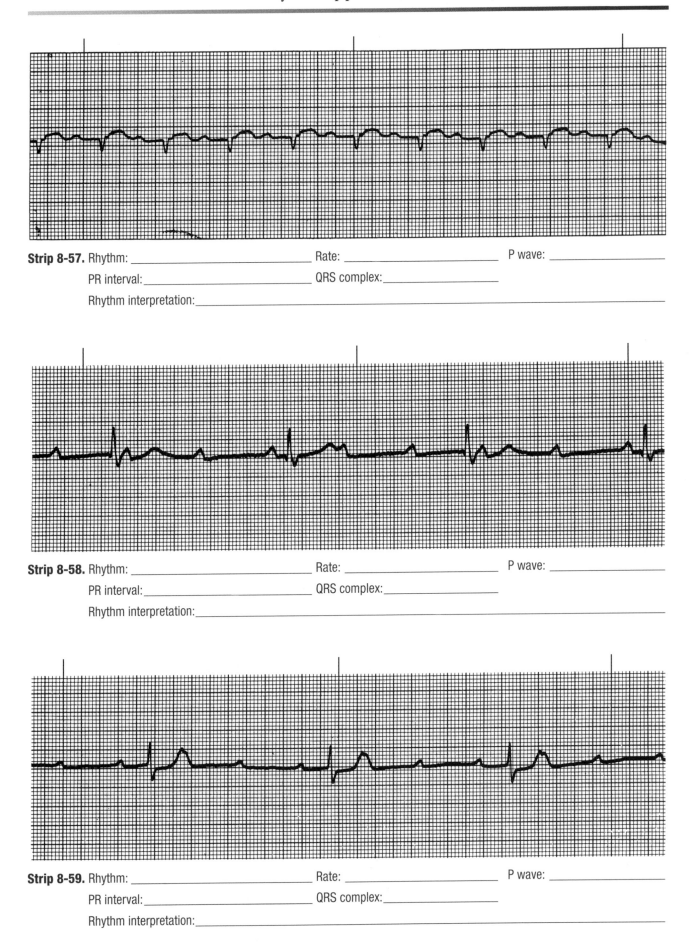

Strip 8-57. Rhythm: _____ Rate: _____ P wave: _____

PR interval: _____ QRS complex: _____

Rhythm interpretation: _____

Strip 8-58. Rhythm: _____ Rate: _____ P wave: _____

PR interval: _____ QRS complex: _____

Rhythm interpretation: _____

Strip 8-59. Rhythm: _____ Rate: _____ P wave: _____

PR interval: _____ QRS complex: _____

Rhythm interpretation: _____

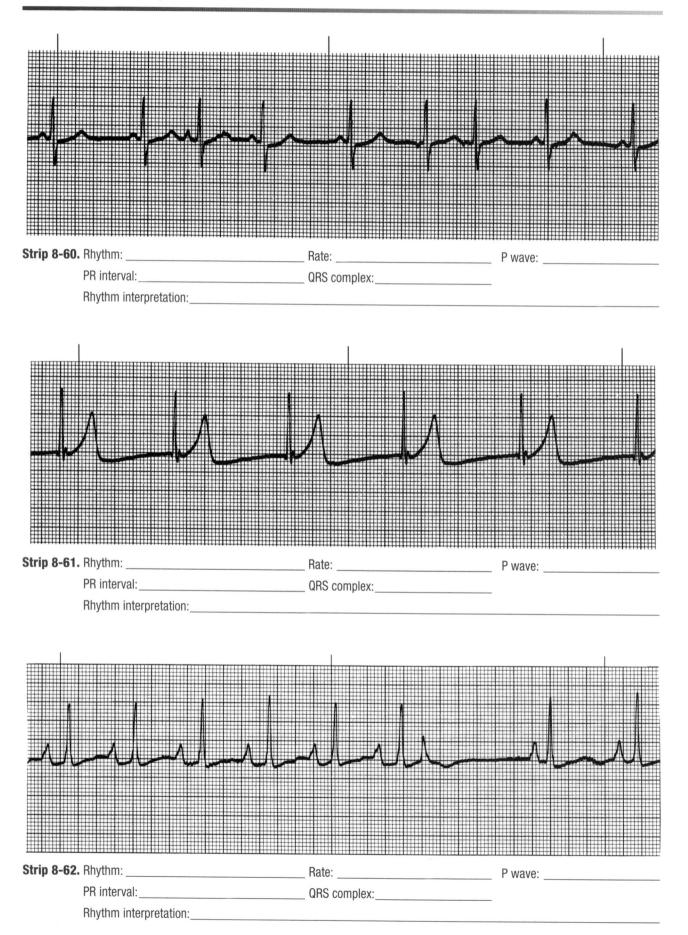

Strip 8-60. Rhythm: _____ Rate: _____ P wave: _____

PR interval: _____ QRS complex: _____

Rhythm interpretation: _____

Strip 8-61. Rhythm: _____ Rate: _____ P wave: _____

PR interval: _____ QRS complex: _____

Rhythm interpretation: _____

Strip 8-62. Rhythm: _____ Rate: _____ P wave: _____

PR interval: _____ QRS complex: _____

Rhythm interpretation: _____

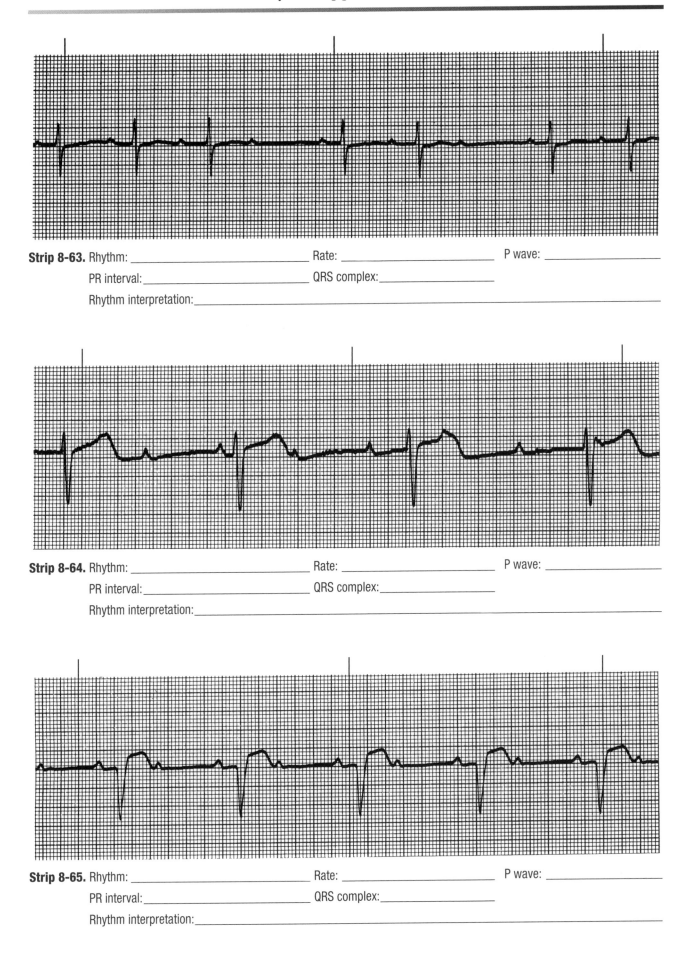

Strip 8-63. Rhythm: _____ Rate: _____ P wave: _____

PR interval: _____ QRS complex: _____

Rhythm interpretation: _____

Strip 8-64. Rhythm: _____ Rate: _____ P wave: _____

PR interval: _____ QRS complex: _____

Rhythm interpretation: _____

Strip 8-65. Rhythm: _____ Rate: _____ P wave: _____

PR interval: _____ QRS complex: _____

Rhythm interpretation: _____

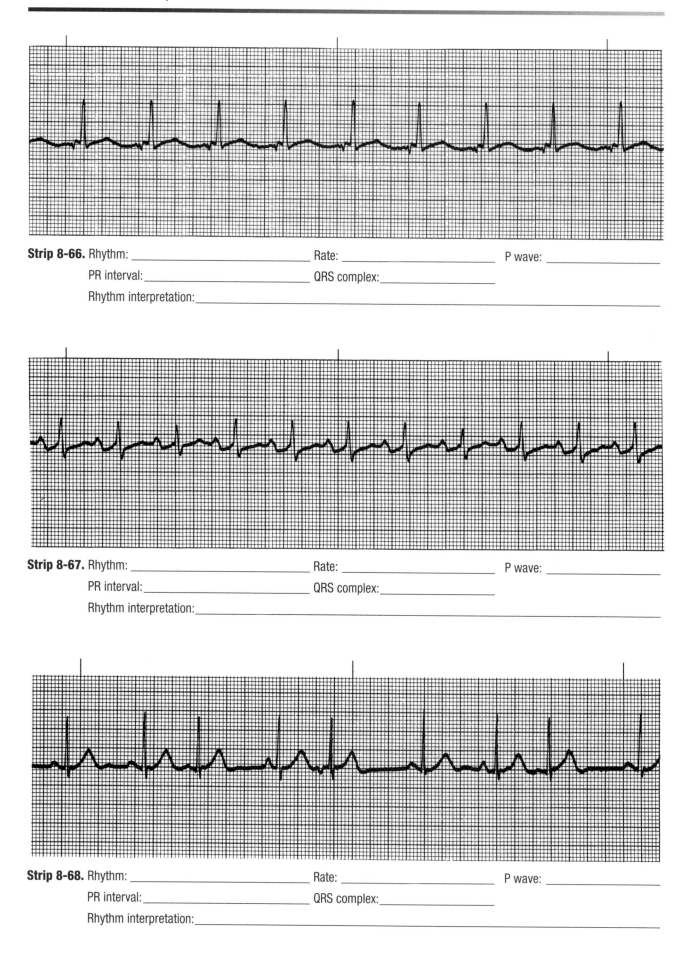

Strip 8-66. Rhythm: _____ Rate: _____ P wave: _____

PR interval: _____ QRS complex: _____

Rhythm interpretation: _____

Strip 8-67. Rhythm: _____ Rate: _____ P wave: _____

PR interval: _____ QRS complex: _____

Rhythm interpretation: _____

Strip 8-68. Rhythm: _____ Rate: _____ P wave: _____

PR interval: _____ QRS complex: _____

Rhythm interpretation: _____

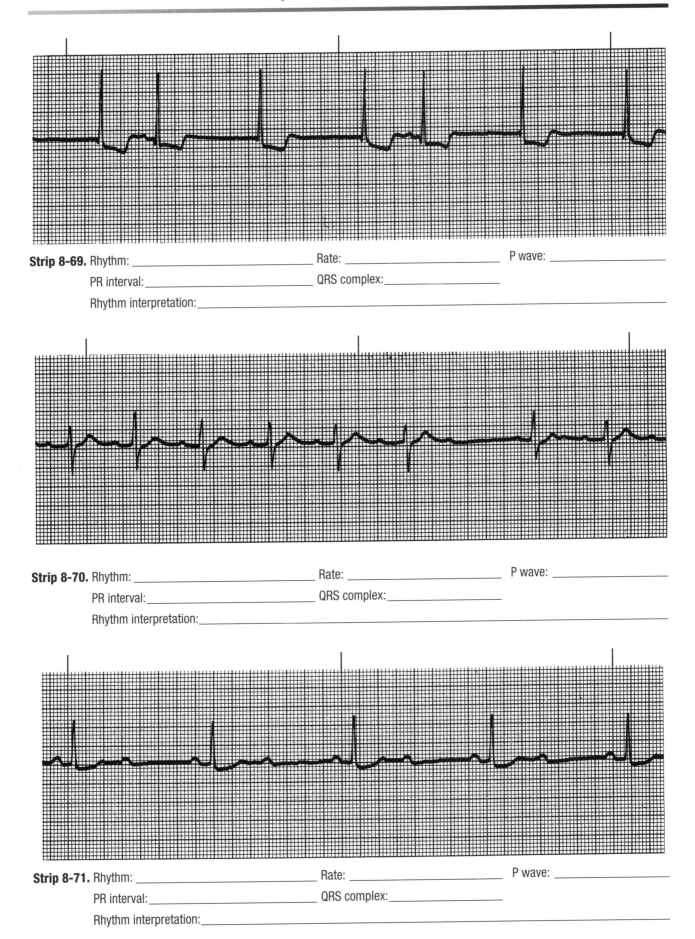

Strip 8-69. Rhythm: _____ Rate: _____ P wave: _____

PR interval: _____ QRS complex: _____

Rhythm interpretation: _____

Strip 8-70. Rhythm: _____ Rate: _____ P wave: _____

PR interval: _____ QRS complex: _____

Rhythm interpretation: _____

Strip 8-71. Rhythm: _____ Rate: _____ P wave: _____

PR interval: _____ QRS complex: _____

Rhythm interpretation: _____

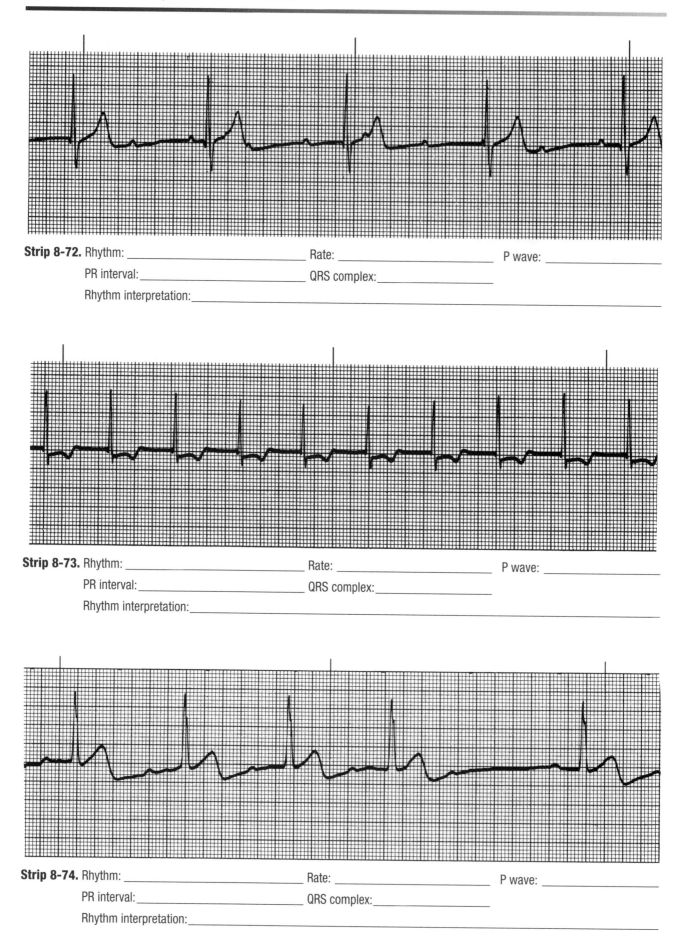

Strip 8-72. Rhythm: _____ Rate: _____ P wave: _____

PR interval: _____ QRS complex: _____

Rhythm interpretation: _____

Strip 8-73. Rhythm: _____ Rate: _____ P wave: _____

PR interval: _____ QRS complex: _____

Rhythm interpretation: _____

Strip 8-74. Rhythm: _____ Rate: _____ P wave: _____

PR interval: _____ QRS complex: _____

Rhythm interpretation: _____

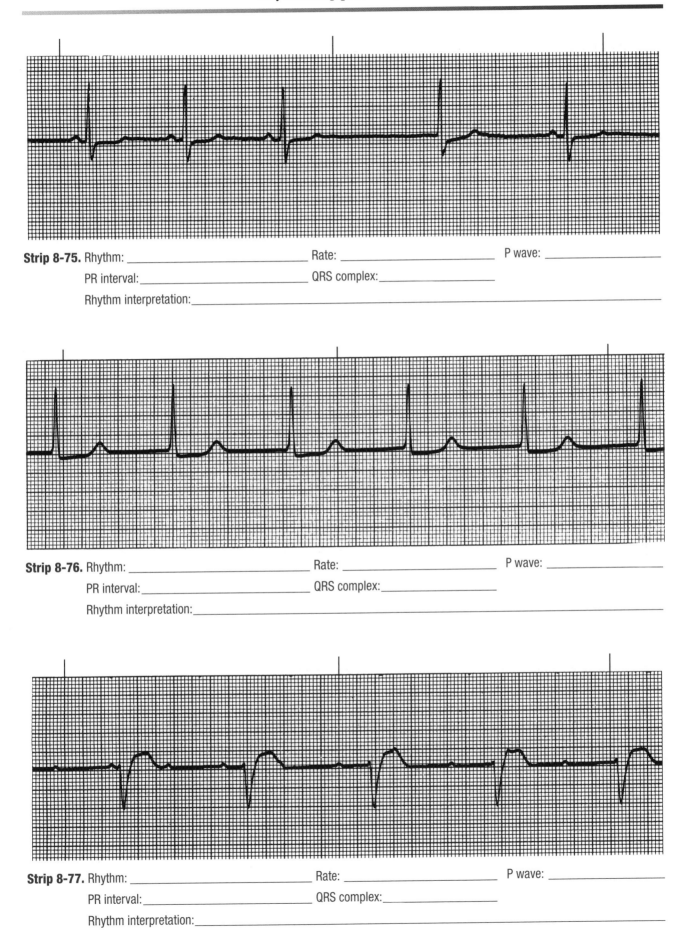

Strip 8-75. Rhythm: _____ Rate: _____ P wave: _____

PR interval: _____ QRS complex: _____

Rhythm interpretation: _____

Strip 8-76. Rhythm: _____ Rate: _____ P wave: _____

PR interval: _____ QRS complex: _____

Rhythm interpretation: _____

Strip 8-77. Rhythm: _____ Rate: _____ P wave: _____

PR interval: _____ QRS complex: _____

Rhythm interpretation: _____

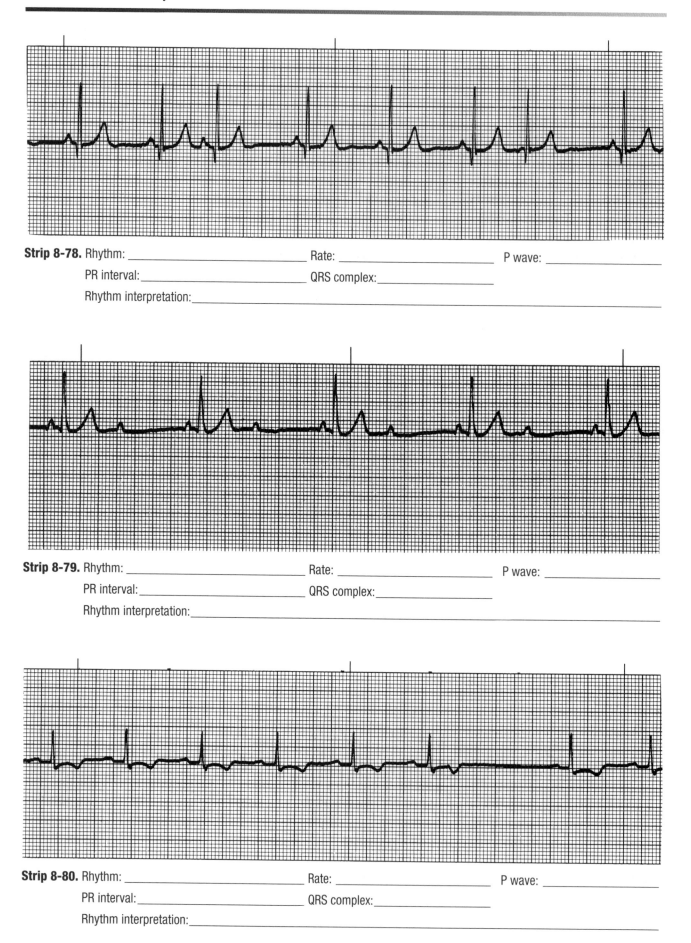

Strip 8-78. Rhythm: _____ Rate: _____ P wave: _____

PR interval:_____ QRS complex:_____

Rhythm interpretation:_____

Strip 8-79. Rhythm: _____ Rate: _____ P wave: _____

PR interval:_____ QRS complex:_____

Rhythm interpretation:_____

Strip 8-80. Rhythm: _____ Rate: _____ P wave: _____

PR interval:_____ QRS complex:_____

Rhythm interpretation:_____

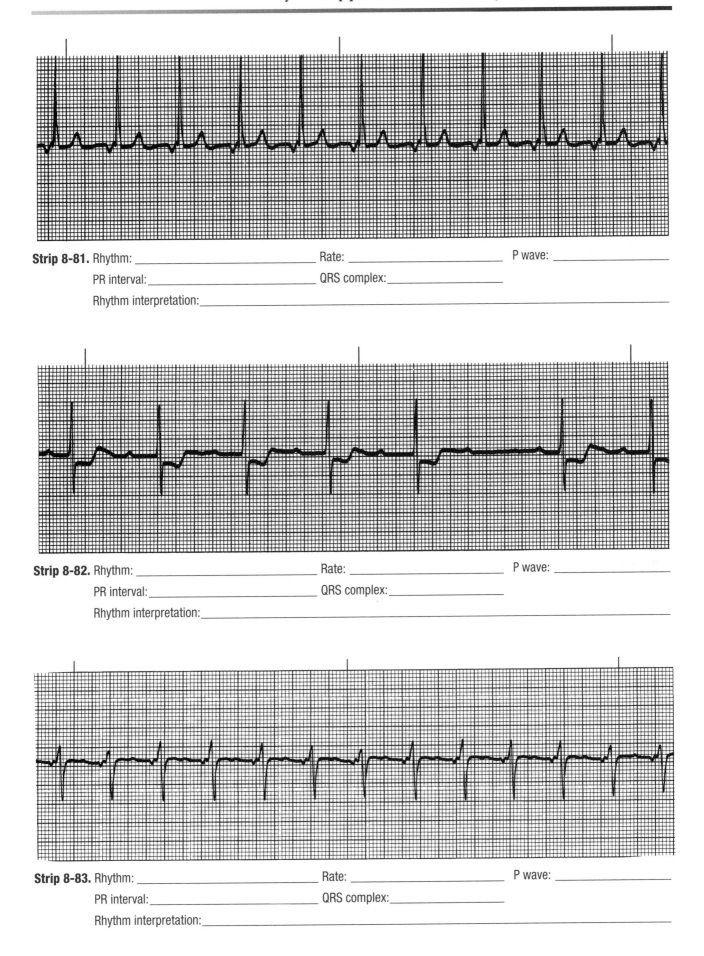

Strip 8-81. Rhythm: _____ Rate: _____ P wave: _____

PR interval: _____ QRS complex: _____

Rhythm interpretation: _____

Strip 8-82. Rhythm: _____ Rate: _____ P wave: _____

PR interval: _____ QRS complex: _____

Rhythm interpretation: _____

Strip 8-83. Rhythm: _____ Rate: _____ P wave: _____

PR interval: _____ QRS complex: _____

Rhythm interpretation: _____

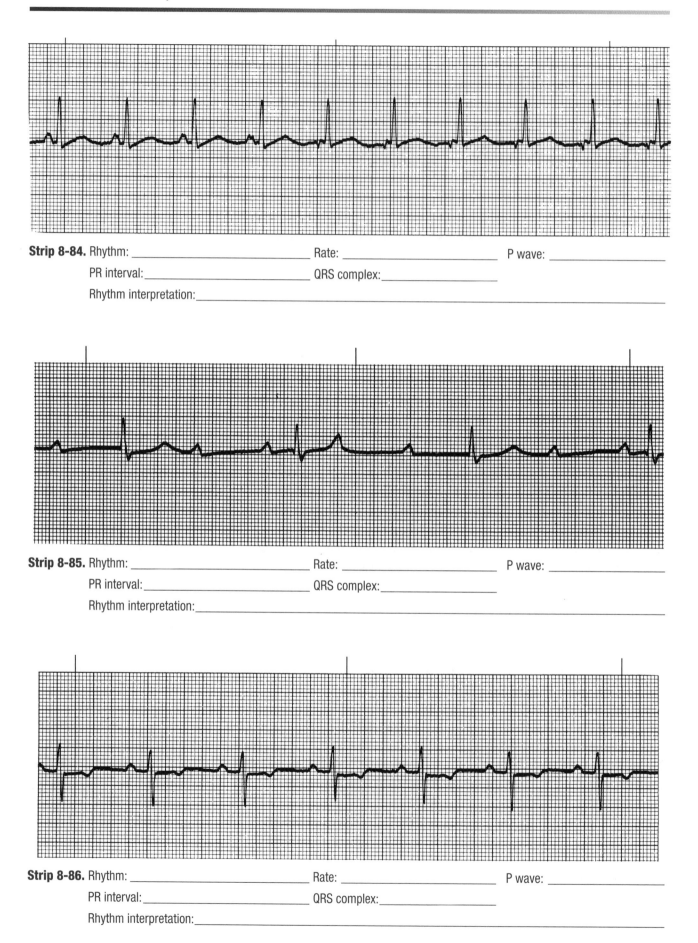

Strip 8-84. Rhythm: _____ Rate: _____ P wave: _____

PR interval:_____ QRS complex:_____

Rhythm interpretation:_____

Strip 8-85. Rhythm: _____ Rate: _____ P wave: _____

PR interval:_____ QRS complex:_____

Rhythm interpretation:_____

Strip 8-86. Rhythm: _____ Rate: _____ P wave: _____

PR interval:_____ QRS complex:_____

Rhythm interpretation:_____

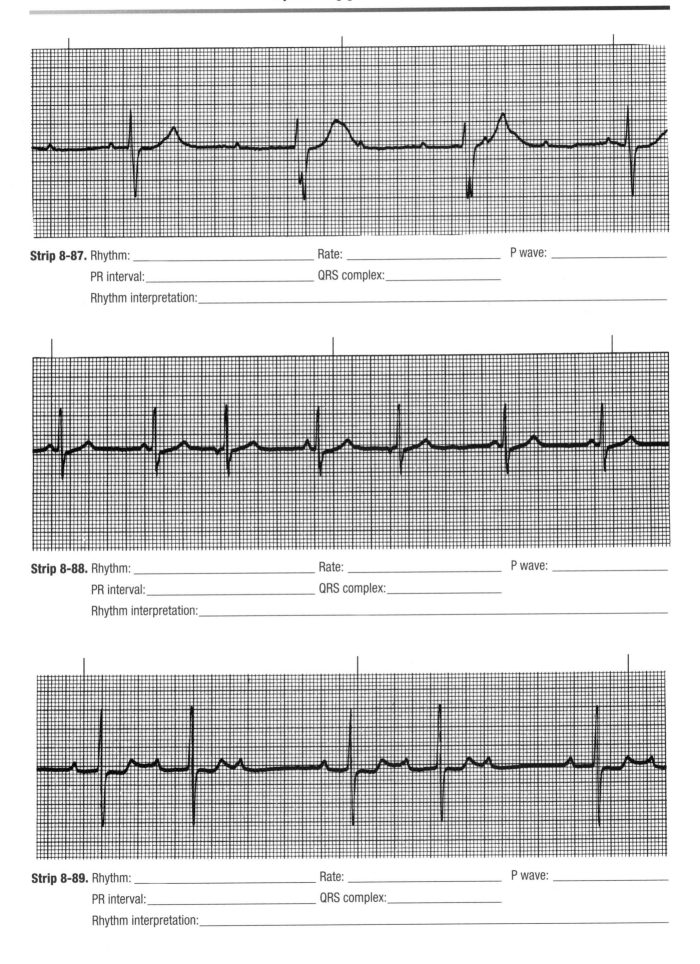

Strip 8-87. Rhythm: _____ Rate: _____ P wave: _____

PR interval: _____ QRS complex: _____

Rhythm interpretation: _____

Strip 8-88. Rhythm: _____ Rate: _____ P wave: _____

PR interval: _____ QRS complex: _____

Rhythm interpretation: _____

Strip 8-89. Rhythm: _____ Rate: _____ P wave: _____

PR interval: _____ QRS complex: _____

Rhythm interpretation: _____

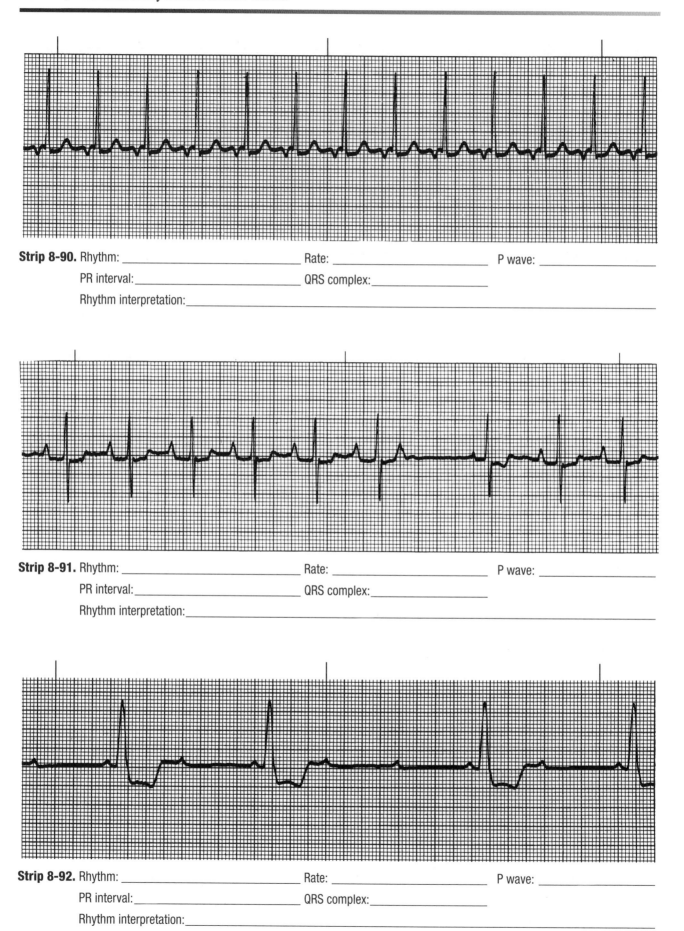

Strip 8-90. Rhythm: _____ Rate: _____ P wave: _____

PR interval: _____ QRS complex: _____

Rhythm interpretation: _____

Strip 8-91. Rhythm: _____ Rate: _____ P wave: _____

PR interval: _____ QRS complex: _____

Rhythm interpretation: _____

Strip 8-92. Rhythm: _____ Rate: _____ P wave: _____

PR interval: _____ QRS complex: _____

Rhythm interpretation: _____

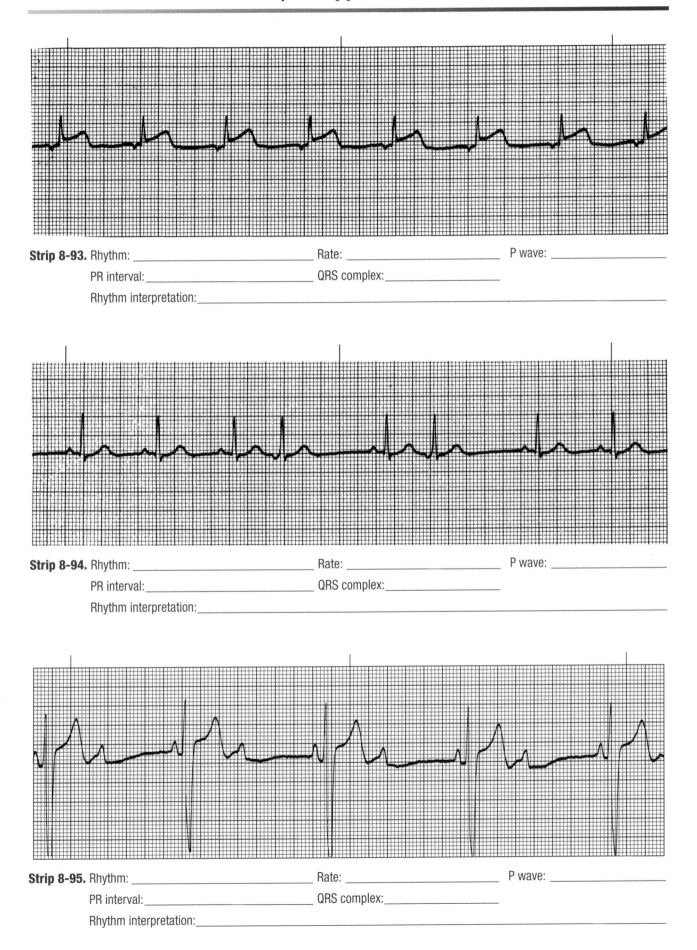

Strip 8-93. Rhythm: _____ Rate: _____ P wave: _____

PR interval: _____ QRS complex: _____

Rhythm interpretation: _____

Strip 8-94. Rhythm: _____ Rate: _____ P wave: _____

PR interval: _____ QRS complex: _____

Rhythm interpretation: _____

Strip 8-95. Rhythm: _____ Rate: _____ P wave: _____

PR interval: _____ QRS complex: _____

Rhythm interpretation: _____

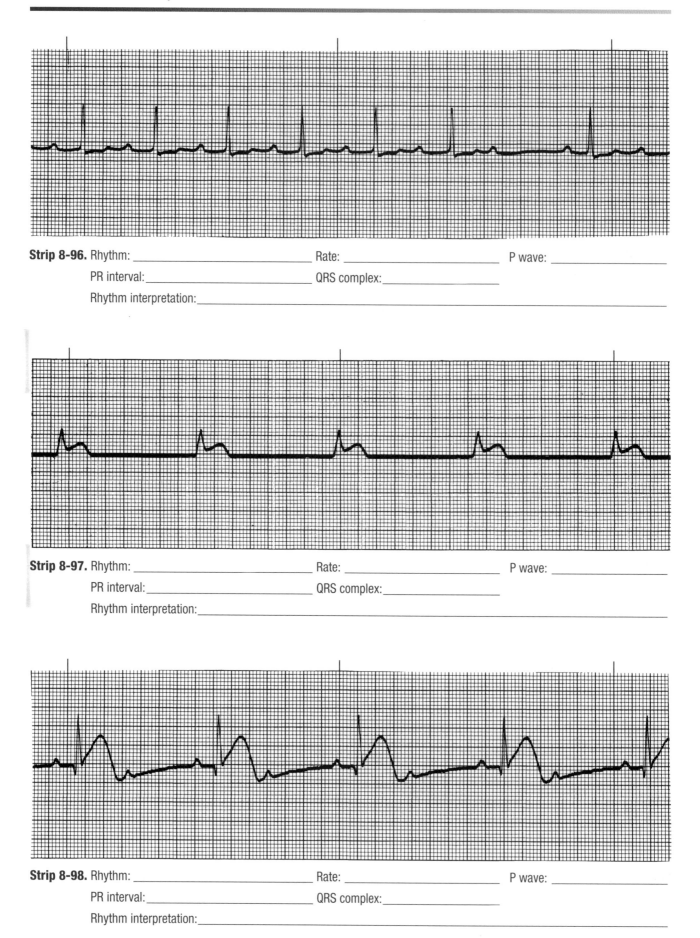

Strip 8-96. Rhythm: _____ Rate: _____ P wave: _____

PR interval: _____ QRS complex: _____

Rhythm interpretation: _____

Strip 8-97. Rhythm: _____ Rate: _____ P wave: _____

PR interval: _____ QRS complex: _____

Rhythm interpretation: _____

Strip 8-98. Rhythm: _____ Rate: _____ P wave: _____

PR interval: _____ QRS complex: _____

Rhythm interpretation: _____

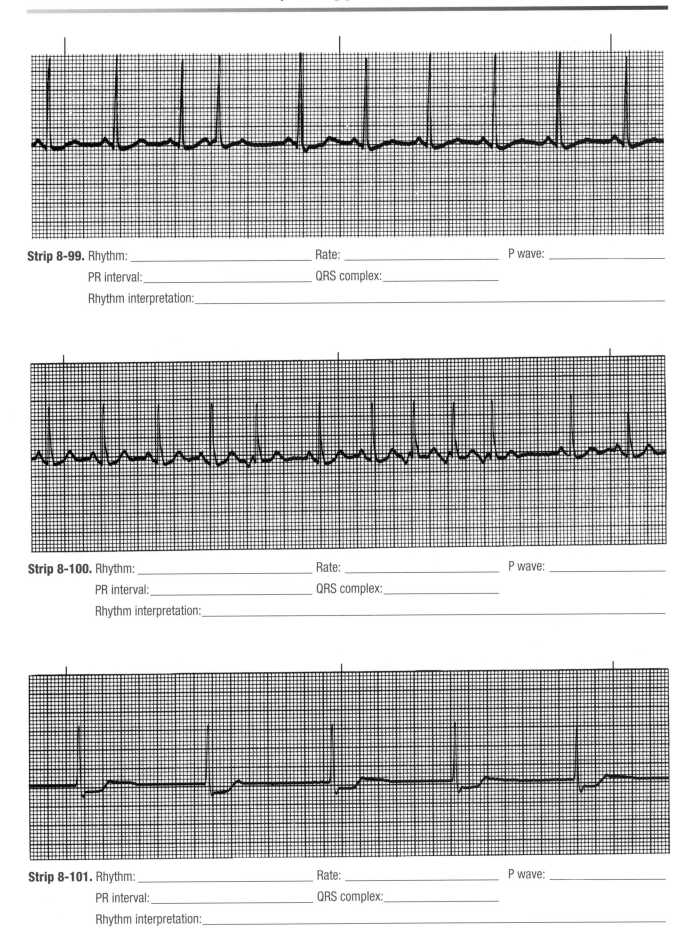

Strip 8-99. Rhythm: _____ Rate: _____ P wave: _____

PR interval:_____ QRS complex:_____

Rhythm interpretation:_____

Strip 8-100. Rhythm: _____ Rate: _____ P wave: _____

PR interval:_____ QRS complex:_____

Rhythm interpretation:_____

Strip 8-101. Rhythm: _____ Rate: _____ P wave: _____

PR interval:_____ QRS complex:_____

Rhythm interpretation:_____

▦ **Skillbuilder practice**

This section contains mixed *sinus, atrial,* and *junctional and AV block* rhythm strips, allowing the student to practice differentiating between two rhythm groups before progressing to a new group. As before, analyze the rhythm strips using the five-step process. Interpret the rhythm by comparing the data collected with the ECG characteristics for each rhythm. All strips are lead II, a positive lead, unless otherwise noted. Check your answers with the answer key in the appendix.

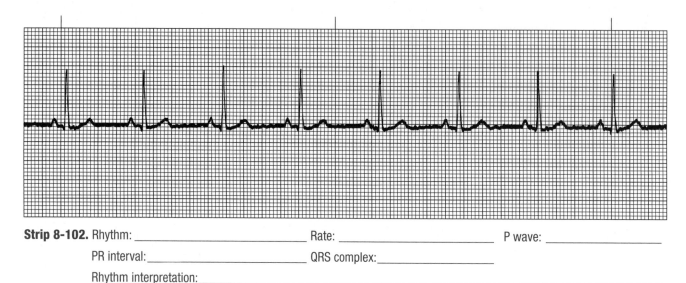

Strip 8-102. Rhythm: _____ Rate: _____ P wave: _____

PR interval:_____ QRS complex:_____

Rhythm interpretation:_____

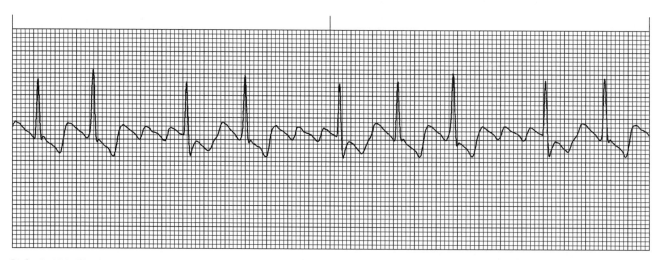

Strip 8-103. Rhythm: _____ Rate: _____ P wave: _____

PR interval:_____ QRS complex:_____

Rhythm interpretation:_____

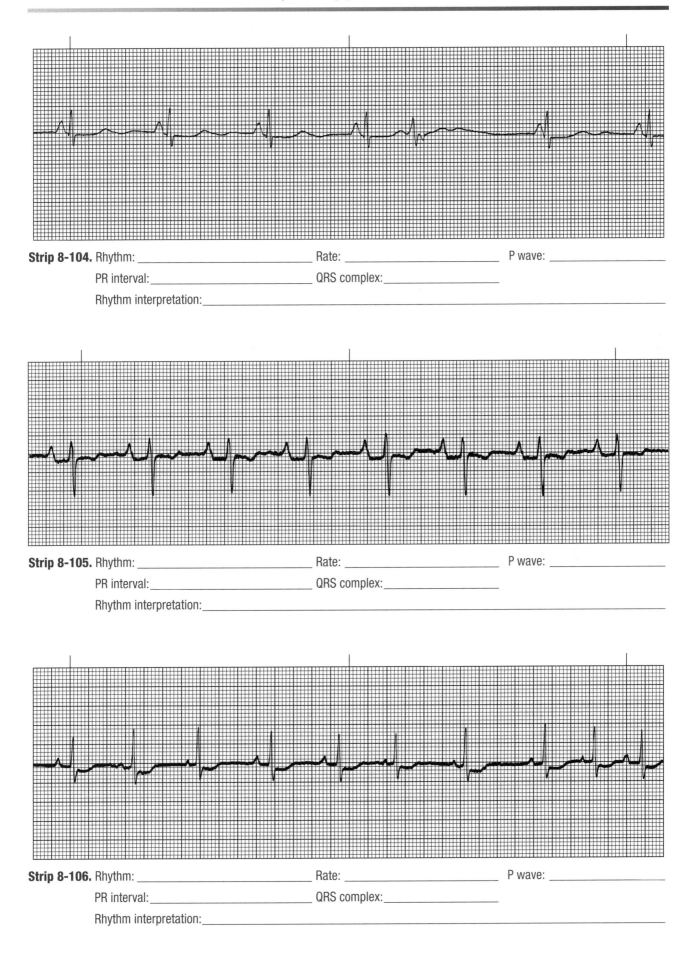

Strip 8-104. Rhythm: _____ Rate: _____ P wave: _____

PR interval: _____ QRS complex: _____

Rhythm interpretation: _____

Strip 8-105. Rhythm: _____ Rate: _____ P wave: _____

PR interval: _____ QRS complex: _____

Rhythm interpretation: _____

Strip 8-106. Rhythm: _____ Rate: _____ P wave: _____

PR interval: _____ QRS complex: _____

Rhythm interpretation: _____

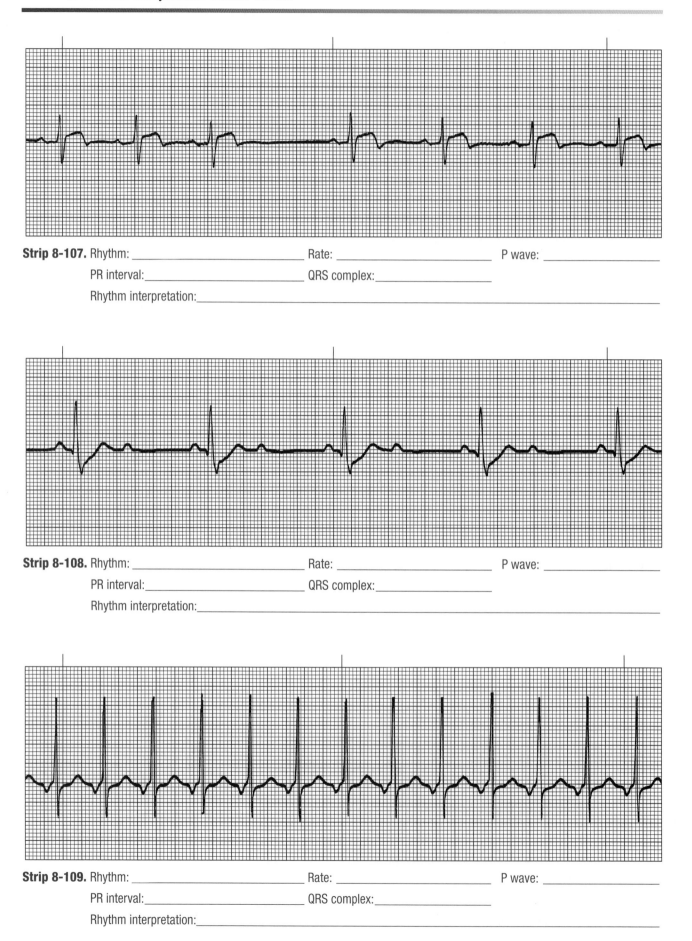

Strip 8-107. Rhythm: _____ Rate: _____ P wave: _____

PR interval:_____ QRS complex:_____

Rhythm interpretation:_____

Strip 8-108. Rhythm: _____ Rate: _____ P wave: _____

PR interval:_____ QRS complex:_____

Rhythm interpretation:_____

Strip 8-109. Rhythm: _____ Rate: _____ P wave: _____

PR interval:_____ QRS complex:_____

Rhythm interpretation:_____

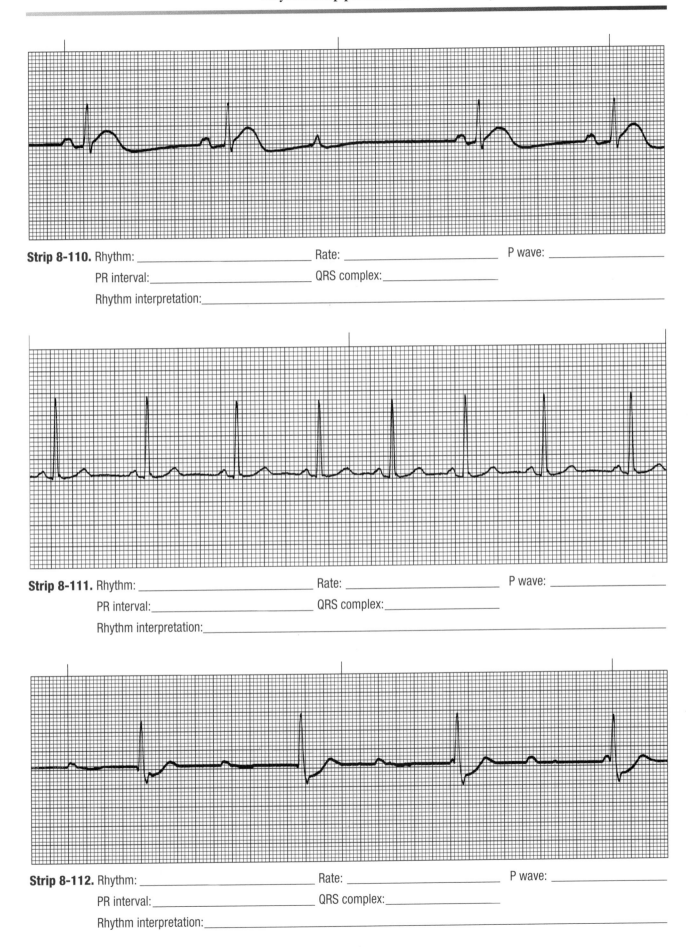

Strip 8-110. Rhythm: _____ Rate: _____ P wave: _____

PR interval:_____ QRS complex:_____

Rhythm interpretation:_____

Strip 8-111. Rhythm: _____ Rate: _____ P wave: _____

PR interval:_____ QRS complex:_____

Rhythm interpretation:_____

Strip 8-112. Rhythm: _____ Rate: _____ P wave: _____

PR interval:_____ QRS complex:_____

Rhythm interpretation:_____

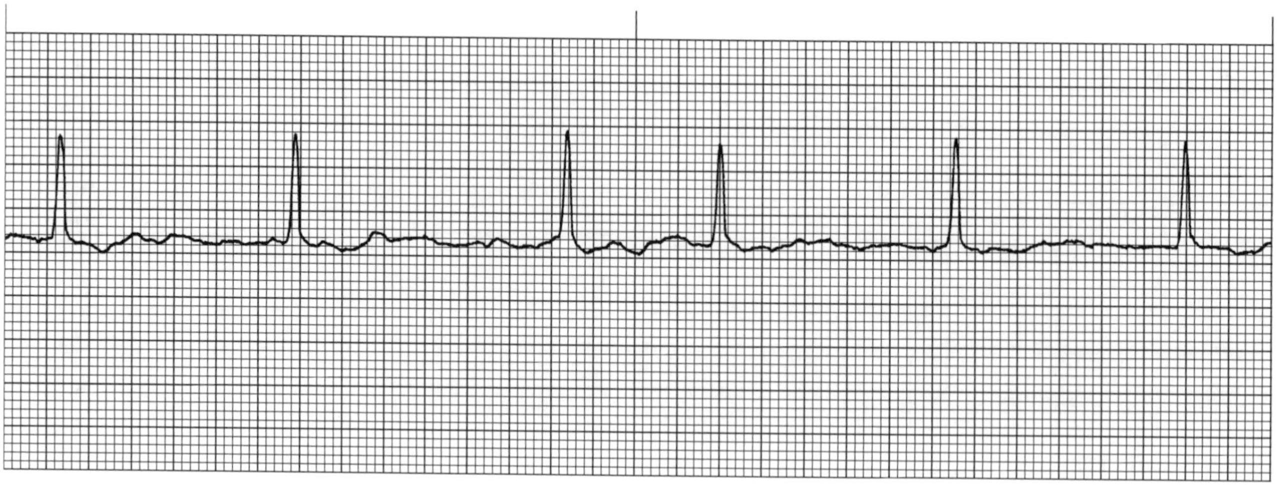

Strip 8-113. Rhythm: _____ Rate: _____ P wave: _____

PR interval: _____ QRS complex: _____

Rhythm interpretation: _____

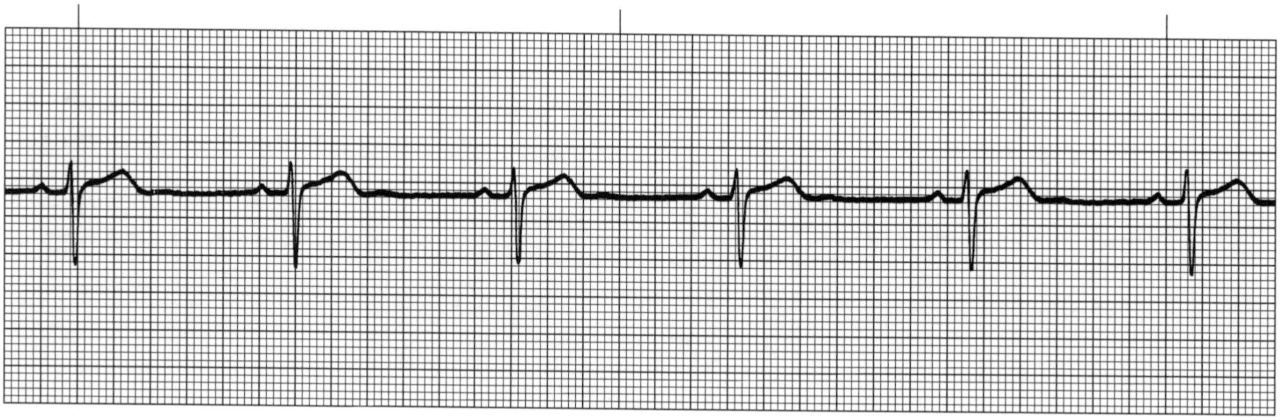

Strip 8-114. Rhythm: _____ Rate: _____ P wave: _____

PR interval: _____ QRS complex: _____

Rhythm interpretation: _____

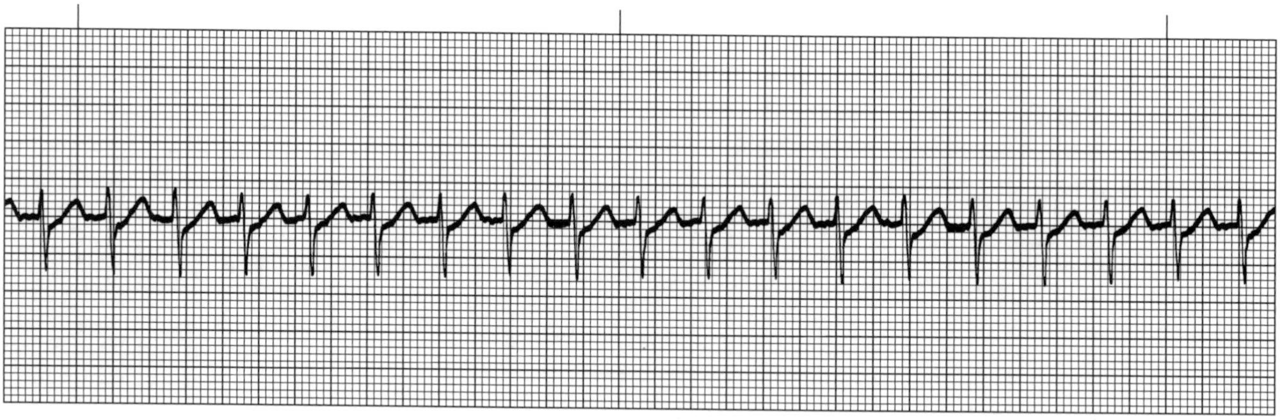

Strip 8-115. Rhythm: _____ Rate: _____ P wave: _____

PR interval: _____ QRS complex: _____

Rhythm interpretation: _____

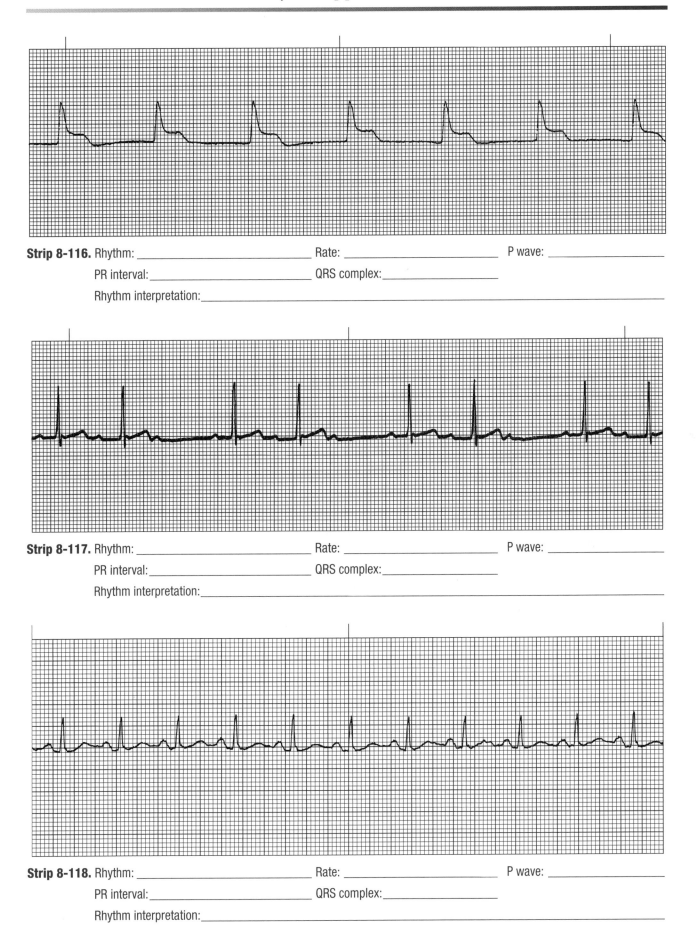

Strip 8-116. Rhythm: _____ Rate: _____ P wave: _____

PR interval: _____ QRS complex: _____

Rhythm interpretation: _____

Strip 8-117. Rhythm: _____ Rate: _____ P wave: _____

PR interval: _____ QRS complex: _____

Rhythm interpretation: _____

Strip 8-118. Rhythm: _____ Rate: _____ P wave: _____

PR interval: _____ QRS complex: _____

Rhythm interpretation: _____

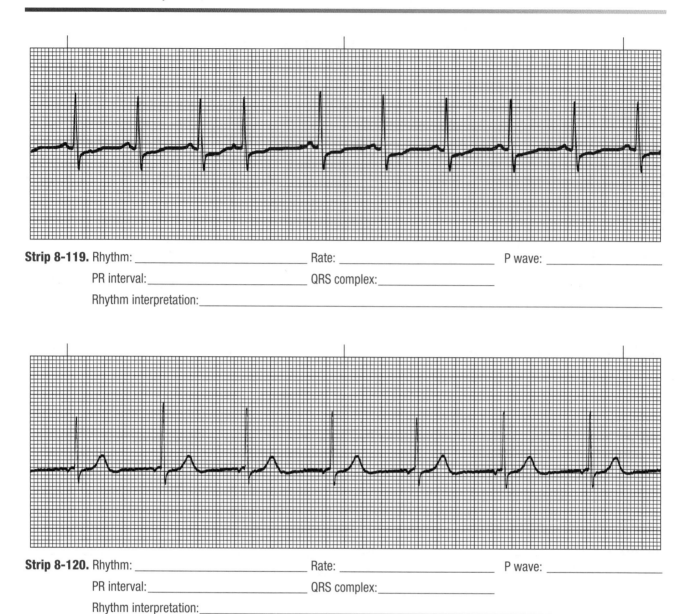

Strip 8-119. Rhythm: _____ Rate: _____ P wave: _____

PR interval: _____ QRS complex: _____

Rhythm interpretation: _____

Strip 8-120. Rhythm: _____ Rate: _____ P wave: _____

PR interval: _____ QRS complex: _____

Rhythm interpretation: _____

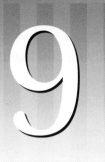

9 Ventricular arrhythmias and bundle-branch block

Overview

The three preceding chapters have focused on *supraventricular* arrhythmias. Supraventricular arrhythmias refer to those rhythms that originate above the bundle branches and include the sinus, atrial, and junctional rhythms. The electrical impulse produced by supraventricular rhythms follows the normal conduction pathway, resulting in simultaneous depolarization of the right and left ventricles. The resulting QRS complex is narrow (0.10 second or less in duration). Ventricular beats and rhythms (Figure 9-1) originate below the bundle of His in a pacemaker site in either the right or left ventricle. When impulses arise in the ventricles, the impulse does not enter the normal conduction pathway, but travels from cell to cell through the myocardium, depolarizing the ventricles asynchronously. Therefore, the ventricles are not stimulated simultaneously and the stimulus spreads through the ventricles in an aberrant manner, resulting in a wide QRS complex of 0.12 second or greater.

Since ventricular depolarization is abnormal, ventricular repolarization will also be abnormal, resulting in changes in the ST segments and T waves. The ST segments and T waves will slope in the opposite direction from the main QRS deflection (if the ectopic QRS complex is predominantly negative, the ST segment is usually elevated and the T wave positive; if the ectopic QRS complex is predominantly positive, the ST segment is usually depressed and the T wave negative). A P wave is not produced in ventricular rhythms.

Ventricular arrhythmias include premature ventricular contractions (PVCs), ventricular tachycardia (VT), ventricular fibrillation (VF), idioventricular rhythm, accelerated idioventricular rhythm, and ventricular standstill. All of these rhythms are associated with a wide QRS complex (except VF and ventricular standstill, which do not have QRS complexes). Because the ventricles are the least efficient of the heart's pacemakers, most of these rhythms are (or have the potential to be) life-threatening and demand prompt recognition and treatment.

The electrical impulse in bundle-branch block originates in the sinus node, not in ventricular tissue, but a discussion of bundle-branch block is included in this rhythm group because of the location of the block within the ventricles and the wide QRS complex.

Bundle-branch block

The intraventricular conduction system consists of the right bundle branch and the left bundle branch, which divides into two fascicles: an anterior fascicle and a posterior fascicle. Block may occur in any part of this conduction system. Normally, the electrical impulses travel through

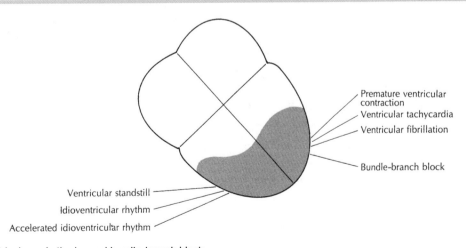

Figure 9-1. Ventricular arrhythmias and bundle-branch block.

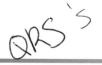

the right bundle branch and the left bundle branch and its fascicles at the same time, causing simultaneous depolarization of the right and left ventricles, resulting in normal depolarization and a QRS duration of 0.10 second or less. When one of the bundle branches is blocked, the electrical impulse travels down the intact bundle, depolarizing that ventricle first, then the impulse progresses through the interventricular septum to depolarize the other ventricle. Depolarization of one ventricle before the other is called *sequential depolarization*. Depolarization of the ventricles is delayed, resulting in a wide QRS complex of 0.12 second or greater. The presence of a bundle-branch block (Figures 9-2 through 9-4 and Box 9-1) can be recognized

Box 9-1.

Bundle-branch block: Identifying ECG features

Rhythm:	Regular
Rate:	That of the underlying rhythm (usually sinus)
P waves:	Sinus
PR interval:	Normal (0.12 to 0.20 second)
QRS complex:	Wide (0.12 second or greater)

by a monitoring lead. Differentiating between right and left bundle-branch block requires a 12-lead electrocardiogram (ECG).

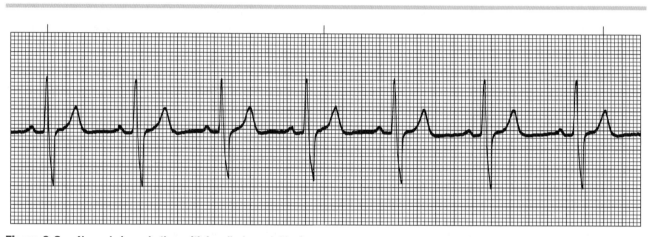

Figure 9-2. **Normal sinus rhythm with bundle-branch block.**

Rhythm:	Regular (off by 2 squares)
Rate:	60 to 65 beats/minute
P waves:	Sinus
PR interval:	0.16 to 0.20 second
QRS complex:	0.12 to 0.14 second.

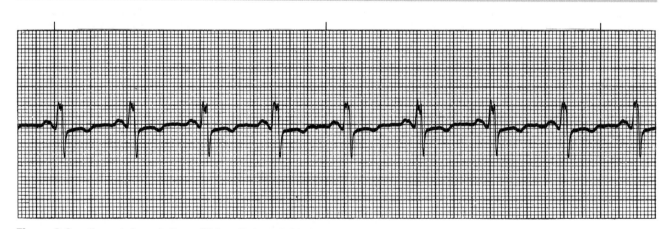

Figure 9-3. **Normal sinus rhythm with bundle-branch block.**

Rhythm:	Regular
Rate:	75 beats/minute
P waves:	Sinus P waves are notched, which could indicate left atrial enlargement.
PR interval:	0.14 to 0.16 second
QRS complex:	0.12 second
Comment:	A notched QRS complex is a common pattern with right bundle-branch block.

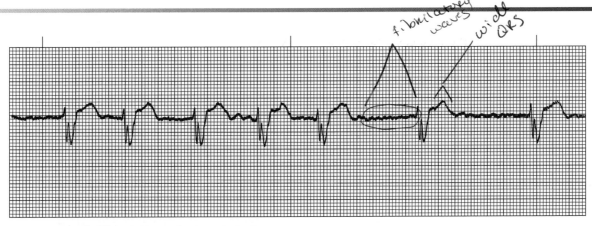

Figure 9.4.   Atrial fibrillation with bundle-branch block.
Rhythm: Irregular
Rate: 70 beats/minute
P waves: Fibrillatory waves present
PR interval: Not measurable
QRS complex: 0.14 to 0.16 second.

Right bundle-branch block (RBBB) may be present in healthy individuals with no apparent underlying heart disease, but more commonly occurs in the presence of coronary artery disease (the most common cause). RBBB may be temporary or chronic. Occasionally, RBBB may appear only when the heart rate exceeds a certain critical level (rate-related BBB). Common causes include anteroseptal myocardial infarction (MI), pulmonary embolism, congestive heart failure, pericarditis, hypertensive heart disease, cardiomyopathy, congenital RBBB, and degenerative disease of the electrical conduction system.

Left bundle-branch block (LBBB) is rarely seen in individuals with healthy hearts. It appears most commonly in elderly individuals with diseased hearts. LBBB may be temporary or chronic, and may be rate-related. The most common cause is hypertensive heart disease. Other causes are the same as with RBBB.

Specific treatment is usually not indicated for a bundle-branch block. Cardiac pacing may be indicated if the bundle-branch block develops as a result of acute MI or in the presence of AV block.

Premature ventricular contractions

A premature ventricular contraction (PVC) (Figures 9-5 through 9-14 and Box 9-2) is a premature, ectopic impulse that arises below the bundle of His in the ventricles. PVCs

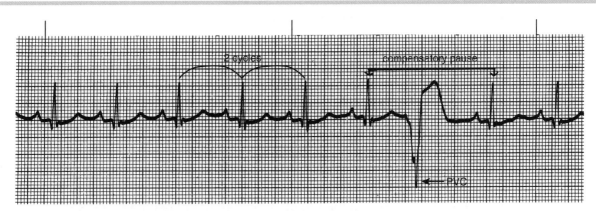

Figure 9-5.   Normal sinus rhythm with one premature ventricular contraction.
Rhythm: Basic rhythm regular; irregular with PVC
Rate: Basic rhythm rate 79 beats/minute
P waves: Sinus P waves with basic rhythm
PR interval: 0.16 to 0.20 second (basic rhythm)
QRS complex: 0.08 to 0.10 second (basic rhythm); 0.14 to 0.16 second (PVC)
Comment: The interval from the beat preceding the PVC to the beat following the PVC is equal to two cardiac cycles and represents a full compensatory pause.

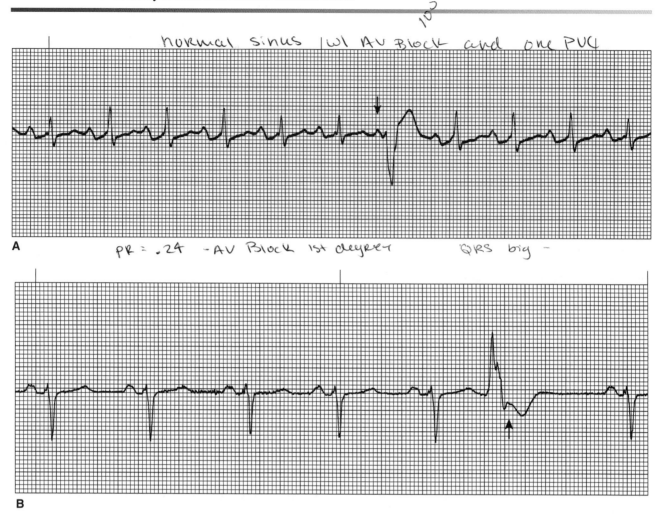

[handwritten: 100]

[handwritten: normal sinus w/ AV Block and one PVC]

A

[handwritten: PR = .24 - AV Block 1st degree   QRS big -]

[handwritten image B annotations]

B

Figure 9-6. **Sinus P waves occurring before and after premature ventricular contractions (PVCs).**
The sinus P waves of the underlying rhythm can be seen just before the PVC in example A and after the PVC in the ST segment in example B. These P waves are associated with the underlying rhythm (not the PVC) and usually are hidden within the wide QRS of the premature ventricular contraction.
Example A: Normal sinus rhythm with first-degree AV block and one PVC.
Example B: Sinus arrhythmia with bundle-branch block and one PVC.

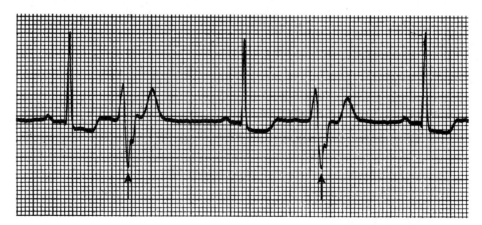

Figure 9-7. Bigeminal premature ventricular contractions.

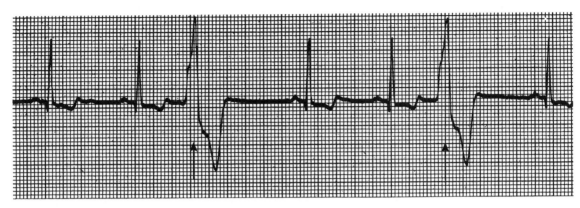

Figure 9-8.   Trigeminal premature ventricular contractions.

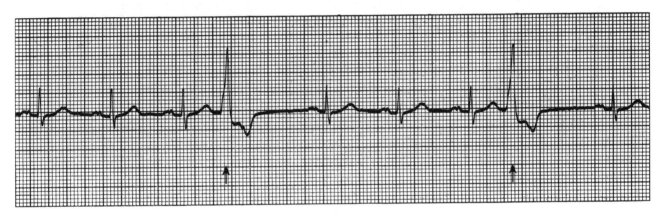

Figure 9-9.   Quadrigeminal premature ventricular contractions.

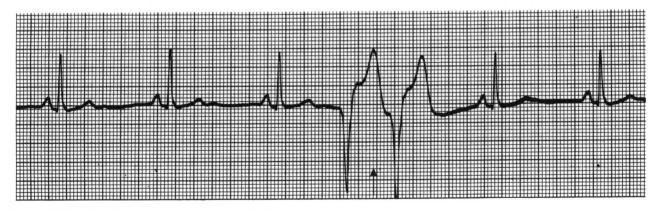

Figure 9-10.   Paired premature ventricular contractions.

occur as a result of reentry in the ventricles, enhanced automaticity of a focus in the ventricles, or triggered activity occurring during ventricular repolarization. PVCs have the following characteristics:

■ The QRS is premature.

■ A P wave isn't associated with the PVC. Normally the P wave of the underlying rhythm (usually sinus) is obscured within the PVC, but sometimes it appears just before or after the PVC in the ST segment or T wave (see Figure 9-6).

■ The QRS is wide (0.12 second or greater) and the morphology is different from the QRS complexes of the underlying rhythm.

■ The ST segment and T wave slope in the opposite direction from the main QRS deflection (if the ectopic QRS complex is predominantly negative, the ST segment is usually elevated and the T waves positive; if the ectopic QRS complex is predominantly positive, the ST segment is usually depressed and the T wave negative).

- The pause associated with the PVC is usually compensatory (the measurement from the beat before the PVC to the beat after the PVC is equal to two R-R intervals of the underlying rhythm, Figure 9-5). The underlying rhythm must be regular to determine a compensatory pause.

PVCs may occur in various patterns. They may appear as a single beat (Figure 9-5), every other beat (bigeminal pattern, Figure 9-7), every third beat (trigeminal pattern, Figure 9-8), every fourth beat (quadrigeminal pattern, Figure 9-9), in pairs (also called couplets, Figure 9-10), or in runs (Figure 9-11). A run of three or more consecutive PVCs constitutes a rhythm. The rate will determine which rhythm is present (idioventricular rhythm, accelerated idioventricular rhythm, or VT).

PVCs that look the same in the same lead are called *unifocal PVCs*. These PVCs originate from a single ectopic focus in the ventricles. PVCs that appear different from one another in the same lead are called *multifocal PVCs* (Figure 9-12). These PVCs usually originate from different ectopic sites, but sometimes may fire from a single site and are

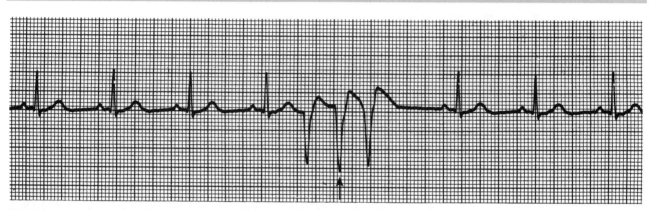

Figure 9-11.   Run of premature ventricular contractions (a burst of ventricular tachycardia).

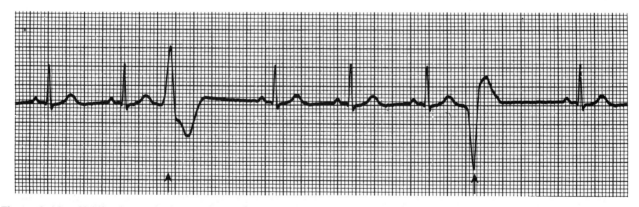

Figure 9-12.   Multifocal premature ventricular contractions.

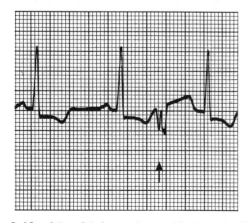

Figure 9-13.   Interpolated premature ventricular contraction.

Box 9-2.
Premature ventricular contraction (PVC): Identifying ECG features

Rhythm:	Underlying rhythm usually regular; irregular with PVC
Rate:	That of underlying rhythm (usually sinus)
P waves:	None associated with PVC; P waves associated with the underlying sinus rhythm can occasionally be seen just before the PVC or after the PVC in the ST segment or T wave; usually these P waves are hidden in the QRS complex
PR interval:	Not measurable
QRS complex:	Premature QRS complex; wide (0.12 second or greater)

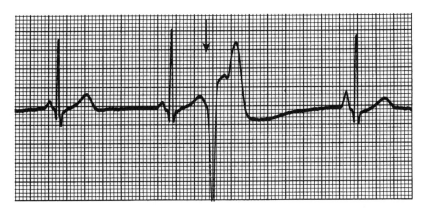

Figure 9-14. R-on-T premature ventricular contraction.

conducted along different routes in the ventricles, resulting in a QRS that differs in morphology in the same lead.

A PVC sandwiched between two normally conducted sinus beats, without greatly disturbing the regularity of the underlying rhythm, is called an *interpolated PVC* (Figure 9-13). The compensatory pause, usually associated with the PVC, is absent.

R-on-T PVC (Figure 9-14) is a term used to describe a PVC which falls on the down slope of the preceding T wave. This period corresponds to the relative refractory period of ventricular repolarization when the myocardium is in its most vulnerable state electrically. During this period, the myocardial cells have repolarized enough to respond to a strong stimulus. Stimulation of the ventricle at this time may precipitate repetitive ventricular contractions, resulting in VT or fibrillation.

PVCs are among the most commonly seen arrhythmias. PVCs may occur in individuals with a healthy heart, but are more common in people with coronary heart disease. PVCs are commonly caused by an increase in sympathetic tone from emotional stress; ingestion of substances such as alcohol, caffeine, or tobacco; mitral valve prolapse, myocardial ischemia or infarction; cardiomyopathy; congestive heart failure; hypoxia; electrolyte imbalances (especially hypokalemia); drug effects (digitalis, epinephrine, norepinephrine); as a reperfusion arrhythmia after thrombolytic therapy or

angioplasty; or following insertion of invasive catheters into the heart, such as pacing leads or a pulmonary artery catheter.

Treatment of PVCs depends on the cause, the patient's symptoms, and the clinical setting. Because occasional PVCs are a normal finding in healthy individuals, no treatment may be indicated, especially if the person is asymptomatic. Initially, a search should be made for possible reversible causes (such as oxygen for hypoxia; replacement of electrolytes; diuretics for heart failure; elimination of certain drugs; avoidance of alcohol, caffeine, or tobacco; and administration of antianxiety medication if indicated). Significant PVCs (more than 6 per minute, multifocal PVCs, paired PVCs, R-on-T PVCs, or PVCs in runs of 3 or more) should be treated with an antiarrhythmic medication, especially in the setting of acute MI or following cardiac surgery because of the increased risk of VT and VF in this setting.

On some occasions a ventricular beat may occur late instead of early. A late ectopic ventricular beat usually occurs after a pause in the underlying rhythm in which the dominant pacemaker (usually the sinus node) fails to initiate an impulse. If the ventricles are not activated by the sinus node, atria, or AV junction within a certain period of time, a focus in the ventricles may "escape" and pace the heart. These are called *ventricular escape beats* (Figure 9-15). The ventricular escape beat is a protective mechanism, protecting the heart from slow rates, and no treatment is required.

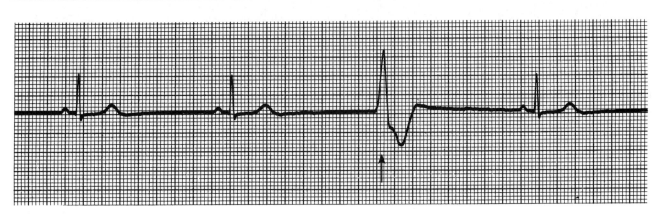

Figure 9-15. Ventricular escape beat.

Ventricular tachycardia

Ventricular tachycardia (VT) (Figures 9-16 through 9-20 and Box 9-3) is an arrhythmia originating in an ectopic focus in the ventricles discharging impulses at a rate of 140 to 250 beats per minute. VT is most likely due to reentry in the ventricles, but can also be caused by enhanced automaticity of a focus in the ventricles or to triggered activity occurring during ventricular repolarization. VT occurs as a series of wide QRS complexes seen in short runs or as a continuous rhythm. Because of the ventricular origin of the impulse, no P waves are produced. The rhythm is usually regular, but may be slightly irregular. The

Ventricular tachycardia (VT): Identifying ECG features

Rhythm:	Regular; can be slightly irregular
Rate:	140 to 250 beats/minute
P waves:	No P waves are associated with VT.
PR interval:	Not measurable
QRS complex:	Wide (0.12 second or greater)

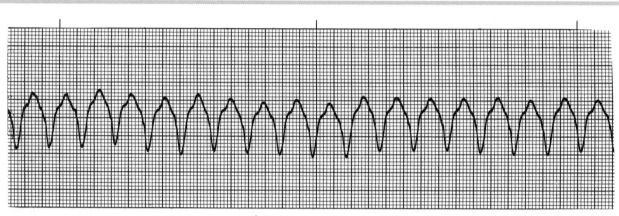

Figure 9-16.   Ventricular tachycardia.

Rhythm:	Regular
Rate:	150 beats/minute
P waves:	None identified
PR interval:	Not measurable
QRS complex:	0.14 to 0.16 second.

pulseless
or pulse

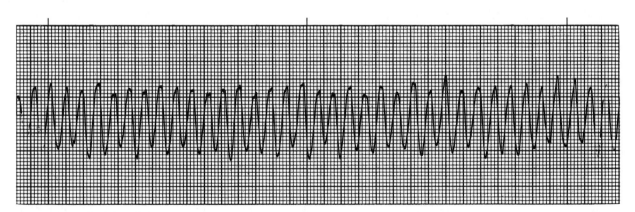

Figure 9-17.   Ventricular flutter.

Rhythm:	Regular
Rate:	375 beats/minute
P waves:	Not seen
PR interval:	Not measurable
QRS complex:	0.12 to 0.14 second
Comment:	Ventricular flutter is a form of ventricular tachycardia. The ventricular rate is so fast the QRS complexes have a sawtooth appearance.

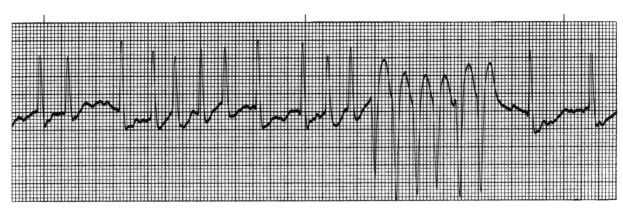

Figure 9-18. Atrial fibrillation with a burst of ventricular tachycardia (VT).

Rhythm:	Basic rhythm irregular; VT regular
Rate:	160 beats/minute (basic rhythm); 250 beats/minute (VT)
P waves:	Fibrillation waves in basic rhythm; none with VT
PR interval:	Not measurable
QRS complex:	0.08 to 0.10 second (basic rhythm); 0.12 second (VT).

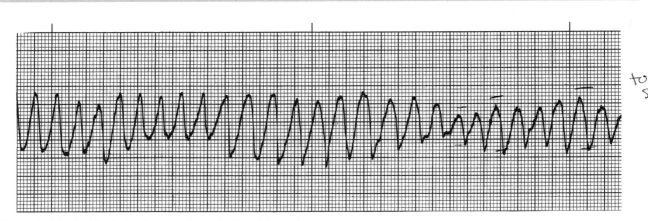

Figure 9-19. Ventricular tachycardia (torsade de pointes).

Rhythm:	Regular
Rate:	250 beats/minute
P waves:	None identified
PR interval:	Not measurable
QRS complex:	0.12 to 0.22 second (some much wider than others)
Comment:	This type of ventricular tachycardia is called *torsade de pointes* (twisting of the points). The QRS changes from negative to positive polarity and appears to twist around the isoelectric line. It is associated with a prolonged QT interval and is refractory to antiarrhythmics. IV magnesium or overdrive pacing has been successful in the treatment of this rhythm.

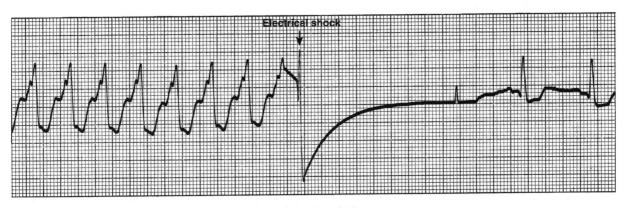

Figure 9-20. Electrical cardioversion of ventricular tachycardia to sinus rhythm.

ST segment and T wave slope in the opposite direction from the main QRS deflection. When the QRS complexes are of the same morphology in the same lead, the rhythm is termed *monomorphic VT*. When the QRS complexes differ in morphology in the same lead, the VT is called *polymorphic VT*.

VT may occasionally occur at rates greater than 250 beats/minute. At such extreme rates the QRS complexes appear sawtooth in appearance and the rhythm is commonly referred to as *ventricular flutter* (Figure 9-17). Ventricular flutter is so rapid that there is virtually no cardiac output. Ventricular flutter is often a precursor to ventricular fibrillation.

VT usually occurs in patients with underlying heart disease. It may be preceded by significant PVCs (more than 6 per minute, paired PVCs, multifocal PVCs), but often occurs without preexisting or precipitating PVCs. The most common cause of sustained VT is coronary artery disease with prior MI. Other causes include myocardial ischemia, acute MI, cardiomyopathy, congestive heart failure, mitral valve prolapse, valvular heart disease, digitalis toxicity, electrolyte imbalances (especially hypokalemia and hypomagnesemia), myocardial contusion, mechanical stimulation of the endocardium by a pacing catheter or pulmonary artery catheter, as an effect of reperfusion following thrombolytic therapy or angioplasty, and drugs that increase sympathetic tone (epinephrine, norepinephrine, dopamine). Certain medications or conditions may prolong the QT interval, causing the ventricles to be particularly vulnerable to a type of polymorphic VT called torsade de pointes (Figure 9-19).

When VT lasts for less than 30 seconds it is called nonsustained VT. VT occurring in short runs of three or more consecutive PVCs at a rate of 140 to 250 beats per minute is considered a "run" or "burst" of nonsustained VT (Figures 9-11 and 9-18). Nonsustained VT, unless frequent, usually doesn't cause symptoms, but it can progress into sustained VT. When VT lasts longer than 30 seconds, it is considered sustained VT. Sustained VT is a life threatening arrhythmia for two major reasons:
1. The rapid ventricular rate and loss of atrial kick reduce cardiac output. This reduction in cardiac output often compounds the already low cardiac output frequently seen in the diseased hearts in which VT tends to occur.
2. The rhythm may degenerate into VF or asystole.

Treatment is based on the patient's presentation. An "unstable" patient refers to an individual who presents with symptoms such as hypotension, chest pain, shortness of breath, signs of decreased perfusion (cool, clammy skin; peripheral cyanosis; decreased level of consciousness; or a decrease in urine output). A "stable" patient refers to an individual with normal blood pressure, no chest pain, and no shortness of breath or signs of decreased perfusion. As part of the initial assessment you should check for a pulse. If there is not a pulse (pulseless VT), the rhythm must be treated as VF. If there is a pulse, protocols for *stable VT* and *unstable VT* are followed.

Treatment protocols: Stable monomorphic VT with pulse

■ Amiodarone (150 mg in 100 mL D_5W) is given as an intravenous piggy-back (IVPB) bolus over 10 minutes. An additional 150 mg IVPB bolus dose can be repeated in 10 minutes for resistant VT. Once the rhythm converts to a stable rhythm, an amiodarone maintenance infusion should be started to prevent reoccurrence of VT. The amiodarone maintenance infusion (900 mg in 500 mL D_5W in a glass bottle) is started at 1 mg per minute for 6 hours, then decreased to 0.5 mg per minute for 18 hours. The total dose of amiodarone (IVPB bolus doses plus maintenance infusion) should not exceed 2.2 g in 24 hours. Oral amiodarone can be started once the maintenance infusion is completed. Elimination of the drug from the body is extremely long (half-life lasts up to 40 days).
■ If the rhythm is unresponsive to amiodarone, sedate the patient and perform synchronized cardioversion beginning at 100 joules biphasic energy dose, increasing in a stepwise fashion with subsequent attempts.

Some physicians prefer to skip drug therapy and go directly to synchronized cardioversion. Figure 9-20 shows cardioversion of VT to sinus rhythm.

Treatment protocols: Unstable monomorphic VT with pulse

■ Sedate the patient (if conscious).
■ Convert the rhythm using synchronized cardioversion beginning at 100 joules biphasic energy dose, increasing in stepwise fashion with subsequent attempts. Once cardioversion has converted the rhythm, a maintenance infusion of amiodarone is usually started at 1 mg per minute for 6 hours, then decreased to 0.5 mg per minute for 18 hours, followed by oral amiodarone once the maintenance infusion is completed.

Treatment of chronic, recurrent VT usually includes therapy with an oral antiarrhythmic. Patients who are refractory to a pharmacologic approach may require further evaluation, which could include specialized electrophysiologic testing and endocardial mapping with long-term options including the use of an implantable cardioverter defibrillator (ICD) or reentry circuit ablation. The ICD is a surgically implanted device developed to deliver an electric shock directly to the heart during a life-threatening tachycardia. Ablation (destruction) of the reentry circuit involves delivering short pulses of radiofrequency current through an intracardiac catheter. It produces a small burn that effectively blocks the part of the circuit supporting the reentrant-type wave.

Torsade de pointes ventricular tachycardia

Torsade de pointes (TdP) (Figure 9-19) is a form of polymorphic VT. This name is derived from a French term meaning "twisting of the points," which describes a QRS complex that changes polarity (from negative to positive and positive to negative) as it twists around the isoelectric line. TdP is an intermediary arrhythmia between VT and VF.

TdP typically occurs when the QT interval of the underlying rhythm is abnormally prolonged, usually 0.5 second or greater. A prolonged QT interval or long QT syndrome (LQTS) is an abnormality of the heart's electrical system. Although the mechanical function of the heart is entirely normal, the electrical problem is thought to be caused by changes in the cardiac ion channels that affect repolarization, causing a lengthened relative refractory period (vulnerable period) that puts the ventricles at risk for TdP and may result in sudden death.

Some causes of TdP VT include bradyarrhythmias (marked sinus bradycardia, third-degree AV block with a slow ventricular response); excessive administration of antiarrhythmics (quinidine, procainamide, disopyramide, amiodarone, sotalol); phenothiazines (prochlorperazine, chloropromazine, thioridazine); psychotropic medications (haloperidol, amitriptyline); electrolyte imbalances (especially hypokalemia, hypomagnesemia, hypocalcemia); liquid protein diets; central nervous system disorders (subarachnoid hemorrhage or intracranial trauma); and congenital LQTS.

The ventricular rate in TdP VT is extremely rapid and the patient usually becomes unstable very quickly. Recognition of TdP is critical not only because of the rapid deterioration of the patient but also because the treatment plan differs greatly from the treatment of monomorphic VT. Amiodarone, a drug used in treating monomorphic VT, can prolong the QT interval and make matters worse in this situation.

Treatment protocols: TdP VT

■ The initial treatment should be immediate unsynchronized shock at 200 joules biphasic energy dose. Due to the variability in the QRS complexes in TdP, it might be difficult or impossible to reliably synchronize to a QRS complex. Although TdP is responsive to electrical therapy, the rhythm has a tendency to recur unless the precipitating factors are eliminated.

■ Magnesium is the pharmacologic treatment of choice for TdP VT. Magnesium is usually very effective even in patients with normal magnesium levels. Magnesium acts as an antiarrhythmic and may terminate or prevent recurrent episodes of TdP. Give a loading dose of 1 to 2 g IV diluted in 10 mL D_5W slowly over 5 minutes. This is followed by a 0.5 to 1 g/hour IV drip. A side effect of magnesium is hypotension, especially if administered rapidly. Magnesium also reduces neuromuscular tone and close monitoring of deep tendon reflexes is suggested.

■ Potassium chloride (like magnesium) is a first-line therapy for TdP. Potassium is essential for maintenance of intracellular tonicity; transmission of nerve impulses; contraction of cardiac, skeletal, and smooth muscles; and maintenance of normal renal function. Depletion usually

results from diuretic therapy, diabetic ketoacidosis, severe diarrhea, or inadequate replacement during prolonged parenteral nutrition therapy. Dosage of potassium depends on the serum potassium level, hospital protocols, and physician orders.

■ Removing or correcting precipitating factors:
1. Bradycardia-induced—Discontinue drugs that decrease heart rate; overdrive pacing or isoproterenol infusion may be used to increase heart rate.
2. Drug-induced — Discontinue drugs that prolong QT interval.
3. Electrolyte-induced — Correct electrolyte abnormalities; magnesium and potassium are considered first-line therapy.

In treatment of congenital prolonged QT syndrome or recurrent TdP VT, an implantable defibrillator ICD can be used as prophylaxis.

Ventricular fibrillation

In ventricular fibrillation (VF) (Figures 9-21 and 9-22 and Box 9-4) a disorganized, chaotic, electrical focus in the ventricles takes over control of the heart. Organized ventricular depolarization and contraction do not occur (there is no QRS complex), but instead the ventricular muscle quivers and is often described as resembling a "bag of worms." The ECG in VF shows characteristic fibrillatory waves that vary in shape and amplitude in an irregular and chaotic pattern.

VF with large amplitude waves is called *coarse VF* (Figure 9-21). If the VF waves are small, the rhythm is called *fine VF* (Figure 9-22). Coarse VF waves are generally more irregular than fine VF waves. Fine VF may resemble ventricular asystole and should be confirmed by examining the rhythm in different leads. The distinction between fine VF and coarse VF is significant because coarse VF usually indicates a more recent onset and is more likely to be reversed by early defibrillation. Fine VF usually indicates that the rhythm has been present longer and may require drug therapy and cardiopulmonary resuscitation (CPR) before defibrillation can be effective. Fine VF will progress to asystole unless the rhythm is treated.

Box 9-4.
Ventricular fibrillation (VF): Identifying ECG features

Rhythm:	None (P wave and QRS complex are absent)
Rate:	None (P wave and QRS complex are absent)
P waves:	Absent; wavy, irregular deflections seen, varying in size, shape, and height and representative of quivering of the ventricles instead of contraction; deflections may be small (described as *fine VF*) or large (described as coarse *VF*)
PR interval:	Not measurable
QRS complex:	Absent

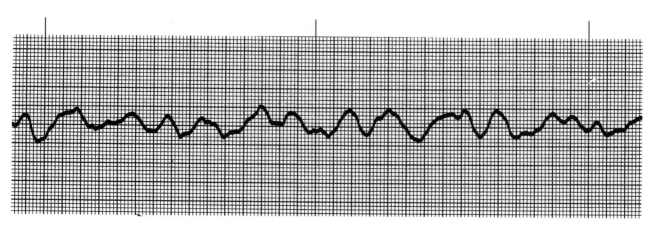

Figure 9-21. Ventricular fibrillation (coarse waveforms).
Rhythm: Chaotic
Rate: 0 beats/minute (no QRS complexes are present)
P waves: None; wave deflections are chaotic and vary in size, shape, and height
PR interval: Not measurable
QRS complex: Absent.

VF is the most common cause of cardiac death in patients with acute MI. Other causes include myocardial ischemia, hypoxia, cardiomyopathy, electrolyte imbalances (especially hypokalemia and hypomagnesemia), digitalis toxicity, excessive doses of antiarrhythmics, cardiac trauma, and mitral valve prolapse. VF may be preceded by significant PVCs or VT, but it may also occur spontaneously without precipitating rhythms. VF may also occur during anesthesia, cardiac catheterization procedures, pacemaker implantation, placement of a pulmonary artery catheter, or after accidental electrocution.

Once VF occurs there is no cardiac output, peripheral pulses and blood pressure are absent, and the patient becomes unconscious immediately. Cyanosis and seizure activity may also be present. Death is imminent unless the rhythm is treated immediately.

Treatment protocols: VF

■ Check the pulse and rapidly assess the patient. If there is a pulse and the patient is conscious, VF isn't the problem. ECG artifacts produced by loose or dry electrodes, patient movement, or muscle tremors may resemble VF.

■ If there is no pulse and the patient is unconscious, defibrillate at 200 joules biphasic energy dose. If the arrest is unwitnessed, perform CPR for 5 cycles (2 minutes) before the initial shock.

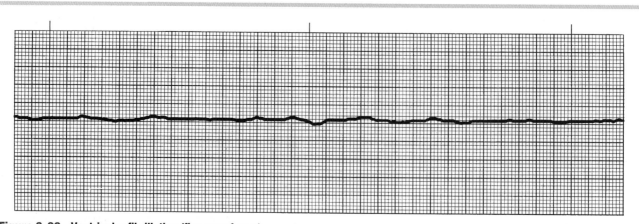

Figure 9-22. Ventricular fibrillation (fine waveforms).
Rhythm: Chaotic
Rate: 0 beats/minute (no QRS complexes are present)
P waves: Absent; wave deflections are chaotic and vary in size, shape, and height
PR interval: Not measurable
QRS complex: Absent.

■ If unsuccessful, start CPR, establish an IV line, and ventilate the patient. Intubate the patient when possible.

■ Administer epinephrine 1 mg IV push and repeat every 3 to 5 minutes. Vasopressin 40 units IV push may be given × 1 dose to replace 1st or 2nd dose epinephrine.

■ Continue CPR for 5 cycles to circulate drug; defibrillate at 360 joules × 1.

■ Consider **one** of the following antiarrhythmics:

1. Amiodarone 300 mg IV push (dilution in 20 mL D₅W is recommended); if VF is refractory or recurs, consider one additional dose of 150 mg IV push in 3 to 5 minutes (dilution in 20 mL D₅W is recommended). If drug therapy is successful, a maintenance infusion of amiodarone can be started at 1 mg per minute for 6 hours followed by 0.5 mg per minute for 18 hours (total dose of IV push and maintenance infusion should not exceed 2.2 g/24 hours). Oral amiodarone can be started following completion of the IV infusion.

2. Lidocaine 1 to 1.5 mg/kg IV push followed by half the initial dose (0.5 to 0.75 mg/kg IV push) every 5 to 10 minutes to a maximum dose of 3 mg/kg. If drug therapy is successful, a maintenance infusion of lidocaine can be started at 1 to 4 mg/minute. The half-life of lidocaine increases after 24 to 48 hours. Therefore, after 24 hours the dosage should be reduced or blood levels monitored. Signs of toxicity include slurred speech, altered consciousness, muscle twitching, seizures, and bradycardia.

Note: All antiarrhythmics have some degree of *proarrhythmic* effects (may induce or worsen ventricular arrhythmias). Use of more than one antiarrhythmic compounds the adverse effects, particularly for bradycardia, hypotension, and TdP. Never use more than one agent unless absolutely necessary.

■ Continue drug therapy, CPR, and defibrillation attempts (drug-CPR-shock pattern) until rhythm resolves or a decision is made to stop resuscitative efforts.

Idioventricular rhythm

Idioventricular rhythm (IVR) (Figure 9-23 and Box 9-5) is a very slow rhythm originating from a focus in the ventricles at a rate of 30 to 40 beats per minutes (sometimes less). Because the impulse originates in the ventricles, there is no P wave and the QRS complex is wide. The rhythm is usually regular. IVR is the normal rhythm of the ventricles.

IVR can occur under either of the following conditions:

■ The heart rate of the dominant pacemaker (usually the sinus node) and the backup pacemaker (usually the AV junction) becomes less than the heart rate of the ventricles.

■ The electrical impulses from the sinus node, the atria, or the AV junction fail to reach the ventricles because of sinus arrest, sinus exit block, or third-degree AV block.

If the ventricles are not activated by the sinus node, the atria, or the AV junction, a focus in the ventricles can "escape" and pace the ventricles. For this reason, IVR is also called ventricular escape rhythm. IVR may occur in short runs of 3 or more consecutive ventricular beats at a rate of 30 to 40 beats per minute and is usually related to increased vagal effect on the higher pacing centers controlling the heart rhythm. Treatment is usually unnecessary. Continuous IVR usually occurs in advanced heart disease and is commonly

Box 9-5.
Idioventricular rhythm: Identifying ECG features

Rhythm:	Regular
Rate:	30 to 40 beats/minute (sometimes less)
P waves:	Absent
PR interval:	Not measurable
QRS complex:	Wide (0.12 second or greater)

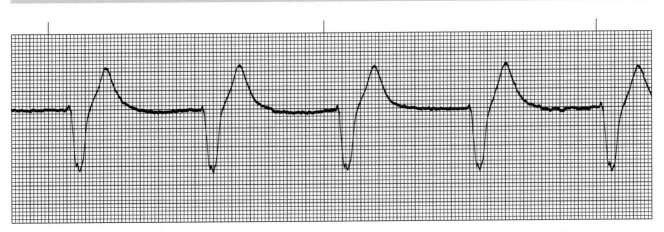

Figure 9-23. Idioventricular rhythm.

Rhythm:	Regular
Rate:	41 beats/minute
P waves:	Absent
PR interval:	Not measurable
QRS complex:	0.22 to 0.24 second.

last fires before asystole

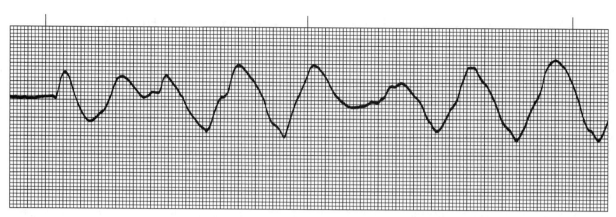

Figure 9-24.   Agonal rhythm, sometimes called "dying heart."

the cardiac rhythm present just before the appearance of the final rhythm, ventricular standstill (asystole). Continuous IVR is generally symptomatic due to the slow rate and the loss of the atrial kick. The rhythm must be treated promptly following the protocols for significant bradycardia (atropine, pacing, and vasopressors to increase blood pressure).

If the rate of IVR falls below 20 beats per minute and the QRS complexes deteriorate into irregular, wide, indistinguishable waveforms, the rhythm is commonly referred to as an *agonal rhythm* or "dying heart"(Figure 9-24). Treatment is usually ineffective at this point.

Accelerated idioventricular rhythm

Accelerated idioventricular rhythm (AIVR) (Figures 9-25 and 9-26 and Box 9-6) originates in an ectopic pacemaker site in the ventricles with a rate between 50 and 100 beats per minute. The term *accelerated* denotes a rhythm that exceeds the inherent idioventricular escape rate of 30 to 40

beats per minute, but isn't fast enough to be VT. AIVR has the same ECG characteristics as IVR (no P waves, wide QRS complex, regular rhythm), but is differentiated by the heart rate. AIVR can occur as a continuous rhythm (Figure 9-25) or in short runs of 3 or more consecutive ventricular beats at a rate of 50 to 100 beats per minute (Figure 9-26).

AIVR is common after acute inferior-wall MI and is frequently a reperfusion rhythm following thrombolytic therapy, angioplasty, or spontaneous reperfusion. AIVR may also be seen with digitalis toxicity.

AIVR is usually well tolerated and is rarely associated with symptoms. If the patient is symptomatic, it is usually related to a decrease in cardiac output from a loss of the atrial kick and not because of the heart rate, which is within a normal range.

Treatment of AIVR with antiarrhythmics is not recommended. Abolishing the ventricular focus may lead to a less desirable rate and rhythm. This rhythm is usually transient, requires no specific therapy, and spontaneously

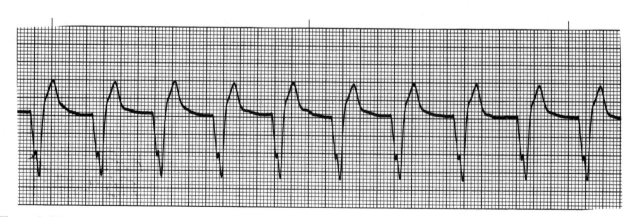

Figure 9-25. Accelerated idioventricular rhythm.

Rhythm:	Regular
Rate:	84 beats/minute
P waves:	None identified
PR interval:	Not measurable
QRS complex:	0.16 second.

episode

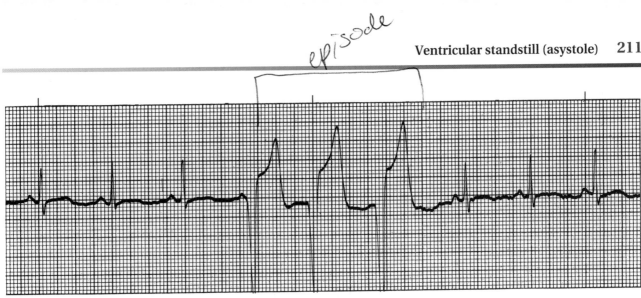

Figure 9-26. Normal sinus rhythm with episode of accelerated idioventricular rhythm (AIVR).
Rhythm: Basic rhythm regular; AIVR basically regular (off by 2 squares)
Rate: 79 beats/minute basic rhythm; around 80 beats/minute AIVR rate
P waves: Sinus P waves with basic rhythm; none with AIVR
PR interval: 0.12 to 0.16 second
QRS complex: 0.06 to 0.08 second (basic rhythm); 0.12 second (AIVR).

Box 9-6.
Accelerated idioventricular rhythm: Identifying ECG features

Rhythm: Regular
Rate: 50 to 100 beats/minute
P waves: Absent
PR interval: Not measurable
QRS complex: Wide (0.12 second or greater)

resolves on its own. A "tincture of time" is most often the best remedy.

Ventricular standstill (asystole)

Ventricular standstill (Figures 9-27 and 9-28 and Box 9-7) is the absence of all electrical activity in the ventricles. When the ventricles are inactive, there are no QRS complexes. The atria, however, may continue to generate electrical activity, producing P waves. Thus, ventricular standstill has two presentations on the ECG tracing: P waves without QRS complexes (Figure 9-27) or a straight line (Figure 9-28).

If P waves are present, some form of advanced heart block (Mobitz II second-degree AV block or third-degree AV block) may have preceded the arrhythmia. Ventricular standstill with a straight line usually occurs following such arrhythmias as VT, VF, IVR, and pulseless electrical activity. Asystole may also occur following termination of a tachyarrhythmia by medications, defibrillation, or cardioversion. Occasionally, ventricular standstill may occur without an obvious precipitating cause. In Figure 9-27, asystole occurred during the pause following a PAC.

Conditions contributing to the development of ventricular standstill include extensive myocardial damage (from

ischemia or infarction), hypoxia, hyperkalemia, hypokalemia, hypothermia, drug overdose, and advanced heart block. Cardiac trauma may also be a contributing factor.

Once ventricular standstill occurs, there is no cardiac output, peripheral pulses and blood pressure are absent, and the patient becomes unconscious immediately. Cyanosis and seizure activity may also be present. Death is imminent unless the arrhythmia is treated immediately. Without cardiac monitoring, ventricular standstill cannot be distinguished from VF at the bedside.

Treatment protocols: Ventricular standstill (asystole)

■ Check pulse and rapidly assess the patient. If there is a pulse and the patient is conscious, ventricular standstill is not the problem.
■ Check monitor lead system (a loose electrode pad or lead wire will show a straight line).
■ Check rhythm in two leads (low amplitude QRS complexes may look like P waves; fine VF may look like a straight line).
■ Start CPR, establish an IV line, and ventilate the patient. Intubate the patient when possible.
■ Give epinephrine 1 mg IV push and repeat every 3 to 5 minutes. Vasopressin 40 units IV push may be given

Box 9-7.
Ventricular standstill: Identifying ECG features

Rhythm: Atrial: If P waves present, will have atrial rhythm
                Ventricular: None
Rate: Atrial: If P waves present, will have atrial rate
                Ventricular: None
P waves: ECG tracings will show either P waves without a QRS complex or a straight line
PR interval: Not measurable
QRS complex: Absent

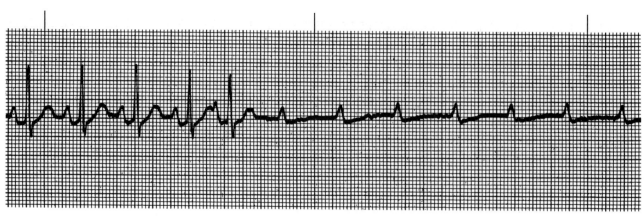

Figure 9-27. Normal sinus rhythm with one premature atrial contraction changing to ventricular standstill.
Rhythm: Basic rhythm regular
Rate: Basic rhythm 100 beats/minute
P waves: Sinus P waves are present
PR interval: 0.16 to 0.18 second (basic rhythm)
QRS complex: 0.06 second (basic rhythm).

× 1 dose to replace first or second dose epinephrine. Continue CPR to circulate the drug.

■ Consider possible causes of the rhythm:
1) Pulmonary embolism
2) Acidosis
3) Tension pneumothorax
4) Cardiac tamponade
5) Hypovolemia (most common cause)
6) Hypoxia
7) Hypothermia or hyperthermia
8) Hypokalemia or hyperkalemia
9) MI
10) Drug overdose

■ Continue administering epinephrine and performing CPR until the rhythm is resolved or a decision is made to discontinue resuscitative efforts.

Prognosis is extremely poor despite resuscitative efforts. The only hope for resuscitation of a person in asystole is to identify and treat a reversible cause. With asystole refractory to treatment, the patient is making the transition from life to death. Medical personnel should try to make that transition as sensitive and dignified as possible.

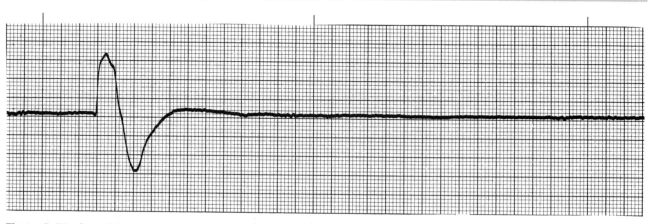

Figure 9-28. One wide ventricular complex changing to ventricular standstill.
Rhythm: 0 beats/minute
Rate: 0 beats/minute
P waves: None identified
PR interval: Not measurable
QRS complex: 0.28 second or wider.

Pulseless electrical activity (PEA)

Pulseless electrical activity (PEA) is a clinical situation (not a specific arrhythmia) in which an organized cardiac rhythm (excluding pulseless VT) is observed on the monitor, but no pulse is palpated. Causes and treatment of PEA are the same as asystole. PEA has a poor prognosis unless the underlying cause can be quickly identified and managed appropriately.

A summary of the identifying ECG features of ventricular arrhythmias and bundle-branch block can be found in Table 9-1.

Table 9-1.

Ventricular arrhythmias and bundle-branch block: Summary of identifying ECG features

Name	Rhythm	Rate (beats/minute)	P waves (lead II)	PR interval	QRS complex
Bundle-branch block	Regular	That of underlying rhythm (usually sinus)	Sinus origin	Normal (0.12 – 0.20 second)	Wide (0.12 second or greater)
Premature ventricular contraction (PVC)	Basic rhythm usually regular; irregular with PVC	That of underlying rhythm (usually sinus)	None associated with PVC; P waves associated with underlying sinus rhythm can sometimes be seen just before PVC or after PVC in ST segment or T wave, but these waves are usually hidden within PVC	Not measurable	Premature QRS complex; abnormal shape; wide (0.12 second or greater)
Ventricular tachycardia (VT)	Regular (can be slightly irregular)	140 to 250	None associated with VT	Not measurable	Wide (0.12 second or greater)
Ventricular fibrillation (VF)	None (P wave and QRS complex are absent)	None (P wave and QRS complex are absent)	Absent; wavy, irregular deflections seen in various sizes, shapes, and heights, representative of ventricular quivering instead of contraction; deflections may be small (described as *fine VF*) or large (described as *coarse VF*)	Not measurable	Absent
Idioventricular rhythm (IVR)	Regular	30 to 40 (sometimes less)	Absent	Not measurable	Wide (0.12 second or greater)
Accelerated IVR	Regular	50 to 100	Absent	Not measurable	Wide (0.12 second or greater)
Ventricular standstill (ventricular asystole)	Atrial: if P waves present, will have atrial rhythm Ventricular: None	Atrial: if P waves present, will have atrial rate Ventricular: None	Tracing will show either P waves without a QRS complex or a straight line	Not measurable	Absent

Rhythm strip practice: Ventricular arrhythmias and bundle-branch block

Analyze the following rhythm strips by following the five basic steps:
- Determine *rhythm regularity*.
- Calculate *heart rate*. (This usually refers to the ventricular rate, but if atrial rate differs you need to calculate both.)
- Identify and examine *P waves*.
- Measure *PR interval*.
- Measure *QRS complex*.

Interpret the rhythm by comparing this data with the ECG characteristics for each rhythm. All rhythm strips are lead II, a positive lead, unless otherwise noted. Check your answers with the answer keys in the appendix.

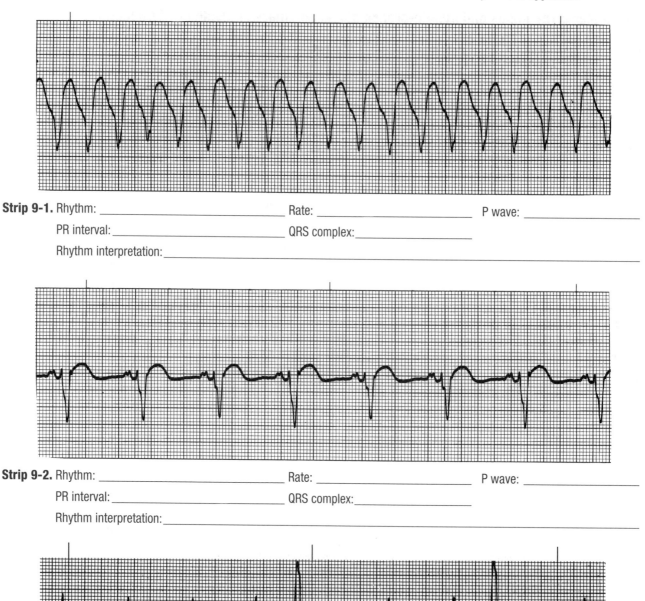

Strip 9-1. Rhythm: _____ Rate: _____ P wave: _____

PR interval: _____ QRS complex: _____

Rhythm interpretation: _____

Strip 9-2. Rhythm: _____ Rate: _____ P wave: _____

PR interval: _____ QRS complex: _____

Rhythm interpretation: _____

Strip 9-3. Rhythm: _____ Rate: _____ P wave: _____

PR interval: _____ QRS complex: _____

Rhythm interpretation: _____

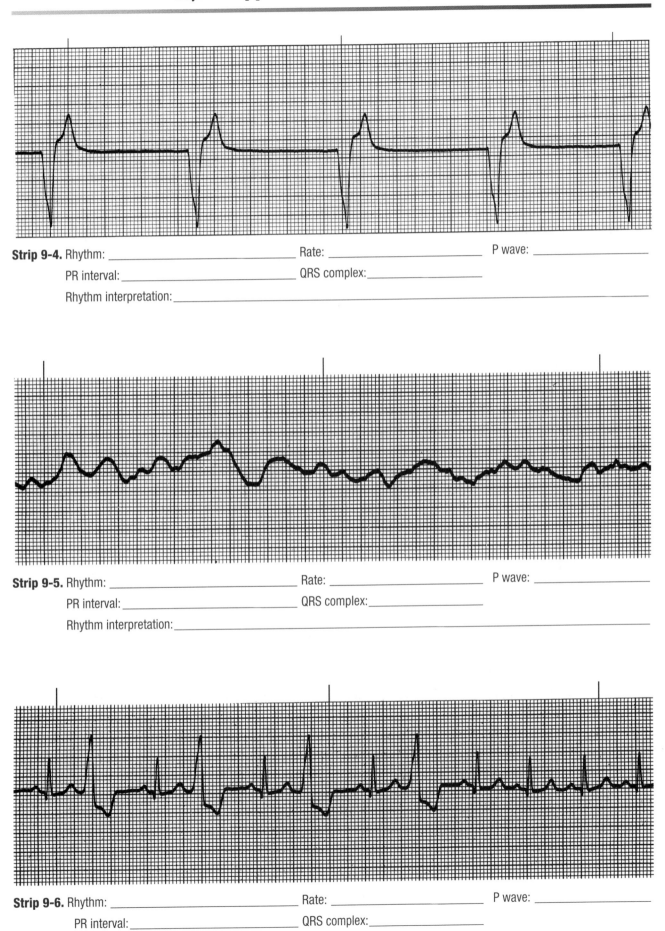

Strip 9-4. Rhythm: _____ Rate: _____ P wave: _____

PR interval: _____ QRS complex: _____

Rhythm interpretation: _____

Strip 9-5. Rhythm: _____ Rate: _____ P wave: _____

PR interval: _____ QRS complex: _____

Rhythm interpretation: _____

Strip 9-6. Rhythm: _____ Rate: _____ P wave: _____

PR interval: _____ QRS complex: _____

Rhythm interpretation: _____

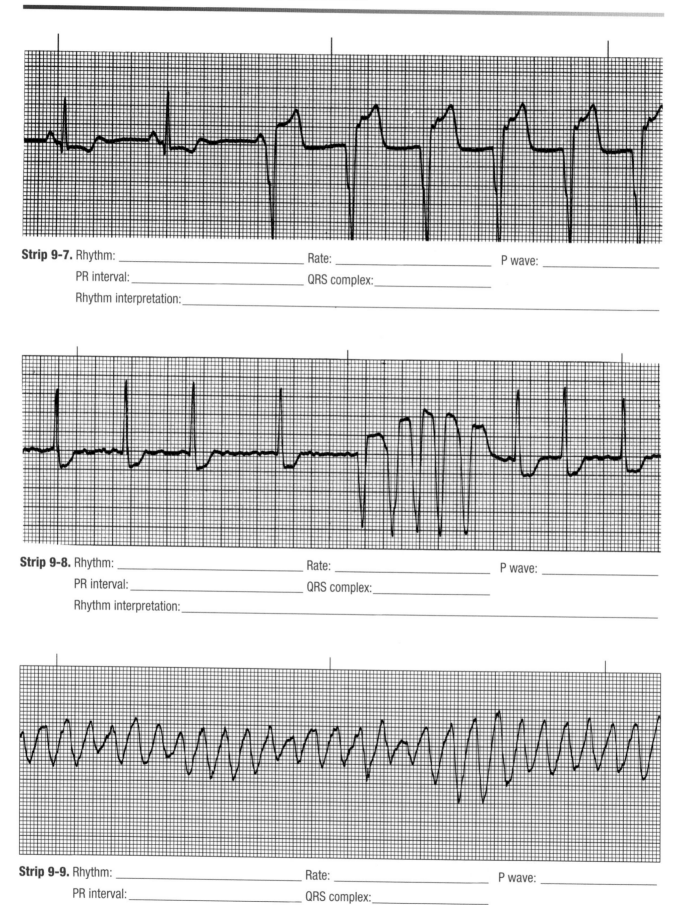

Strip 9-7. Rhythm: _____ Rate: _____ P wave: _____

PR interval: _____ QRS complex: _____

Rhythm interpretation: _____

Strip 9-8. Rhythm: _____ Rate: _____ P wave: _____

PR interval: _____ QRS complex: _____

Rhythm interpretation: _____

Strip 9-9. Rhythm: _____ Rate: _____ P wave: _____

PR interval: _____ QRS complex: _____

Rhythm interpretation: _____

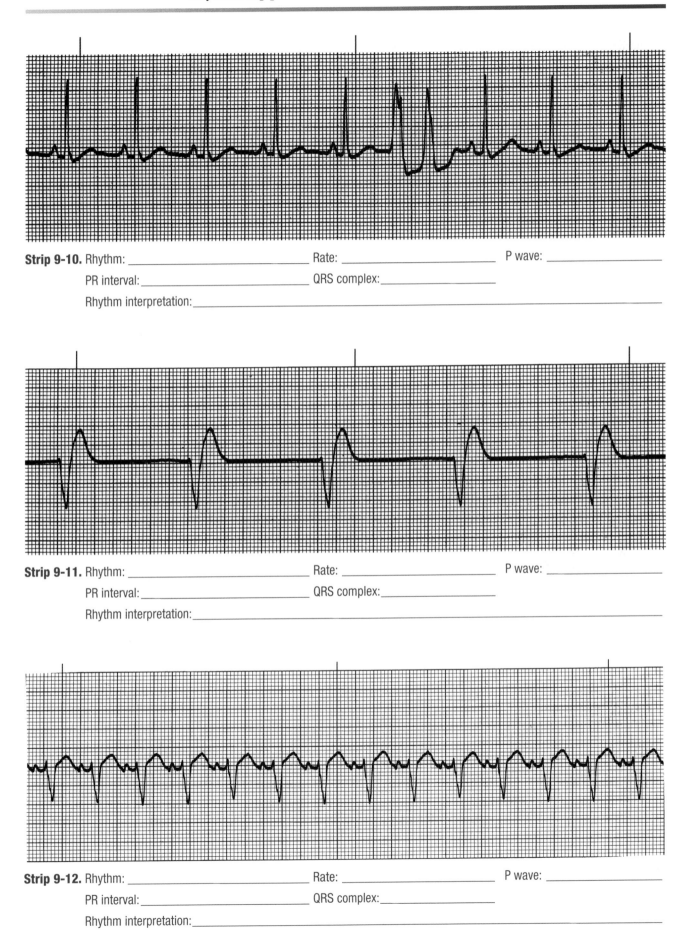

Strip 9-10. Rhythm: _____ Rate: _____ P wave: _____

PR interval: _____ QRS complex: _____

Rhythm interpretation: _____

Strip 9-11. Rhythm: _____ Rate: _____ P wave: _____

PR interval: _____ QRS complex: _____

Rhythm interpretation: _____

Strip 9-12. Rhythm: _____ Rate: _____ P wave: _____

PR interval: _____ QRS complex: _____

Rhythm interpretation: _____

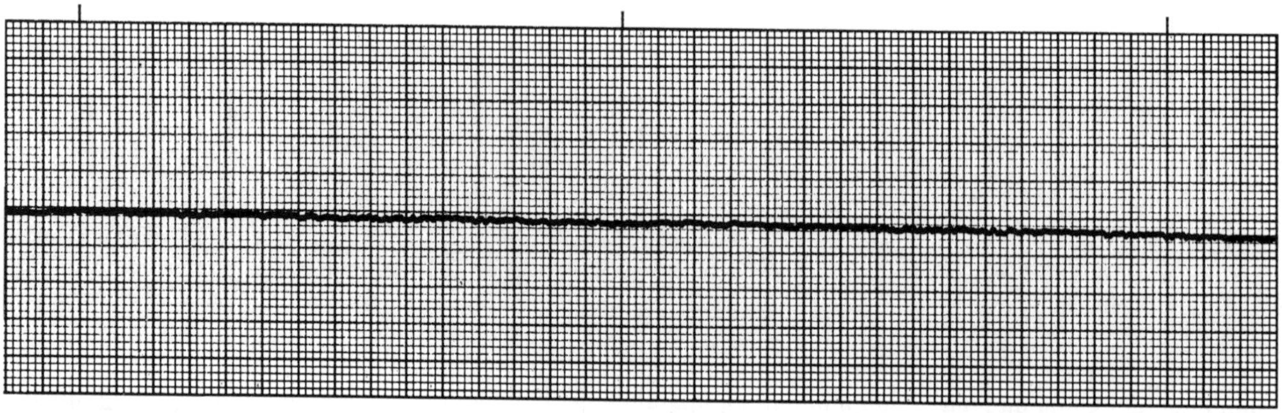

Strip 9-13. Rhythm: _____ Rate: _____ P wave: _____

PR interval: _____ QRS complex: _____

Rhythm interpretation: _____

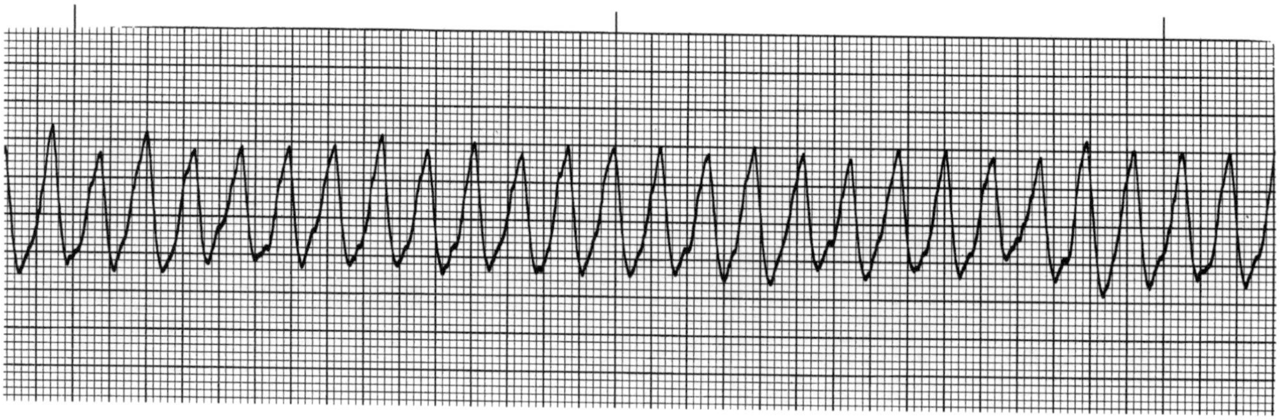

Strip 9-14. Rhythm: _____ Rate: _____ P wave: _____

PR interval: _____ QRS complex: _____

Rhythm interpretation: _____

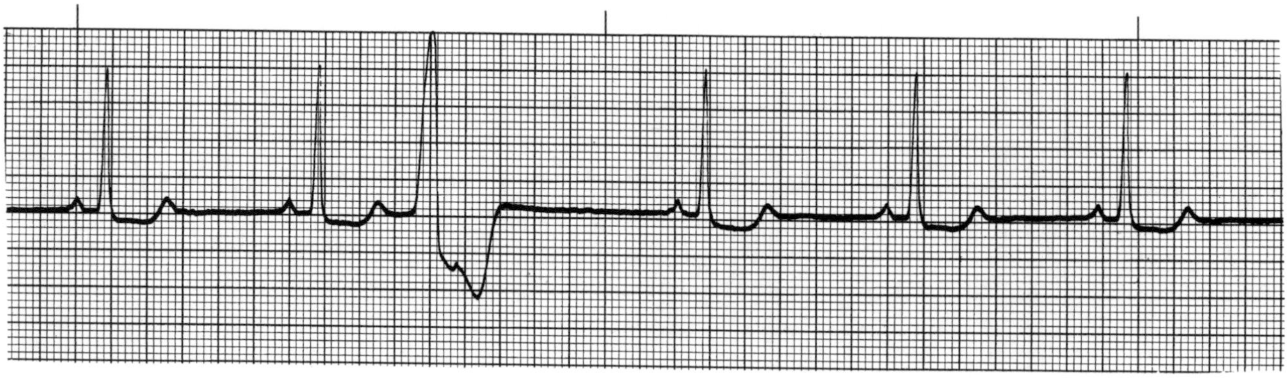

Strip 9-15. Rhythm: _____ Rate: _____ P wave: _____

PR interval: _____ QRS complex: _____

Rhythm interpretation: _____

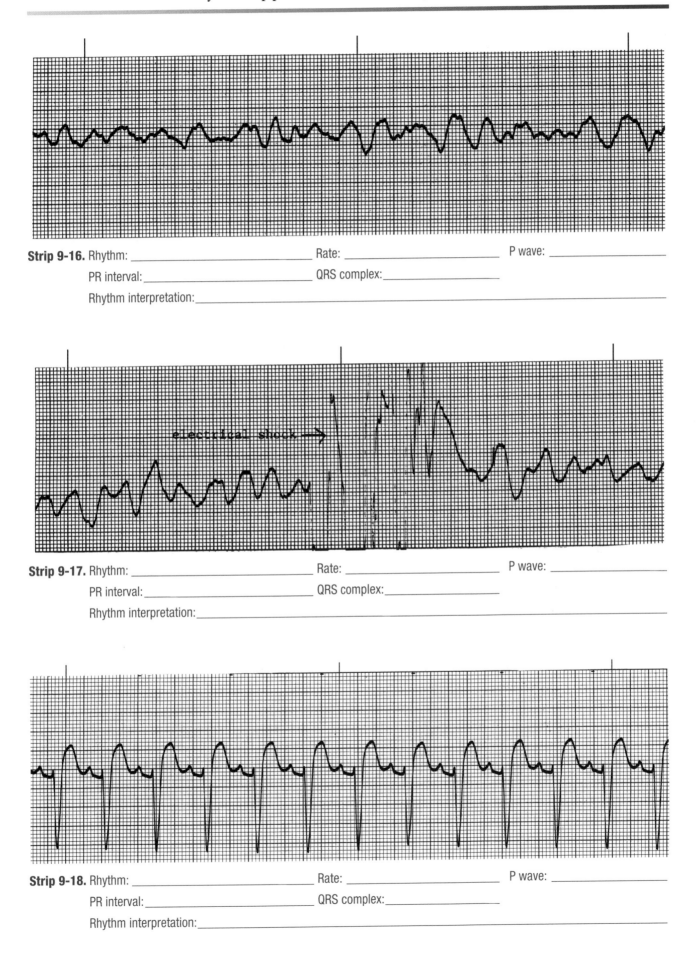

Strip 9-16. Rhythm: _____ Rate: _____ P wave: _____

PR interval: _____ QRS complex: _____

Rhythm interpretation: _____

Strip 9-17. Rhythm: _____ Rate: _____ P wave: _____

PR interval: _____ QRS complex: _____

Rhythm interpretation: _____

Strip 9-18. Rhythm: _____ Rate: _____ P wave: _____

PR interval: _____ QRS complex: _____

Rhythm interpretation: _____

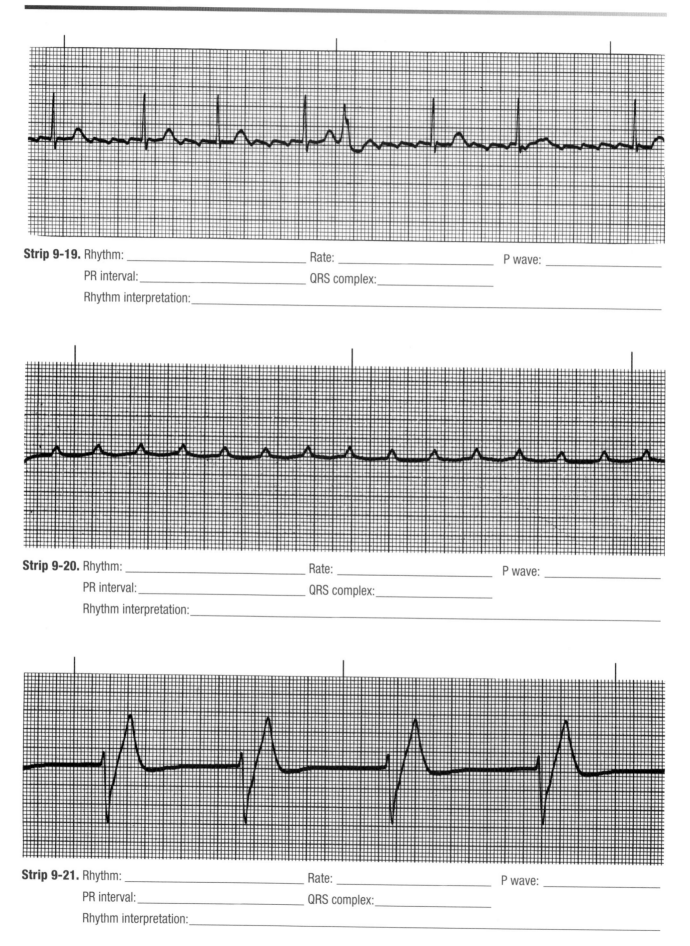

Strip 9-19. Rhythm: _____ Rate: _____ P wave: _____

PR interval: _____ QRS complex: _____

Rhythm interpretation: _____

Strip 9-20. Rhythm: _____ Rate: _____ P wave: _____

PR interval: _____ QRS complex: _____

Rhythm interpretation: _____

Strip 9-21. Rhythm: _____ Rate: _____ P wave: _____

PR interval: _____ QRS complex: _____

Rhythm interpretation: _____

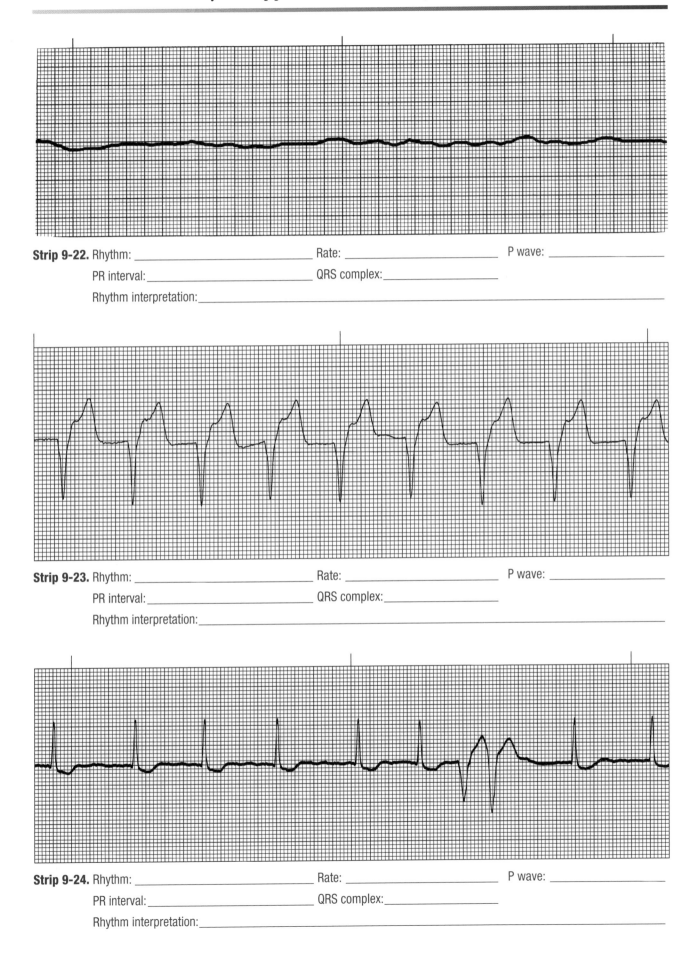

Strip 9-22. Rhythm: _____ Rate: _____ P wave: _____

PR interval: _____ QRS complex: _____

Rhythm interpretation: _____

Strip 9-23. Rhythm: _____ Rate: _____ P wave: _____

PR interval: _____ QRS complex: _____

Rhythm interpretation: _____

Strip 9-24. Rhythm: _____ Rate: _____ P wave: _____

PR interval: _____ QRS complex: _____

Rhythm interpretation: _____

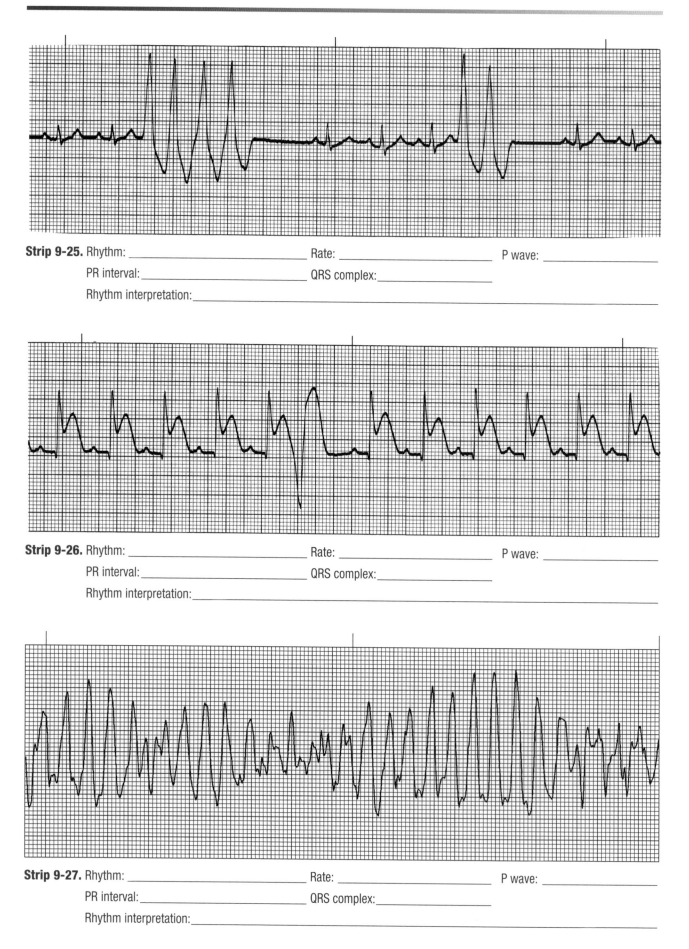

Strip 9-25. Rhythm: _____ Rate: _____ P wave: _____

PR interval: _____ QRS complex: _____

Rhythm interpretation: _____

Strip 9-26. Rhythm: _____ Rate: _____ P wave: _____

PR interval: _____ QRS complex: _____

Rhythm interpretation: _____

Strip 9-27. Rhythm: _____ Rate: _____ P wave: _____

PR interval: _____ QRS complex: _____

Rhythm interpretation: _____

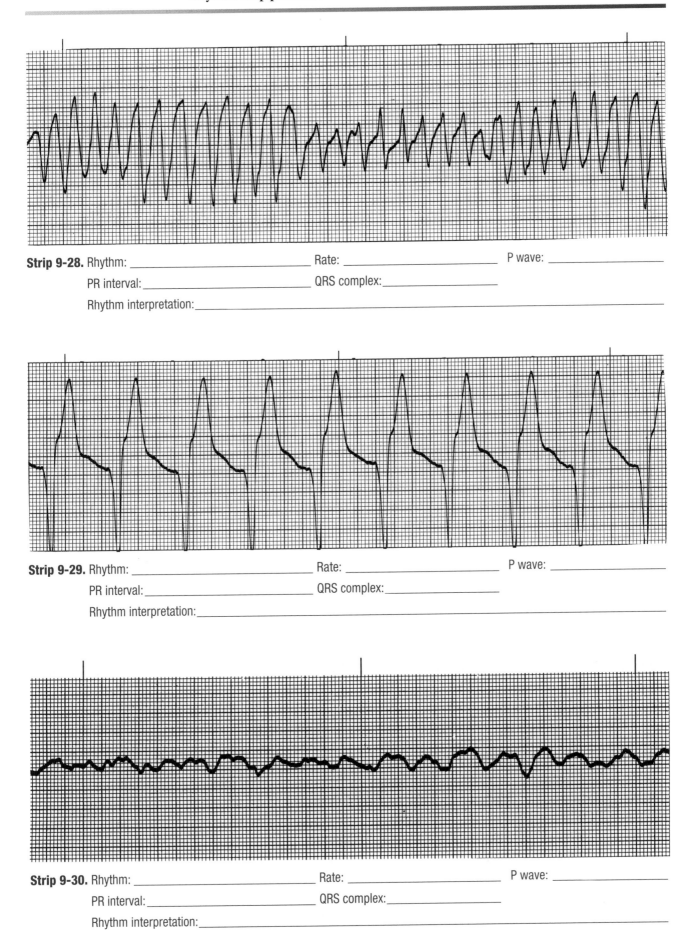

Strip 9-28. Rhythm: _____ Rate: _____ P wave: _____

PR interval: _____ QRS complex: _____

Rhythm interpretation: _____

Strip 9-29. Rhythm: _____ Rate: _____ P wave: _____

PR interval: _____ QRS complex: _____

Rhythm interpretation: _____

Strip 9-30. Rhythm: _____ Rate: _____ P wave: _____

PR interval: _____ QRS complex: _____

Rhythm interpretation: _____

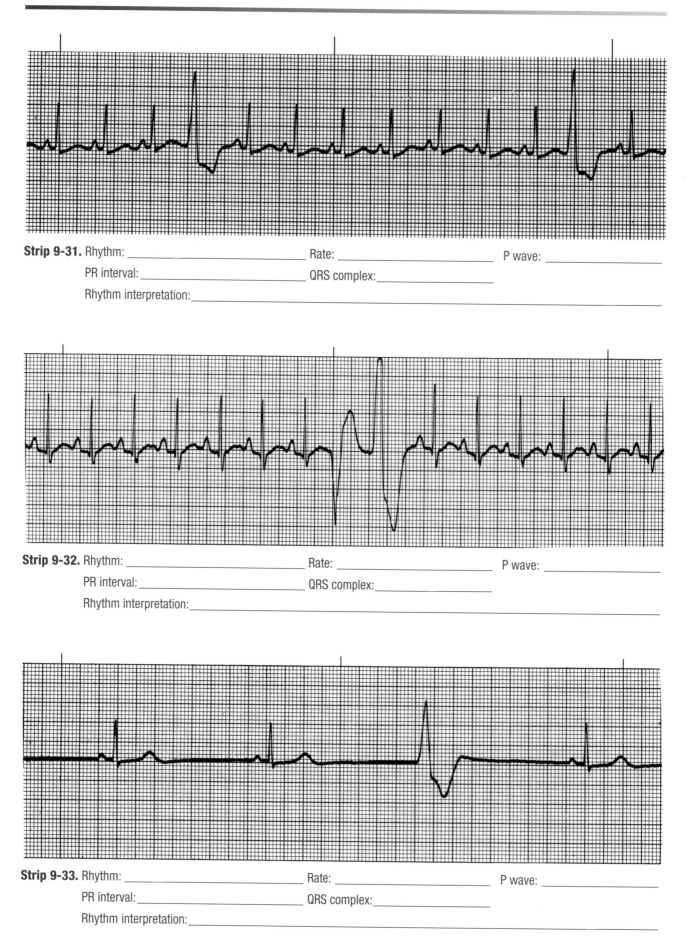

Strip 9-31. Rhythm: _____ Rate: _____ P wave: _____

PR interval: _____ QRS complex: _____

Rhythm interpretation: _____

Strip 9-32. Rhythm: _____ Rate: _____ P wave: _____

PR interval: _____ QRS complex: _____

Rhythm interpretation: _____

Strip 9-33. Rhythm: _____ Rate: _____ P wave: _____

PR interval: _____ QRS complex: _____

Rhythm interpretation: _____

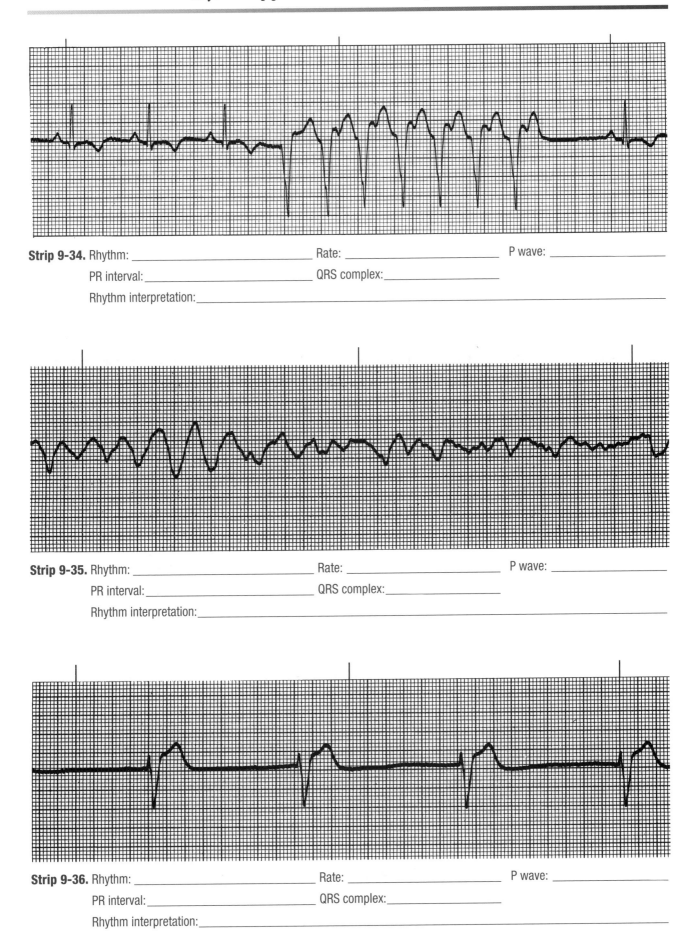

Strip 9-34. Rhythm: _____ Rate: _____ P wave: _____

PR interval: _____ QRS complex: _____

Rhythm interpretation: _____

Strip 9-35. Rhythm: _____ Rate: _____ P wave: _____

PR interval: _____ QRS complex: _____

Rhythm interpretation: _____

Strip 9-36. Rhythm: _____ Rate: _____ P wave: _____

PR interval: _____ QRS complex: _____

Rhythm interpretation: _____

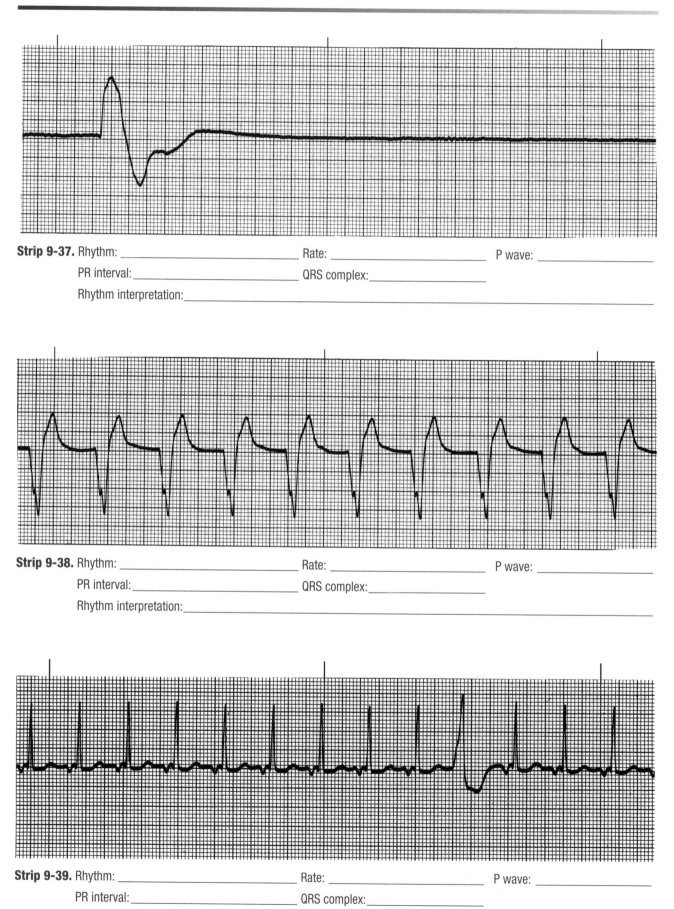

Strip 9-37. Rhythm: _____ Rate: _____ P wave: _____

PR interval: _____ QRS complex: _____

Rhythm interpretation: _____

Strip 9-38. Rhythm: _____ Rate: _____ P wave: _____

PR interval: _____ QRS complex: _____

Rhythm interpretation: _____

Strip 9-39. Rhythm: _____ Rate: _____ P wave: _____

PR interval: _____ QRS complex: _____

Rhythm interpretation: _____

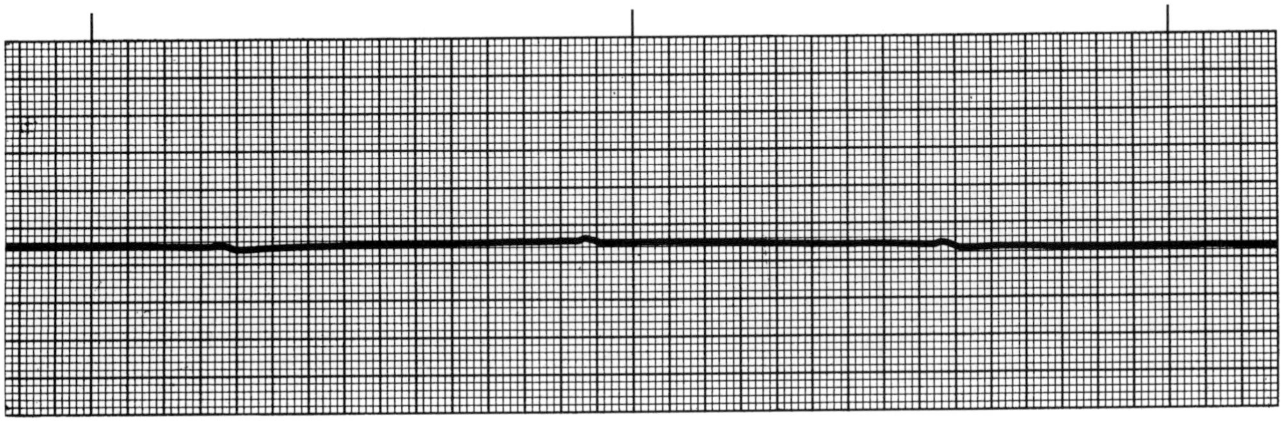

Strip 9-40. Rhythm: _____ Rate: _____ P wave: _____

PR interval: _____ QRS complex: _____

Rhythm interpretation: _____

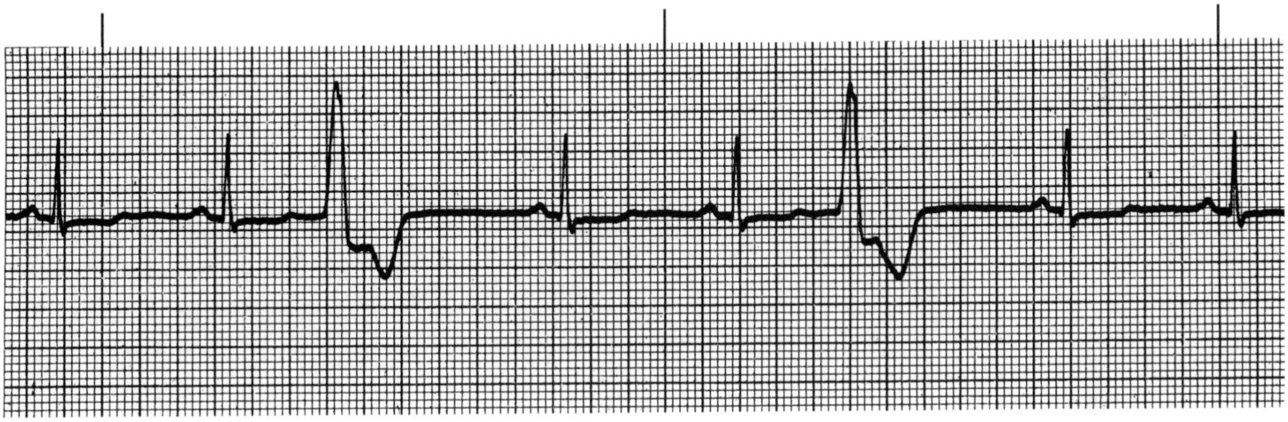

Strip 9-41. Rhythm: _____ Rate: _____ P wave: _____

PR interval: _____ QRS complex: _____

Rhythm interpretation: _____

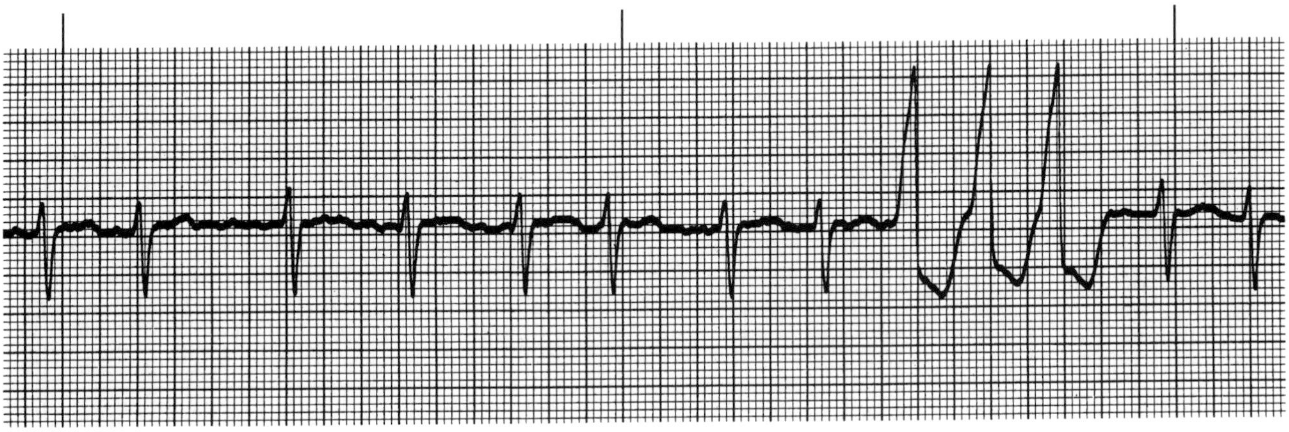

Strip 9-42. Rhythm: _____ Rate: _____ P wave: _____

PR interval: _____ QRS complex: _____

Rhythm interpretation: _____

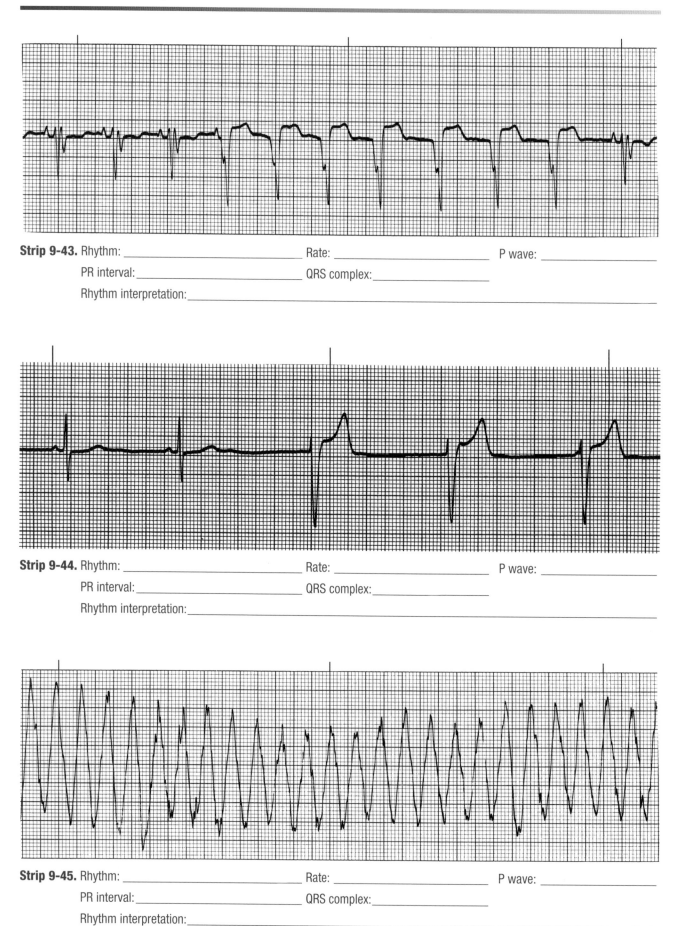

Strip 9-43. Rhythm: _____ Rate: _____ P wave: _____

PR interval: _____ QRS complex: _____

Rhythm interpretation: _____

Strip 9-44. Rhythm: _____ Rate: _____ P wave: _____

PR interval: _____ QRS complex: _____

Rhythm interpretation: _____

Strip 9-45. Rhythm: _____ Rate: _____ P wave: _____

PR interval: _____ QRS complex: _____

Rhythm interpretation: _____

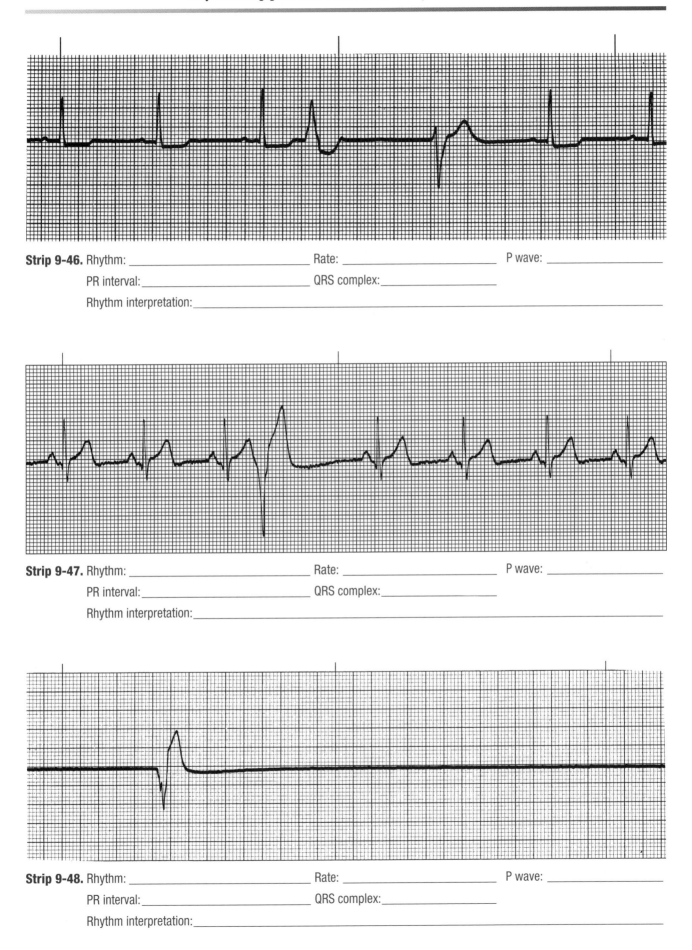

Strip 9-46. Rhythm: _____ Rate: _____ P wave: _____

PR interval: _____ QRS complex: _____

Rhythm interpretation: _____

Strip 9-47. Rhythm: _____ Rate: _____ P wave: _____

PR interval: _____ QRS complex: _____

Rhythm interpretation: _____

Strip 9-48. Rhythm: _____ Rate: _____ P wave: _____

PR interval: _____ QRS complex: _____

Rhythm interpretation: _____

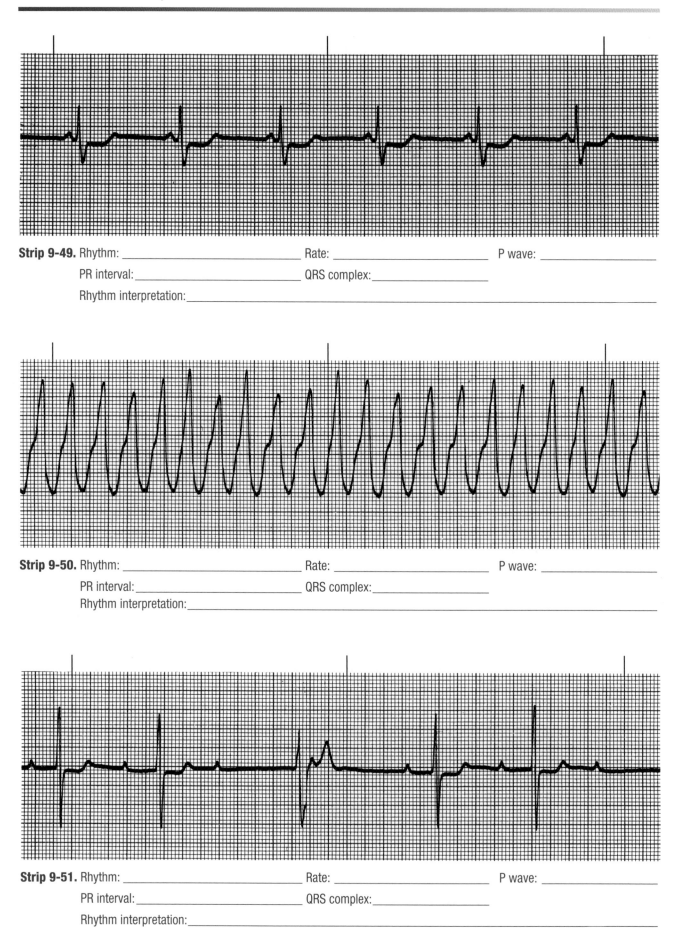

Strip 9-49. Rhythm: _____ Rate: _____ P wave: _____

PR interval: _____ QRS complex: _____

Rhythm interpretation: _____

Strip 9-50. Rhythm: _____ Rate: _____ P wave: _____

PR interval: _____ QRS complex: _____

Rhythm interpretation: _____

Strip 9-51. Rhythm: _____ Rate: _____ P wave: _____

PR interval: _____ QRS complex: _____

Rhythm interpretation: _____

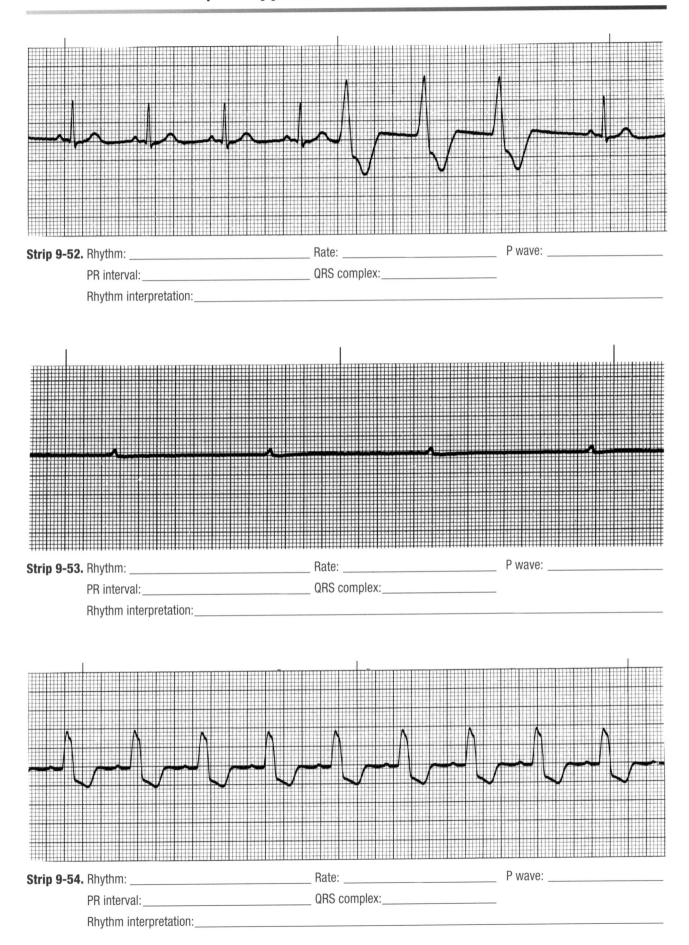

Strip 9-52. Rhythm: _____ Rate: _____ P wave: _____

PR interval: _____ QRS complex: _____

Rhythm interpretation: _____

Strip 9-53. Rhythm: _____ Rate: _____ P wave: _____

PR interval: _____ QRS complex: _____

Rhythm interpretation: _____

Strip 9-54. Rhythm: _____ Rate: _____ P wave: _____

PR interval: _____ QRS complex: _____

Rhythm interpretation: _____

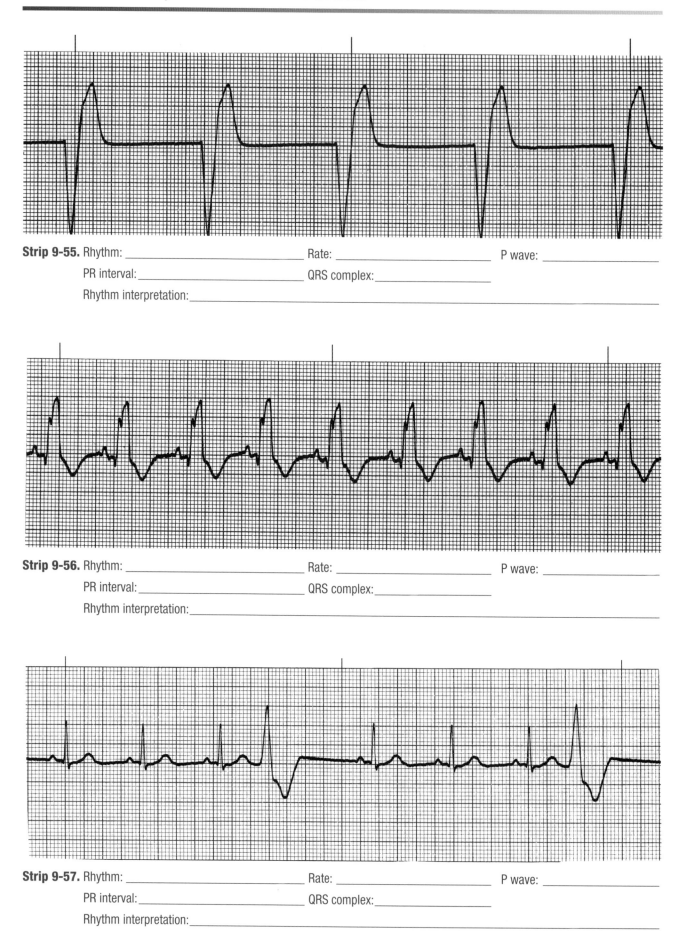

Strip 9-55. Rhythm: _____ Rate: _____ P wave: _____

PR interval: _____ QRS complex: _____

Rhythm interpretation: _____

Strip 9-56. Rhythm: _____ Rate: _____ P wave: _____

PR interval: _____ QRS complex: _____

Rhythm interpretation: _____

Strip 9-57. Rhythm: _____ Rate: _____ P wave: _____

PR interval: _____ QRS complex: _____

Rhythm interpretation: _____

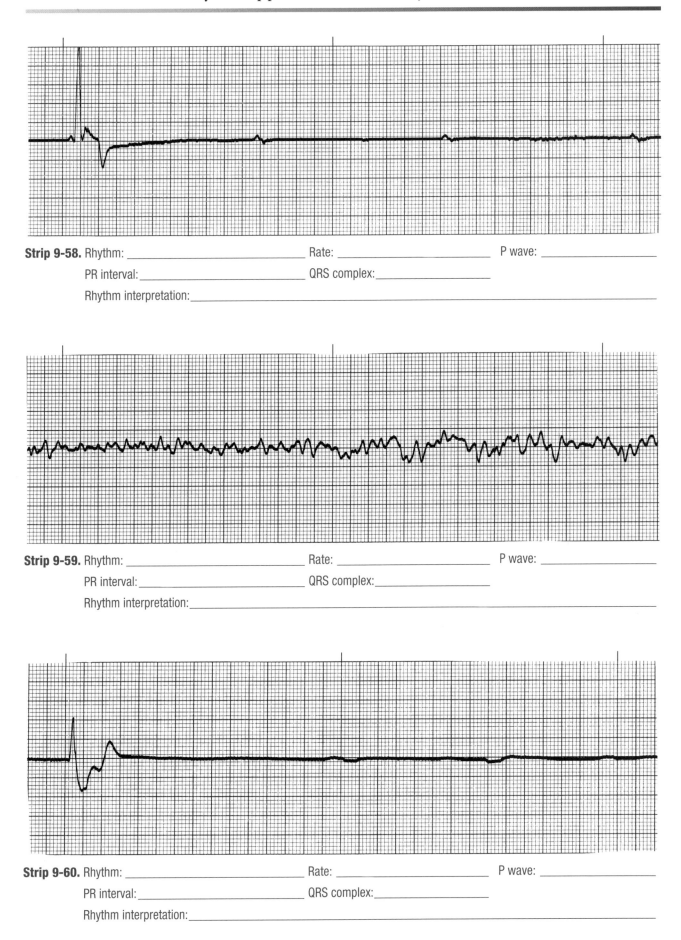

Strip 9-58. Rhythm: _____ Rate: _____ P wave: _____

PR interval: _____ QRS complex: _____

Rhythm interpretation: _____

Strip 9-59. Rhythm: _____ Rate: _____ P wave: _____

PR interval: _____ QRS complex: _____

Rhythm interpretation: _____

Strip 9-60. Rhythm: _____ Rate: _____ P wave: _____

PR interval: _____ QRS complex: _____

Rhythm interpretation: _____

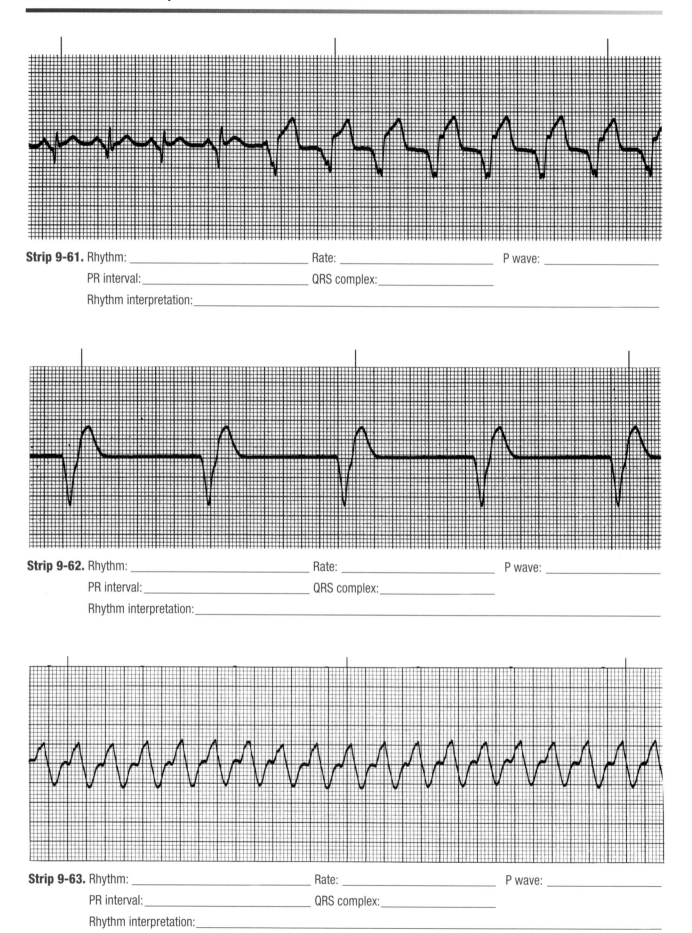

Strip 9-61. Rhythm: _____ Rate: _____ P wave: _____

PR interval: _____ QRS complex: _____

Rhythm interpretation: _____

Strip 9-62. Rhythm: _____ Rate: _____ P wave: _____

PR interval: _____ QRS complex: _____

Rhythm interpretation: _____

Strip 9-63. Rhythm: _____ Rate: _____ P wave: _____

PR interval: _____ QRS complex: _____

Rhythm interpretation: _____

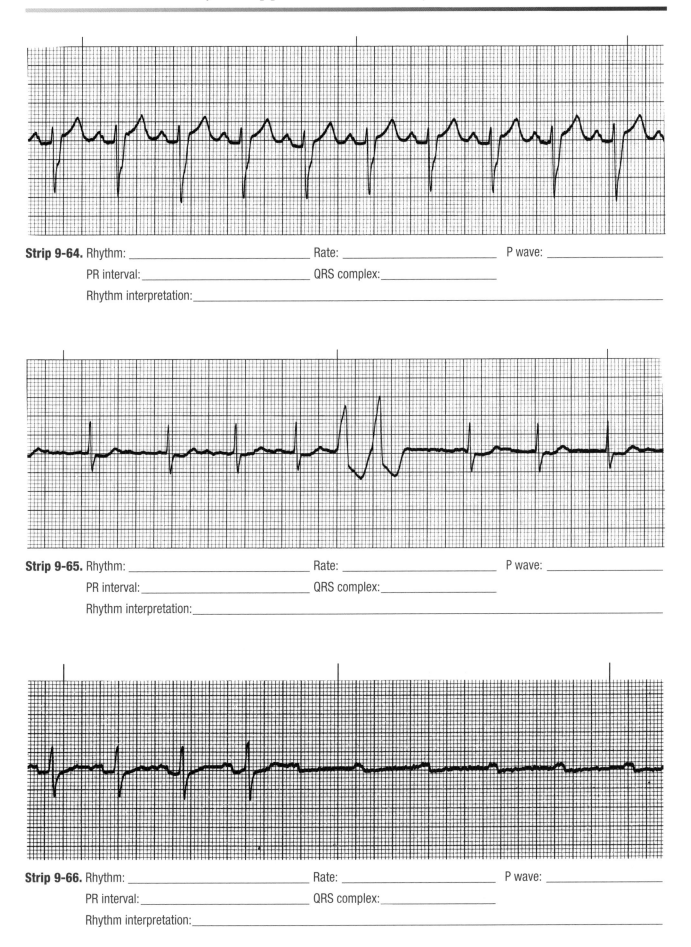

Strip 9-64. Rhythm: _____ Rate: _____ P wave: _____

PR interval: _____ QRS complex: _____

Rhythm interpretation: _____

Strip 9-65. Rhythm: _____ Rate: _____ P wave: _____

PR interval: _____ QRS complex: _____

Rhythm interpretation: _____

Strip 9-66. Rhythm: _____ Rate: _____ P wave: _____

PR interval: _____ QRS complex: _____

Rhythm interpretation: _____

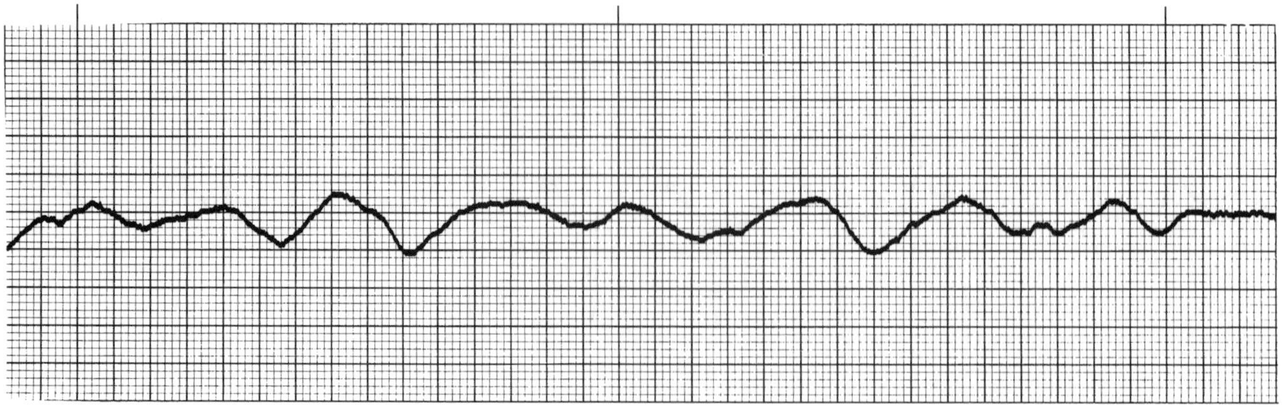

Strip 9-67. Rhythm: _____ Rate: _____ P wave: _____

PR interval: _____ QRS complex: _____

Rhythm interpretation: _____

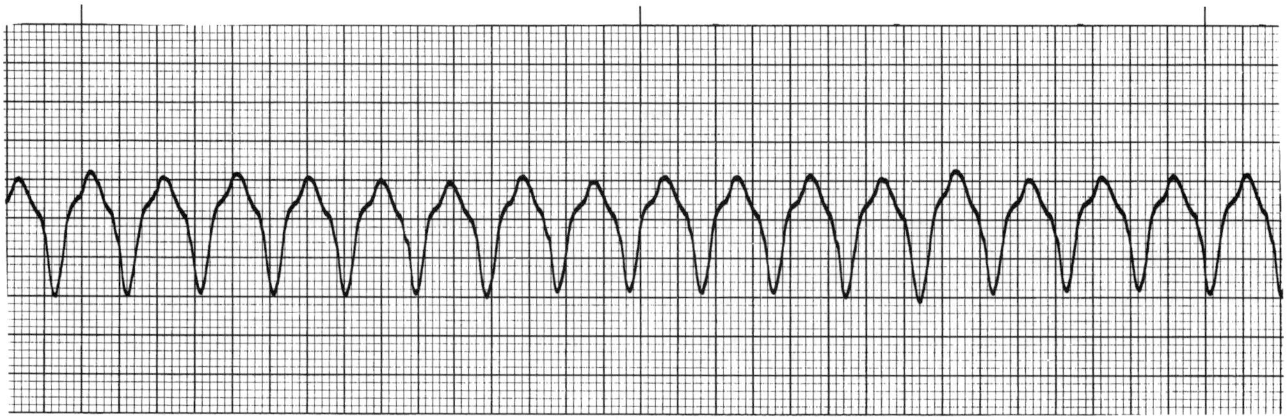

Strip 9-68. Rhythm: _____ Rate: _____ P wave: _____

PR interval: _____ QRS complex: _____

Rhythm interpretation: _____

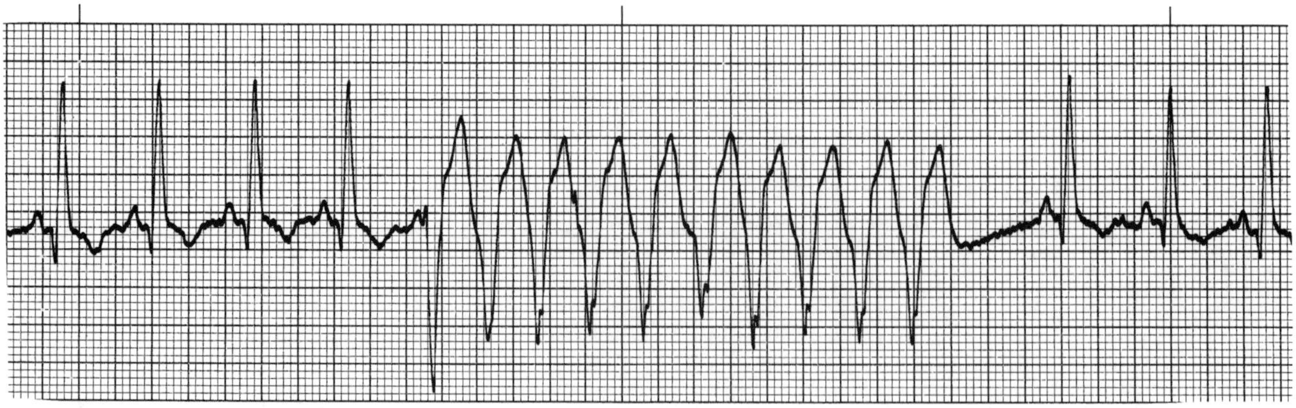

Strip 9-69. Rhythm: _____ Rate: _____ P wave: _____

PR interval: _____ QRS complex: _____

Rhythm interpretation: _____

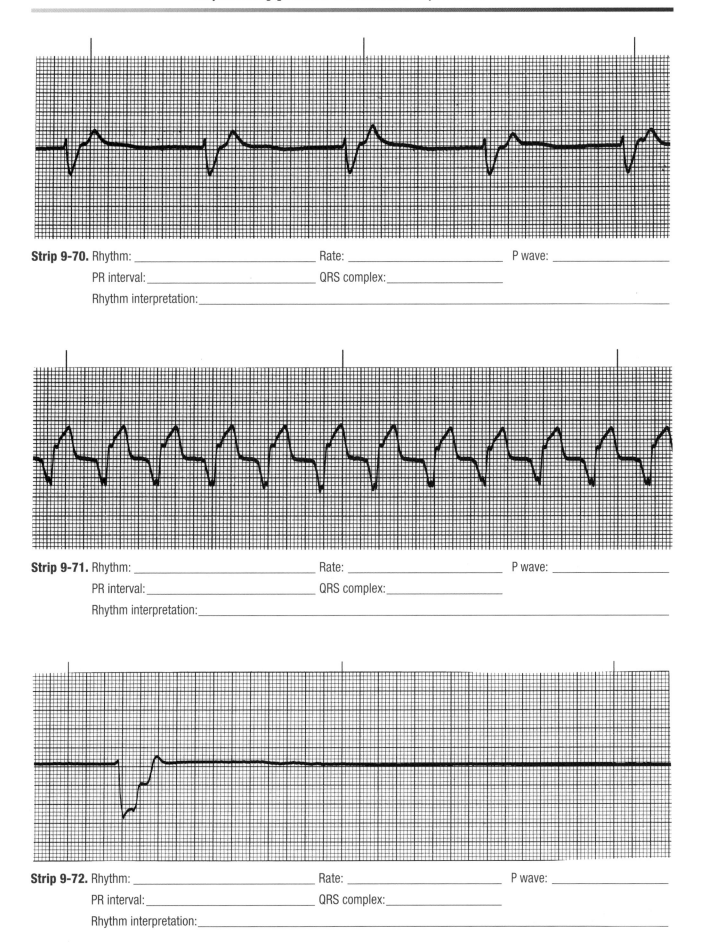

Strip 9-70. Rhythm: _____ Rate: _____ P wave: _____

PR interval: _____ QRS complex: _____

Rhythm interpretation: _____

Strip 9-71. Rhythm: _____ Rate: _____ P wave: _____

PR interval: _____ QRS complex: _____

Rhythm interpretation: _____

Strip 9-72. Rhythm: _____ Rate: _____ P wave: _____

PR interval: _____ QRS complex: _____

Rhythm interpretation: _____

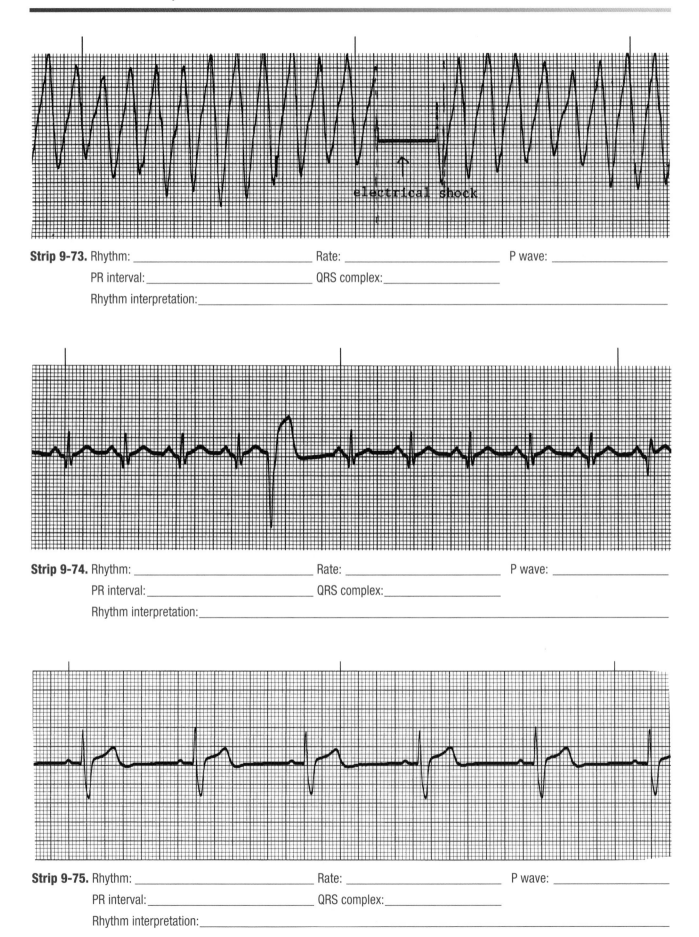

electrical shock

Strip 9-73. Rhythm: _____ Rate: _____ P wave: _____

PR interval: _____ QRS complex: _____

Rhythm interpretation: _____

Strip 9-74. Rhythm: _____ Rate: _____ P wave: _____

PR interval: _____ QRS complex: _____

Rhythm interpretation: _____

Strip 9-75. Rhythm: _____ Rate: _____ P wave: _____

PR interval: _____ QRS complex: _____

Rhythm interpretation: _____

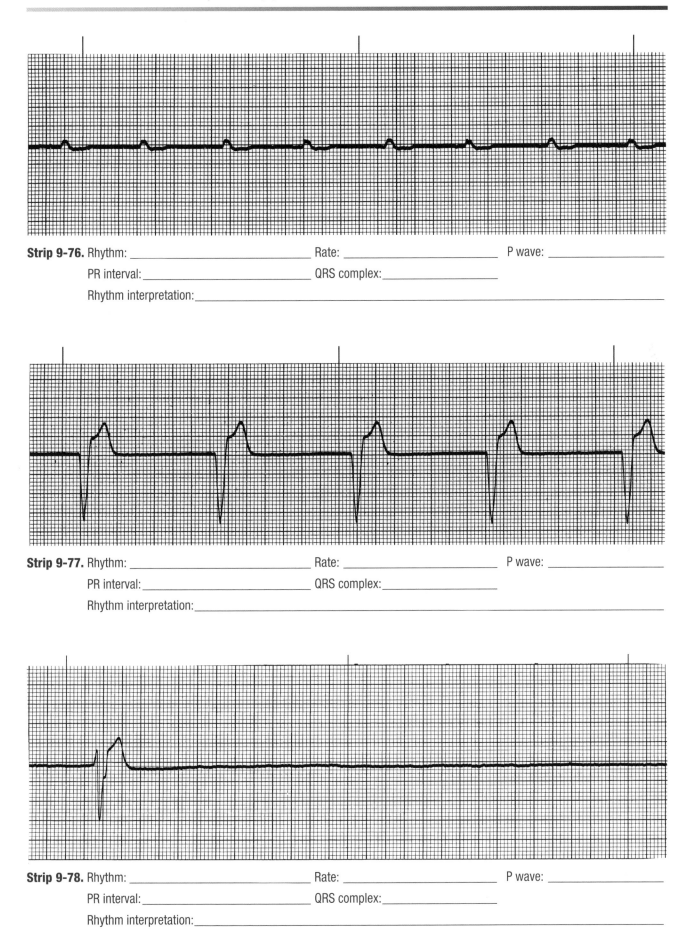

Strip 9-76. Rhythm: _____ Rate: _____ P wave: _____

PR interval: _____ QRS complex: _____

Rhythm interpretation: _____

Strip 9-77. Rhythm: _____ Rate: _____ P wave: _____

PR interval: _____ QRS complex: _____

Rhythm interpretation: _____

Strip 9-78. Rhythm: _____ Rate: _____ P wave: _____

PR interval: _____ QRS complex: _____

Rhythm interpretation: _____

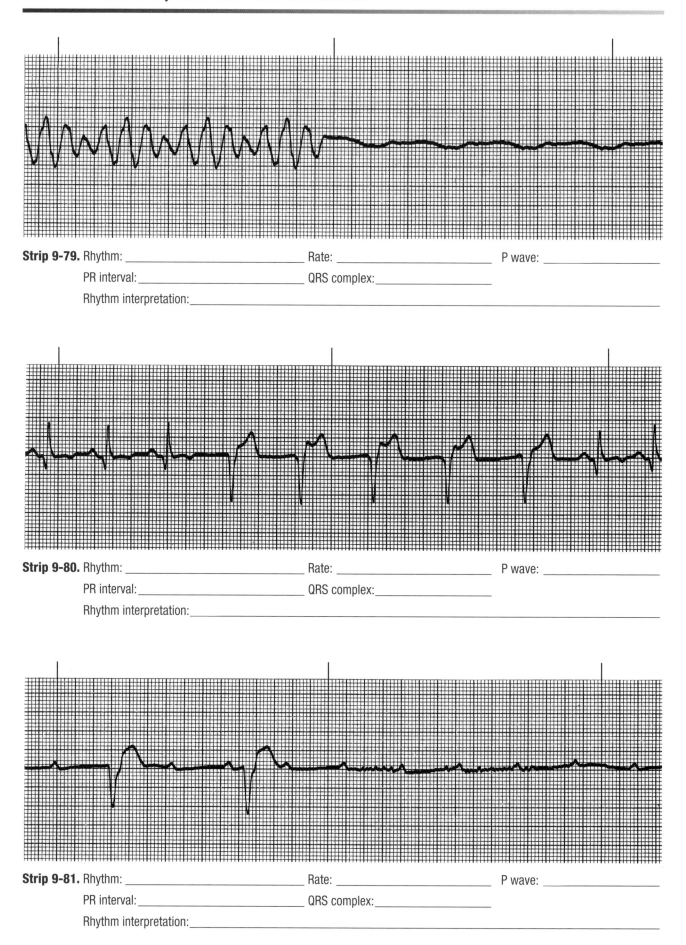

Strip 9-79. Rhythm: _____ Rate: _____ P wave: _____

PR interval: _____ QRS complex: _____

Rhythm interpretation: _____

Strip 9-80. Rhythm: _____ Rate: _____ P wave: _____

PR interval: _____ QRS complex: _____

Rhythm interpretation: _____

Strip 9-81. Rhythm: _____ Rate: _____ P wave: _____

PR interval: _____ QRS complex: _____

Rhythm interpretation: _____

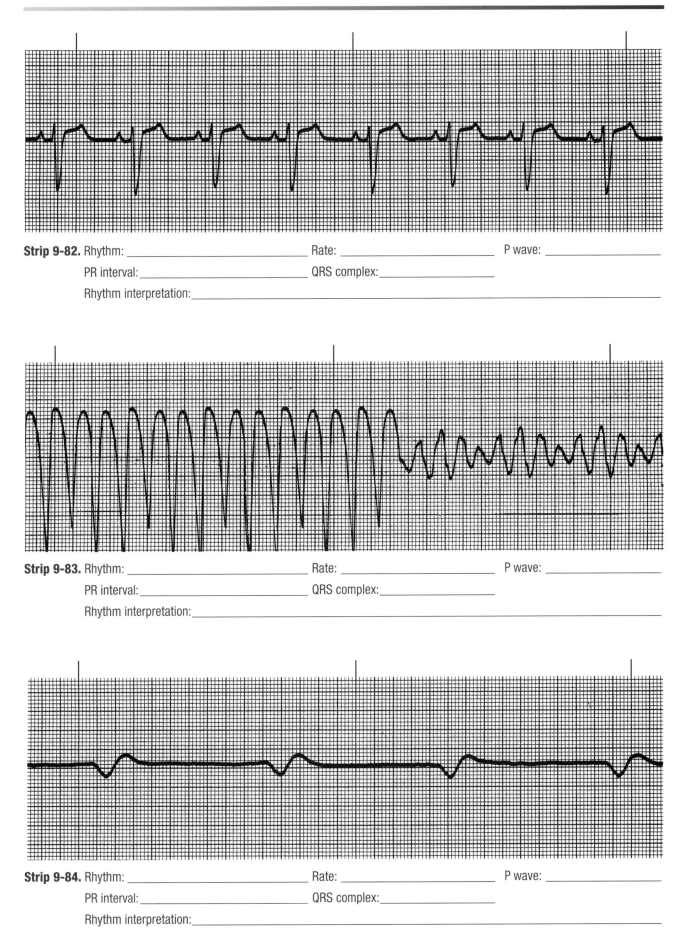

Strip 9-82. Rhythm: _____ Rate: _____ P wave: _____

PR interval: _____ QRS complex: _____

Rhythm interpretation: _____

Strip 9-83. Rhythm: _____ Rate: _____ P wave: _____

PR interval: _____ QRS complex: _____

Rhythm interpretation: _____

Strip 9-84. Rhythm: _____ Rate: _____ P wave: _____

PR interval: _____ QRS complex: _____

Rhythm interpretation: _____

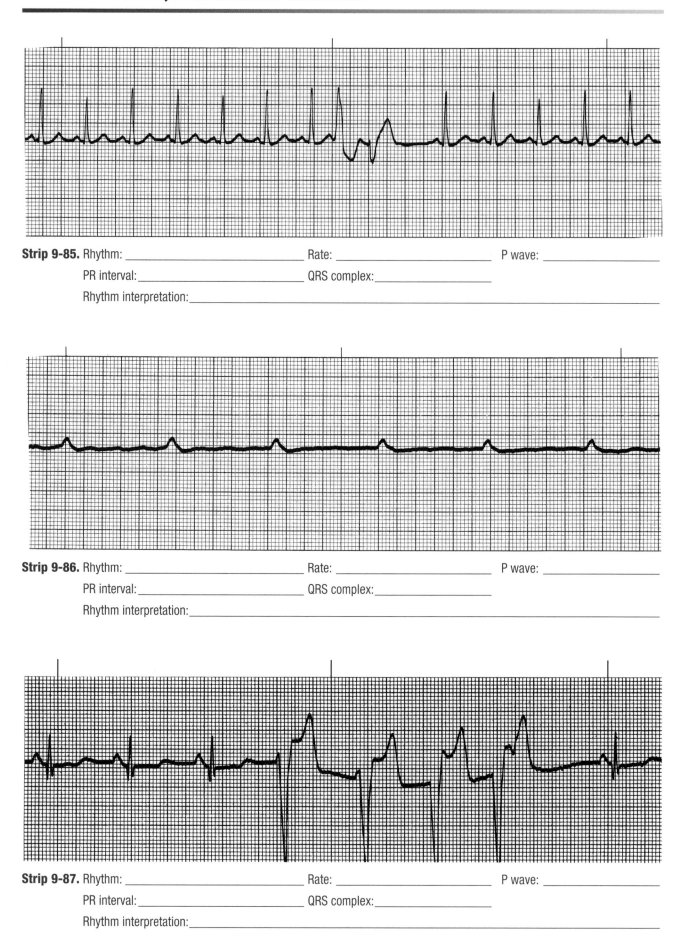

Strip 9-85. Rhythm: _____ Rate: _____ P wave: _____

PR interval: _____ QRS complex: _____

Rhythm interpretation: _____

Strip 9-86. Rhythm: _____ Rate: _____ P wave: _____

PR interval: _____ QRS complex: _____

Rhythm interpretation: _____

Strip 9-87. Rhythm: _____ Rate: _____ P wave: _____

PR interval: _____ QRS complex: _____

Rhythm interpretation: _____

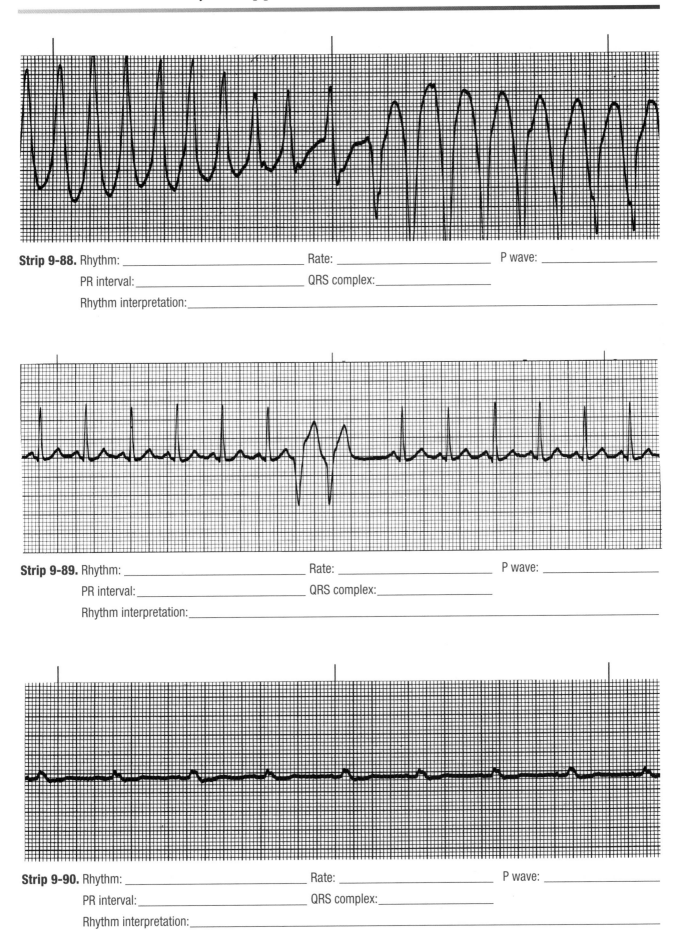

Strip 9-88. Rhythm: _____ Rate: _____ P wave: _____

PR interval: _____ QRS complex: _____

Rhythm interpretation: _____

Strip 9-89. Rhythm: _____ Rate: _____ P wave: _____

PR interval: _____ QRS complex: _____

Rhythm interpretation: _____

Strip 9-90. Rhythm: _____ Rate: _____ P wave: _____

PR interval: _____ QRS complex: _____

Rhythm interpretation: _____

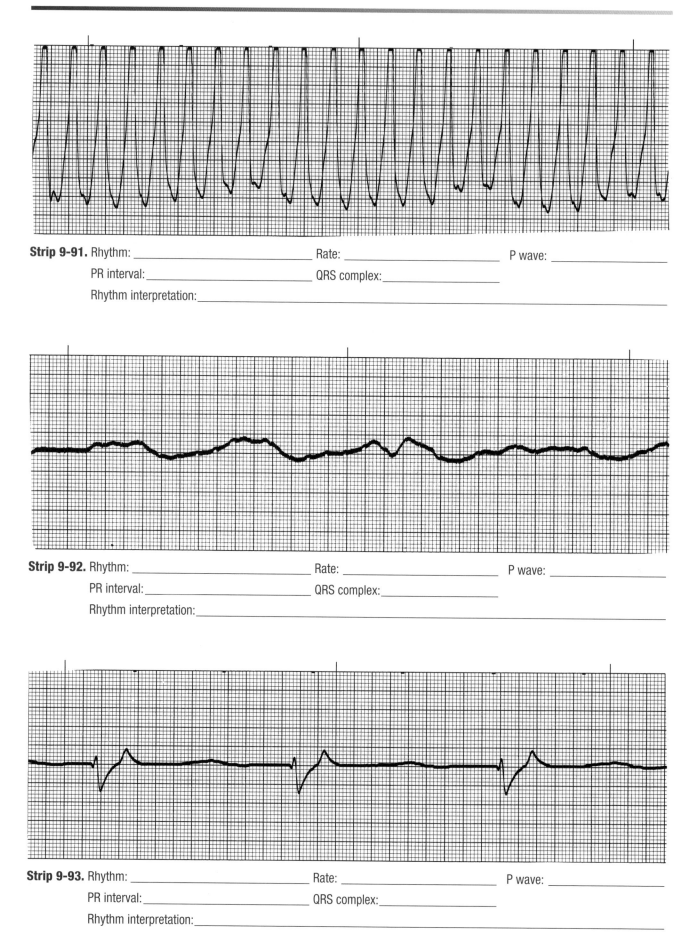

Strip 9-91. Rhythm: _____ Rate: _____ P wave: _____

PR interval: _____ QRS complex: _____

Rhythm interpretation: _____

Strip 9-92. Rhythm: _____ Rate: _____ P wave: _____

PR interval: _____ QRS complex: _____

Rhythm interpretation: _____

Strip 9-93. Rhythm: _____ Rate: _____ P wave: _____

PR interval: _____ QRS complex: _____

Rhythm interpretation: _____

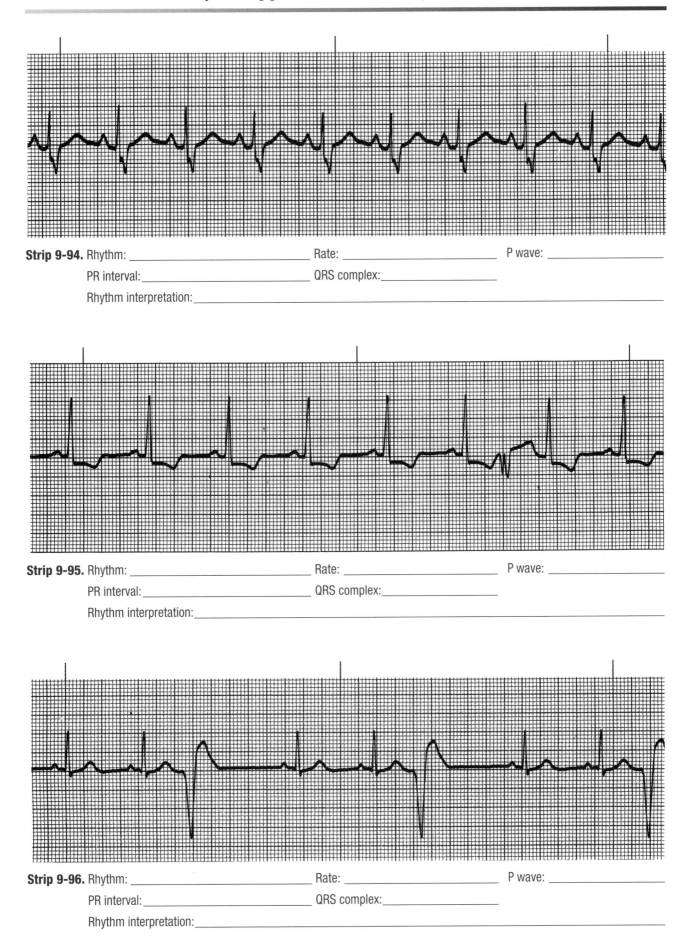

Strip 9-94. Rhythm: _____ Rate: _____ P wave: _____

PR interval: _____ QRS complex: _____

Rhythm interpretation: _____

Strip 9-95. Rhythm: _____ Rate: _____ P wave: _____

PR interval: _____ QRS complex: _____

Rhythm interpretation: _____

Strip 9-96. Rhythm: _____ Rate: _____ P wave: _____

PR interval: _____ QRS complex: _____

Rhythm interpretation: _____

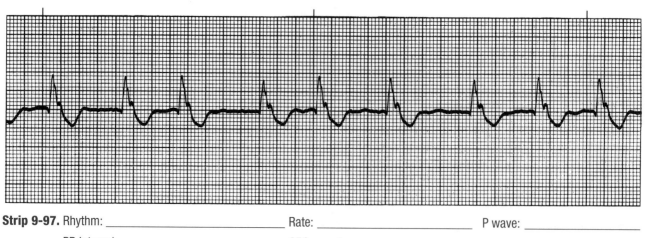

Strip 9-97. Rhythm: _____ Rate: _____ P wave: _____

PR interval: _____ QRS complex: _____

Rhythm interpretation: _____

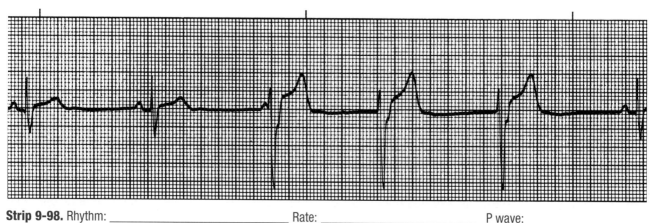

Strip 9-98. Rhythm: _____ Rate: _____ P wave: _____

PR interval: _____ QRS complex: _____

Rhythm interpretation: _____

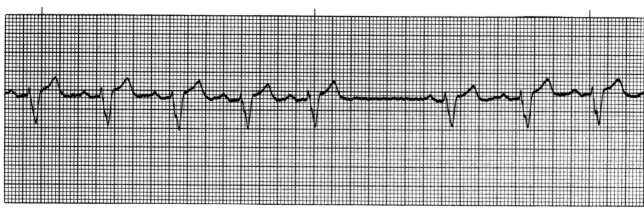

Strip 9-99. Rhythm: _____ Rate: _____ P wave: _____

PR interval: _____ QRS complex: _____

Rhythm interpretation: _____

Strip 9-100. Rhythm: _____ Rate: _____ P wave: _____

PR interval: _____ QRS complex: _____

Rhythm interpretation: _____

⊞ Skillbuilder practice

This section contains *mixed sinus, atrial, and junctional and AV block*, and *ventricular rhythm strips*, allowing the student to practice differentiating between two rhythm groups before progressing to the Posttest. As before, analyze the rhythm strips using the five-step process. Interpret the rhythm by comparing the data collected with the ECG characteristics for each rhythm. All strips are lead II, a positive lead, unless otherwise noted. Check your answers with the answer key in the appendix.

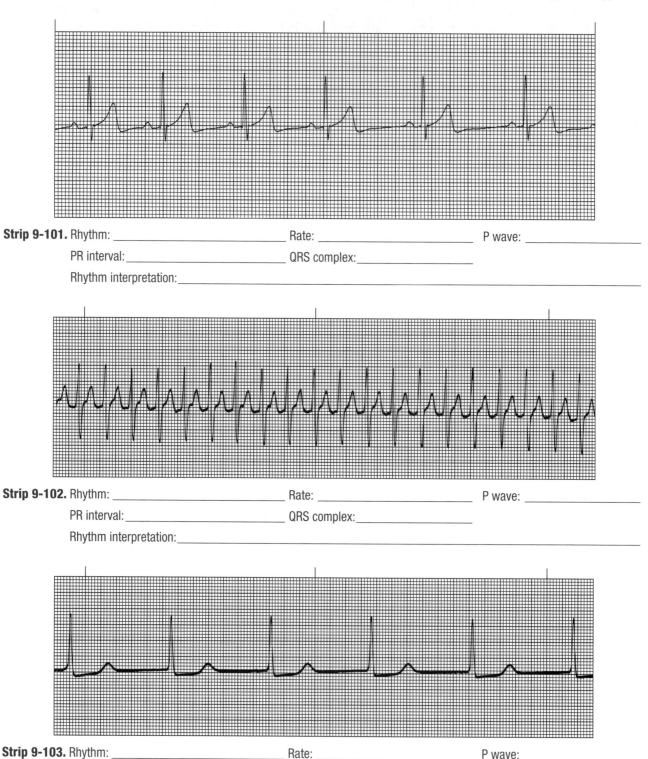

Strip 9-101. Rhythm: _____ Rate: _____ P wave: _____

PR interval: _____ QRS complex: _____

Rhythm interpretation: _____

Strip 9-102. Rhythm: _____ Rate: _____ P wave: _____

PR interval: _____ QRS complex: _____

Rhythm interpretation: _____

Strip 9-103. Rhythm: _____ Rate: _____ P wave: _____

PR interval: _____ QRS complex: _____

Rhythm interpretation: _____

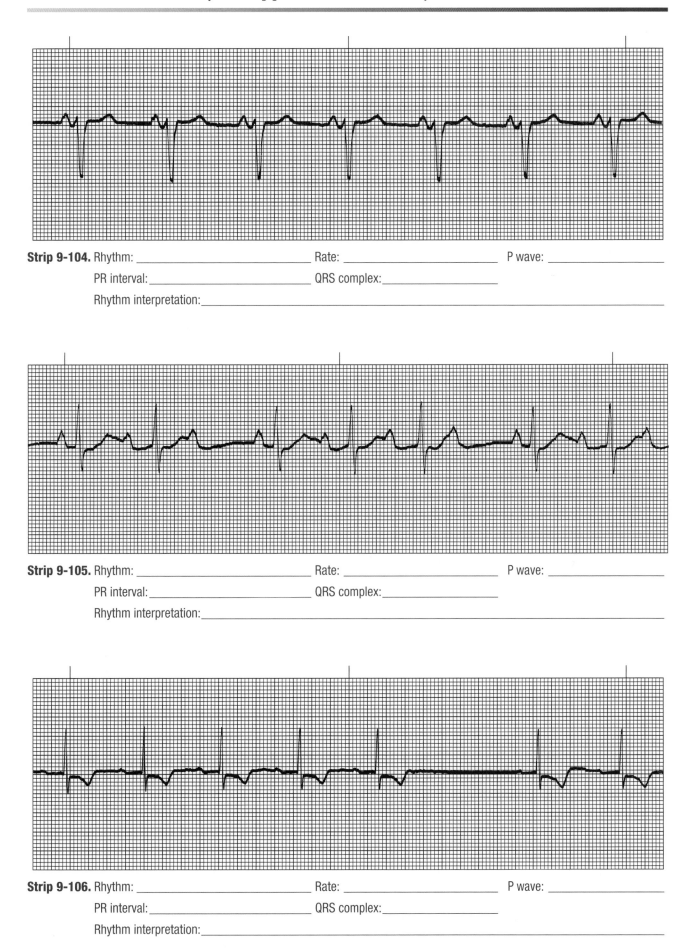

Strip 9-104. Rhythm: _____ Rate: _____ P wave: _____

PR interval: _____ QRS complex: _____

Rhythm interpretation: _____

Strip 9-105. Rhythm: _____ Rate: _____ P wave: _____

PR interval: _____ QRS complex: _____

Rhythm interpretation: _____

Strip 9-106. Rhythm: _____ Rate: _____ P wave: _____

PR interval: _____ QRS complex: _____

Rhythm interpretation: _____

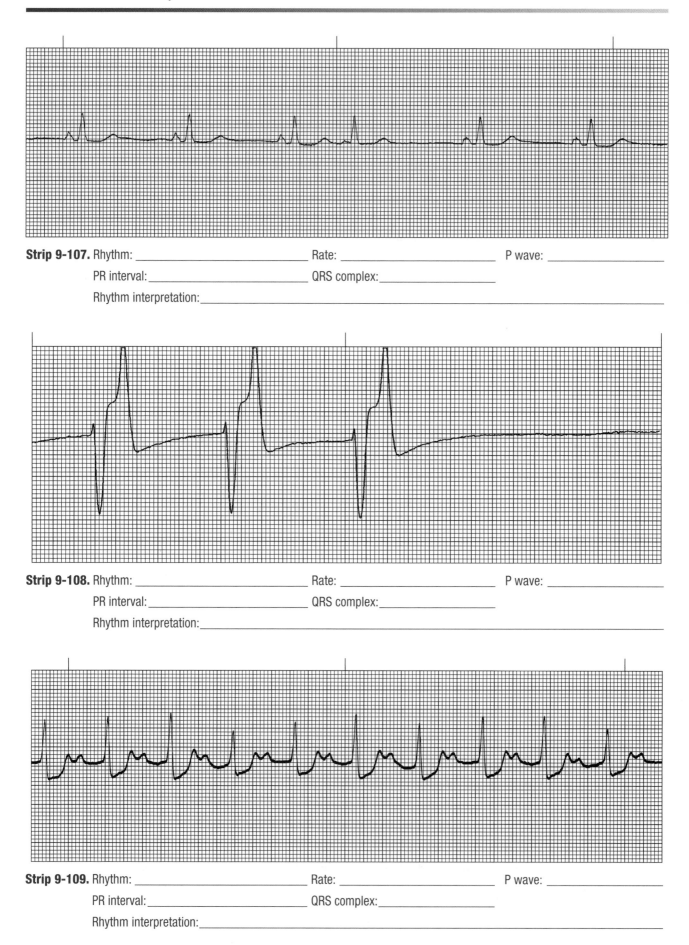

Strip 9-107. Rhythm: _____ Rate: _____ P wave: _____

PR interval: _____ QRS complex: _____

Rhythm interpretation: _____

Strip 9-108. Rhythm: _____ Rate: _____ P wave: _____

PR interval: _____ QRS complex: _____

Rhythm interpretation: _____

Strip 9-109. Rhythm: _____ Rate: _____ P wave: _____

PR interval: _____ QRS complex: _____

Rhythm interpretation: _____

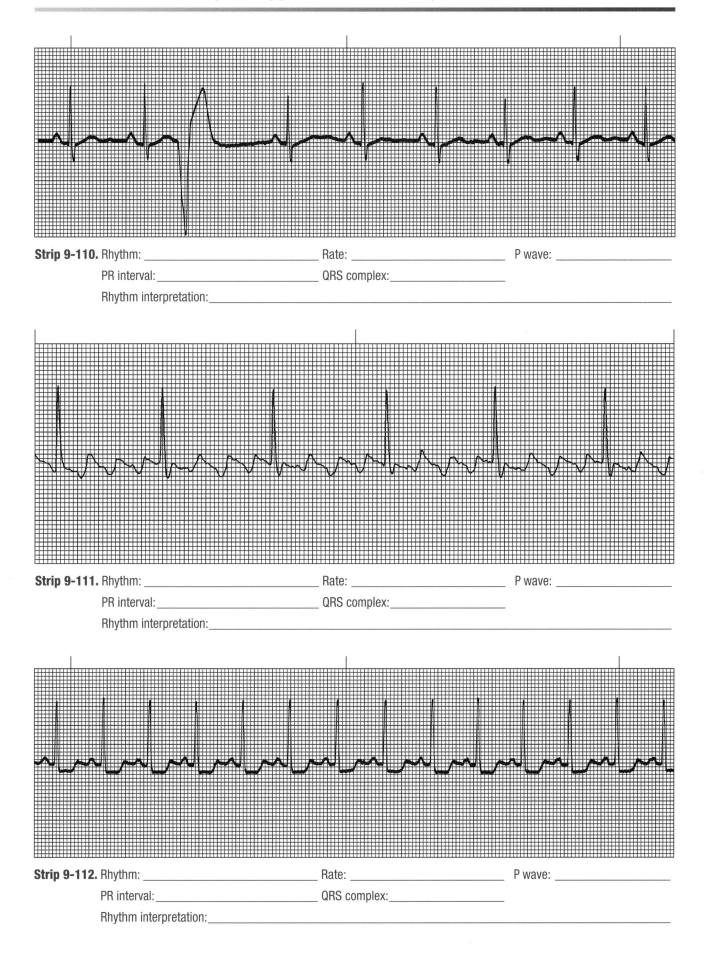

Strip 9-110. Rhythm: _____ Rate: _____ P wave: _____

PR interval:_____ QRS complex:_____

Rhythm interpretation:_____

Strip 9-111. Rhythm: _____ Rate: _____ P wave: _____

PR interval:_____ QRS complex:_____

Rhythm interpretation:_____

Strip 9-112. Rhythm: _____ Rate: _____ P wave: _____

PR interval:_____ QRS complex:_____

Rhythm interpretation:_____

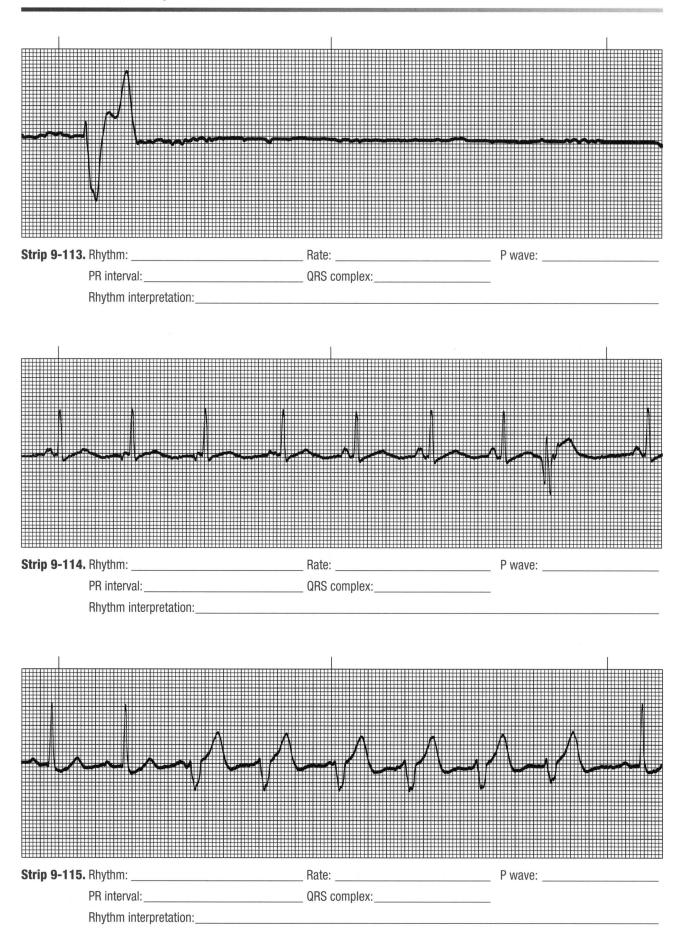

Strip 9-113. Rhythm: _____ Rate: _____ P wave: _____

PR interval: _____ QRS complex: _____

Rhythm interpretation: _____

Strip 9-114. Rhythm: _____ Rate: _____ P wave: _____

PR interval: _____ QRS complex: _____

Rhythm interpretation: _____

Strip 9-115. Rhythm: _____ Rate: _____ P wave: _____

PR interval: _____ QRS complex: _____

Rhythm interpretation: _____

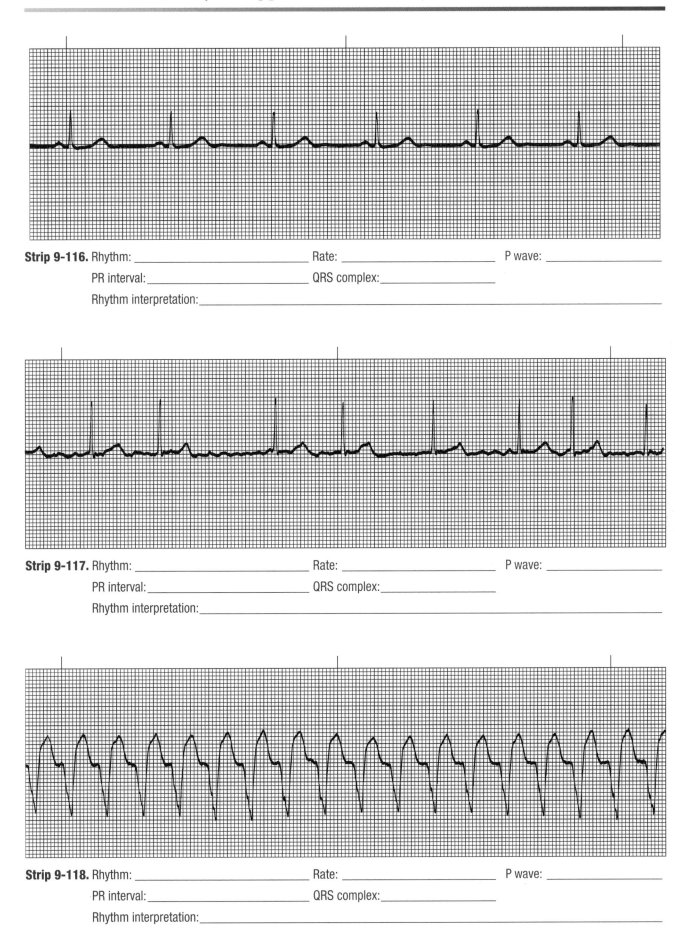

Strip 9-116. Rhythm: _____ Rate: _____ P wave: _____

PR interval: _____ QRS complex: _____

Rhythm interpretation: _____

Strip 9-117. Rhythm: _____ Rate: _____ P wave: _____

PR interval: _____ QRS complex: _____

Rhythm interpretation: _____

Strip 9-118. Rhythm: _____ Rate: _____ P wave: _____

PR interval: _____ QRS complex: _____

Rhythm interpretation: _____

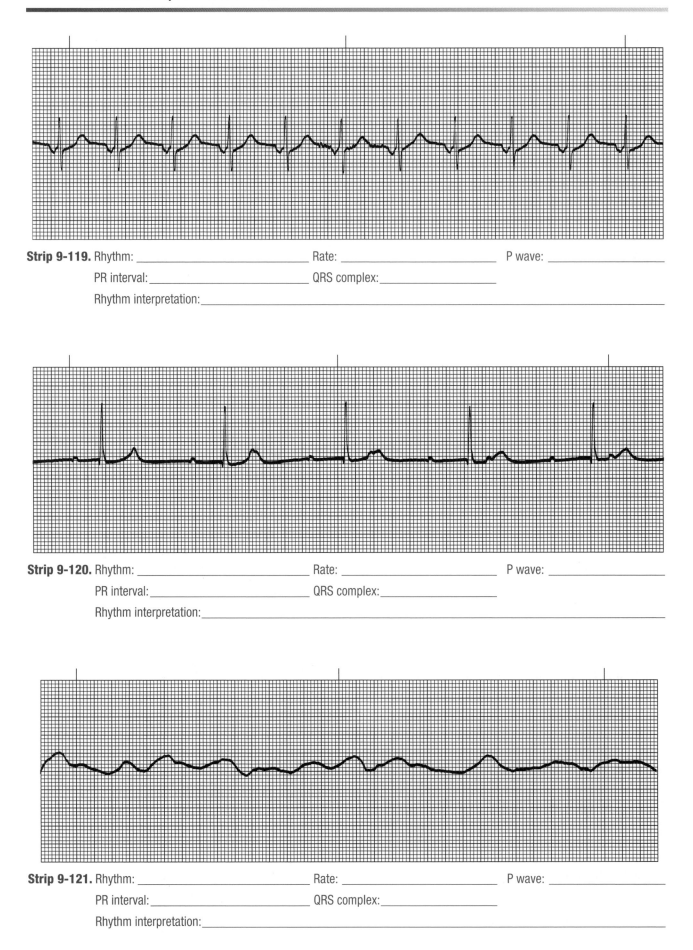

Strip 9-119. Rhythm: _____ Rate: _____ P wave: _____

PR interval: _____ QRS complex: _____

Rhythm interpretation: _____

Strip 9-120. Rhythm: _____ Rate: _____ P wave: _____

PR interval: _____ QRS complex: _____

Rhythm interpretation: _____

Strip 9-121. Rhythm: _____ Rate: _____ P wave: _____

PR interval: _____ QRS complex: _____

Rhythm interpretation: _____

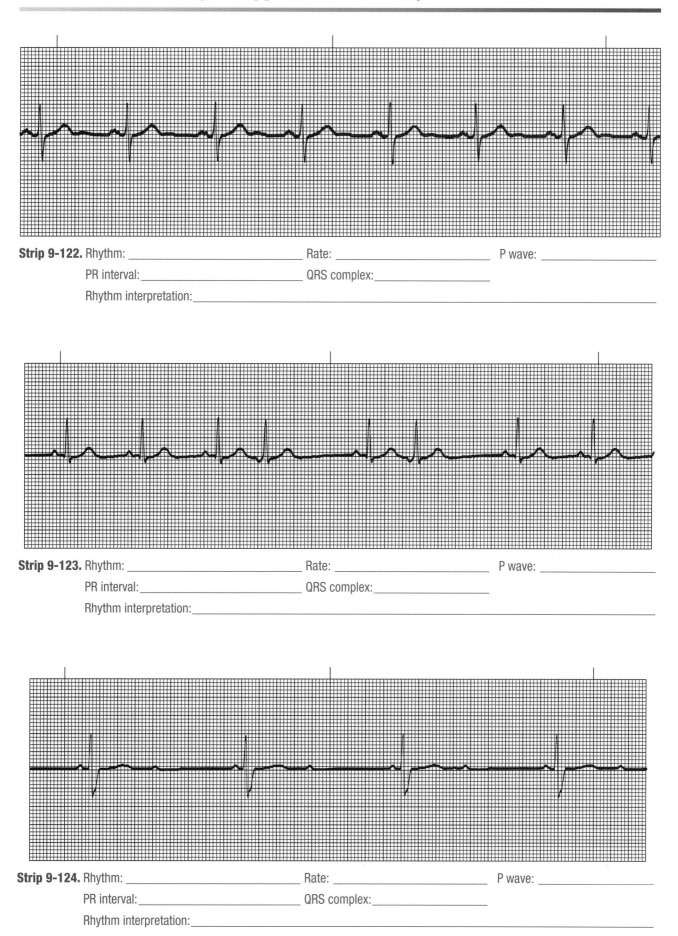

Strip 9-122. Rhythm: _____ Rate: _____ P wave: _____

PR interval: _____ QRS complex: _____

Rhythm interpretation: _____

Strip 9-123. Rhythm: _____ Rate: _____ P wave: _____

PR interval: _____ QRS complex: _____

Rhythm interpretation: _____

Strip 9-124. Rhythm: _____ Rate: _____ P wave: _____

PR interval: _____ QRS complex: _____

Rhythm interpretation: _____

10 Pacemakers

Overview

An artificial pacemaker is an electronic device that generates and transmits an electrical stimulus to the atria, the ventricles, or both, resulting in depolarization, followed by muscle contraction. The use of artificial pacemakers may be necessitated when there is a significant malfunction of the heart's electrical system, usually involving the sinus node, the atria, or the atrioventricular (AV) conduction pathways. The result may be a slow, fast, or irregular rhythm, which can affect the heart's pumping ability and may lead to a decrease in cardiac output and in the quality of life. Some indications for pacing include:

- **Sinoatrial dysfunction**
  1. Sinus bradycardia
  2. Sinus arrest
  3. Sinus exit block
  4. Atrial flutter or fibrillation
  5. Sick sinus syndrome (rhythms in which there is marked bradycardia alternating with periods of tachycardia, especially atrial flutter or fibrillation; also called tachy-brady syndrome).
  6. Chronotropic incompetence (sinus node is not capable of increasing its rate in response to activity
- **AV block**
  1. Second-degree AV block, Mobitz II
  2. Third-degree AV block
- **Hypersensitive carotid sinus** — Stimulation of the carotid sinus that causes episodes of asystole resulting in recurrent syncope; stimulators may include turning the head from side to side, or wearing a tight necktie or collar.

Pacemakers may be inserted on a temporary or permanent basis depending on the clinical situation. Temporary pacing is appropriate in emergent situations (transient symptomatic bradycardias or AV block associated with myocardial ischemia or drug toxicity). Temporary pacing may also be used to provide prophylactic therapy for high-risk patients during cardiac catheterization, during and after cardiac surgery, and to override tachyarrhythmias (overdrive pacing). Permanent pacemaker implantation is considered for unresolved rhythms or conditions in which clinical symptoms are present and for which long-term pacing is indicated.

A pacemaker system (Figure 10-1) consists of a pulse generator and a pacing lead:

- **Pulse generator** — The pulse generator houses a battery, a lead connector, and electronic circuitry for pacemaker settings.
- **Pacing lead** — The pacing lead has one or two metal poles (electrodes) at the tip of the catheter that come in contact with the endocardium (Figure 10-1). A lead with only one electrode at its tip is called a unipolar pacing system. A lead with two electrodes at its tip is called a bipolar pacing system. The pacing lead serves as a transmission line between the pulse generator and the endocardium. Electrical impulses are transmitted from the pulse generator (through the pacing lead) to the endocardium, while information about intrinsic electrical activity is relayed from the electrode tip (through the pacing lead) back to the generator. If the generator responds by sending a pacing impulse to the heart, it is called triggering. If a pacing impulse is not sent to the heart, this is called inhibition. Many permanent pacing leads are constructed with fixation devices (screws, tines, or barbs) that help guarantee long-term contact with the endocardium. Temporary pacing leads are not constructed with fixation devices so they can be easily removed when pacing is no longer required.

Pacemakers can function in a fixed rate mode or a demand mode:

- **Fixed rate mode (asynchronous)** — Fixed rate pacemakers initiate impulses at a set rate, regardless of the patient's intrinsic heart rate. This mode of pacing is known as asynchronous pacing because it's not synchronized to sense the patient's own heart rhythm. This may result in competition between the patient's natural (intrinsic) rhythm and that produced by the pacemaker. Ventricular tachycardia or ventricular fibrillation may be induced if the pacing stimulus falls during the vulnerable period of the cardiac cycle. Fixed rate pacemakers are rarely used today.
- **Demand mode (synchronous)** — A demand pacemaker paces only when the heart fails to depolarize on its own (fires only "on demand"). Demand pacemakers are designed with a sensing mechanism that inhibits discharge when the patient's heart rate is adequate and a pacing mechanism that triggers the pacemaker to fire when no intrinsic activity occurs within a preset period. This mode of pacing is called synchronous pacing because

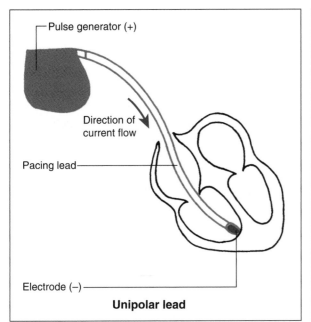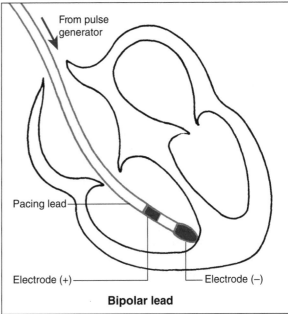

Figure 10-1. Unipolar and bipolar pacing leads.

it is synchronized to sense the patient's cardiac rhythm. Demand pacing is the most commonly used pacemaker mode today.

A pacemaker system may be single- or dual-chamber:

■ **Single-chamber** — A single-chamber pacemaker system uses one lead inserted into either the right atrium or the right ventricle. This pacemaker can sense and pace only the chamber into which it is inserted.

If a single-chamber atrial pacemaker senses a P wave, the pacemaker is inhibited from firing an electrical stimulus. If it does not sense a P wave, the pacemaker sends an electrical stimulus to the atrium. Stimulation of the atrium produces a *pacemaker spike* (a vertical line on the ECG), followed by a P wave (Figure 10-2, example A).

If a single-chamber ventricular pacemaker senses a QRS complex, the pacemaker is inhibited from firing an electrical stimulus. If it does not sense a QRS complex, the pacemaker sends an electrical stimulus to the ventricle. Stimulation of the ventricle produces a pacemaker spike followed by a wide QRS complex, resembling a ventricular ectopic beat (Figure 10-2, example B). Single-chamber ventricular pacing is the most commonly used temporary type of pacing and is also frequently used for permanent pacing. Single-chamber atrial or ventricular pacing can be used with epicardial pacing wires.

■ **Dual-chamber** — A dual-chamber pacemaker system uses two leads, one going to the right atrium and the other

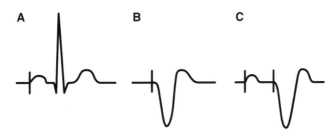

Figure 10-2. Single-chamber and dual-chamber pacing examples.
(A) The single-chamber atrial pacemaker looks for a P wave and fires into the atrium if no P wave is sensed; the pacing spike is followed by a P wave.
(B) The single-chamber ventricular pacemaker looks for a QRS complex and fires into the ventricle if no QRS is sensed; the pacing spike is followed by a wide QRS complex.
(C) The dual-chamber pacemaker looks for a P wave; if no P wave is sensed, the pacemaker delivers a stimulus into the atrium; the pacing spike is followed by a P wave. After a programmed electronic PR interval (the AV interval), if no QRS is sensed, a second stimulus is delivered into the ventricle; the pacing spike is followed by a wide QRS complex.

to the right ventricle. The dual-chamber pacemaker can sense and pace in both chambers.

If a dual-chamber pacemaker senses a P wave, the pacemaker is inhibited from firing an electrical stimulus. If the pacemaker does not sense a P wave, the pacemaker sends an electrical stimulus to the atrium. Stimulation of the atrium produces a pacemaker spike, followed by a P wave. The pacemaker is programmed to wait, simulating an electronic PR interval. In pacing terminology the artificial PR interval is called the *AV interval*. If a dual-chamber pacemaker senses a QRS complex, it is inhibited from firing an electrical stimulus. If the pacemaker does not sense a QRS complex, the pacemaker will send an electrical stimulus to the ventricle. Stimulation of the ventricle produces a pacemaker spike followed by a wide QRS complex. Figure 10-2, example C, shows stimulation of the atria and the ventricle by a dual-chamber pacemaker.

Dual-chamber pacemakers are often called AV sequential pacemakers because of their ability to stimulate the atria and ventricles in sequence (first the atria, then the ventricles), mimicking normal heart physiology and thus preserving the atrial kick.

Dual-chamber pacemakers are frequently used with permanent pacing and can also be used with epicardial pacing. Dual-chamber temporary pacing can be done, but it is difficult to place temporary atrial wires and it is not as reliable as ventricular pacing.

Temporary pacemakers

Temporary pacing can be accomplished with transcutaneous (external), transvenous, or epicardial methods:

■ *Transcutaneous pacing (TCP)* — TCP refers to the delivery of a pacing stimulus to the heart through pads placed on the patient's outer chest (Figure 10-3). Requirements for TCP include pacing pads, a pacing cable, and a defibrillator monitor with pacing capabilities. TCP is recommended as the initial pacing method of choice in emergent

cardiac situations. External pacemakers are noninvasive, effective, and quick and easy to apply. TCP provides only ventricular pacing.

TCP is indicated as a treatment for symptomatic bradyarrhythmias (sinus bradycardia, slow atrial flutter or fibrillation, Mobitz II second-degree AV block, or third-degree AV block). TCP is not effective in rhythms without meaningful contractile activity such as ventricular standstill and pulseless electrical activity (PEA) that occur in the setting of cardiac arrest. This is because the primary problem in these situations is the inability of the myocardium to contract when appropriately stimulated.

External pacemakers should not be relied upon for an extended period of time. They should be used only as a temporary measure in emergency situations until transvenous access is available or the cause of the bradyarrhythmia is resolved. Transvenous pacing is still the treatment of choice for patients requiring a temporary but longer period of pacemaker support.

The technique of TCP involves:

1. **Attach pacing pads to chest.** TCP involves attaching two large pacing pads to the skin surface of the patient's chest. Multifunction pads have the capability to monitor the heart rhythm, externally pace, and defibrillate through one set of pads. The pads have conductive gel on the inner surface to help transmit the electrical current through the chest wall. The large surface area of the pad and the conductive gel also help minimize the possibility of skin burns from the procedure. If possible, excess hair should be clipped before the pads are applied to maximize contact with the skin surface.

Most manufacturers recommend the pads be placed in an anterior-posterior position. The anterior pad (labeled "front") is placed to the left of the sternum, halfway between the xiphoid process and the left nipple. In the female patient, the anterior pad should be positioned under the left breast. The posterior pad (labeled "back") is placed on the left posterior chest directly behind the anterior pad.

Successful TCP requires a higher electrical current output (mA) than conventional transvenous pacing to overcome the resistance of the chest wall. Placement of the pacing pads affects the amount of current required to depolarize the ventricle. The placement that offers the most direct pathway to the heart usually requires the lowest mA in order to pace the heart. Currents of 50 mA or more may be associated with discomfort and sedation may be required.

2. **Connect pacing pads to defibrillator or monitor.** Connect the pacing pads to a pacing cable and a defibrillator monitor system with pacing capabilities.

3. **Initiate pacing.** Set the defibrillator or monitor to pace setting. Set the pacing rate first (usually 70), then slowly increase the mA until consistent ventricular capture is seen on the monitor (a pacing spike followed by a wide QRS complex, Figure 10-4). If capture is lost during pacing, the mA may have to be increased.

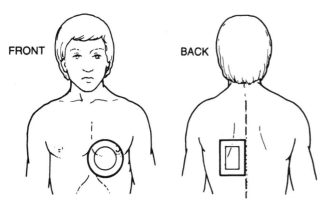

FRONT   **BACK**

Figure 10-3. External pacing pad placement (anterior-posterior position).

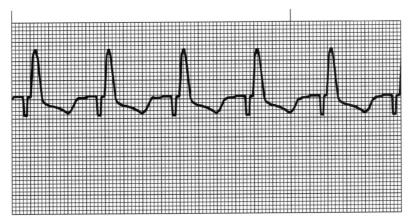

Figure 10-4. Electrical capture of the ventricle with an external pacemaker. This figure shows a square pacing spike (Zoll monitor-defibrillator with external pacemaker). Other external pacemakers may have a different pacing artifact.

Verify that electrical capture (seen on the monitor) is associated with mechanical capture (verified by palpable pulses). Evaluate pulses on the patient's right side to avoid confusion between the presence of an actual pulse and skeletal muscle contractions caused by the external pacemaker.

■ *Transvenous pacing* — Transvenous pacing refers to the delivery of a pacing stimulus to the heart through a vein (transvenous approach). Requirements for transvenous pacing include an external pulse generator, a pacing lead wire, and a bridging cable to connect the two (Figure 10-5).

Some indications for transvenous pacing include symptomatic bradyarrhythmias (sinus bradycardia, Mobitz II second-degree AV block, and third-degree AV block), prophylactic therapy during cardiac catheterization for high-risk patients, and overdrive pacing of tachyarrhythmias. Transvenous pacing is usually not effective when meaningful contractile activity is absent (ventricular standstill and PEA). For significant unresolved rhythm or conduction disorders, permanent pacing is required.

Temporary pulse generators are externally controlled by manipulating dials on the face of the unit. Removable batteries are contained within the generator housing. Prior to insertion of a pacing lead, prepare the equipment. Insert a new 9-volt battery into the battery compartment; set pacing rate at 100 beats per minute, the mA to 5, and the sensitivity knob to maximum clockwise position for demand (synchronous) pacing. Insert the end of the bridging cable into matching terminals on the pulse generator, and turn pulse generator on to verify proper functioning of the battery and unit.

The preferred routes of access for transvenous pacing are the right internal jugular vein, the right subclavian, and the right femoral vein. The pacing lead is inserted into the vein of choice and guided into the heart using fluoroscopy. Once the wire is visualized in the right atrium, a balloon

at the tip of the pacing catheter is inflated and the wire is floated through the tricuspid valve into the apex of the right ventricle for single-chamber ventricular pacing. Even though single-chamber atrial pacing and dual-chamber pacing can be done, single-chamber ventricular pacing is the most reliable and preferred choice for transvenous pacing. Once proper placement is verified, the balloon is deflated. The distal tail of the pacing catheter is connected to the negative connection of the bridging cable and the proximal tail is connected to the positive connection of the bridging cable.

Using the dials on the external pulse generator, adjust the pacemaker settings:

1. **Determine voltage threshold.** This is the smallest amount of voltage (mA) required to pace the heart. While watching the cardiac monitor, gradually turn down the mA until capture is lost (usually 0.7 to 1.0 mA) and then gradually turn up the mA until capture is regained. The point at which capture is regained is the threshold. Set the mA at twice threshold level.

2. **Set pacing rate.** This is determined by the physician (usually 70 beats per minute).

3. **Set sensitivity.** Sensitivity is usually maintained at maximum clockwise position (5 o'clock).

The number of temporary transvenous pacing leads being placed is decreasing, largely due to the improved reperfusion management of acute MI and improved access to permanent pacing systems.

■ *Epicardial pacing* — Epicardial pacing refers to the delivery of a pacing stimulus to the heart through wires placed on the epicardial surface of the atrium, ventricle, or both, during cardiac surgery. Two wires are attached to the atrium for single-chamber atrial pacing (one wire serves as ground) or to the ventricle for single-chamber ventricular pacing, or two wires are attached to both chambers for dual-chamber pacing. The wires are loosely sutured to the outer surface of the heart and pulled through the chest wall where they are attached to a bridging cable and an

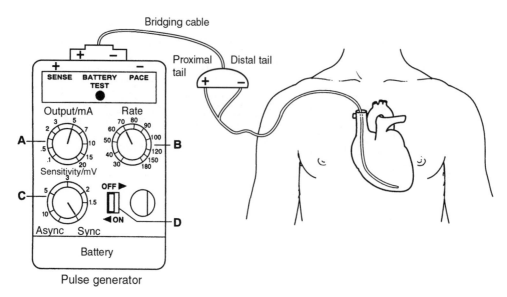

Figure 10-5.   Temporary transvenous pacemaker system.
A. Output or mA dial
  1. Controls the amount of electrical energy delivered to endocardium.
  2. Increase mA by turning dial clockwise to higher number; decrease mA by turning dial counterclockwise to lower number.
B. Rate dial
  1. Determines the heart rate in beats/minute at which the stimulus is to be delivered.
C. Sensitivity or mV dial
  1. Controls the ability of the generator to sense the electrical activity.
  2. In maximum clockwise position (5 o'clock), provides demand (synchronous) pacing.
  3. In maximum counterclockwise position (7 o'clock), provides fixed rate (asynchronous) pacing.
  4. Increase sensitivity (mV) by turning mV dial clockwise to lower number; decrease sensitivity by turning dial counterclockwise to higher number.
D. On/off control
  1. Activates/inactivates the pulse generator.

external pulse generator. Atrial wires usually exit to the right of the sternum and ventricular wires exit to the left. When no longer needed, the wires are gently pulled out through the wound.

Epicardial pacing is used after cardiac surgery to treat symptomatic bradyarrhythmias, as a prophylactic measure for high-risk patients, and to treat tachyarrhythmias using overdrive pacing techniques.

Permanent pacemakers

A permanent pacemaker system (Figure 10-6) refers to an implanted generator and a lead wire (or wires) that is introduced into the heart through a central vein (often the subclavian). The implant procedure is relatively simple, usually performed under local anesthesia and conscious sedation, and lasts about 1 hour. The procedure is facilitated by fluoroscopy, which enables the physician to view

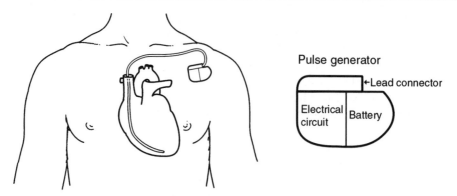

Figure 10-6.   Permanent pacemaker system.

the passage of the lead wire. After satisfactory placement of the pacing lead is confirmed, the lead is connected to the pacemaker generator. The generator is placed in the subcutaneous tissue just below the left or right clavicle. Generally the patient's nondominant side is chosen to minimize interference with the patient's daily activities.

The major reason for implanting a pacemaker is the presence of a symptomatic bradycardia. Symptomatic bradycardia is a term used to define a bradycardic rhythm that is directly responsible for symptoms such as syncope, transient dizziness, confusion, fatigue, exercise intolerance, congestive heart failure, dyspnea, and hypotension.

Permanent pacemaker technology has undergone major advances since pacemakers were first introduced in the 1950s. Early pacemakers paced a single chamber (the right ventricle) at a fixed rate. Today's pacemakers function as demand pacemakers, sensing the patient's natural beats and pacing the heart "on demand" (pacing only when needed). Most of the permanent pacemakers used today are the dual-chamber demand type. Although these dual-chamber models are more expensive, they maintain AV synchrony (the atria pace first, then the ventricles), preserving the atrial kick and often providing patients with a higher quality of life. Studies have shown that unnecessary pacing of the right ventricle can lead to heart failure and an increased incidence of atrial fibrillation. The newer dual-chamber devices can keep the amount of right ventricular pacing to a minimum and thus prevent worsening of the heart disease.

Permanent pacemakers are also available for specific conditions or needs:

■ **Rate-responsive pacemaker** — This pacemaker has sensors that detect changes in the patient's physical activity and automatically adjust the pacing rate to meet the body's metabolic needs. Rate-responsive pacing mimics the heart's normal rhythm, enabling patients to participate in more activities.

■ **Biventricular pacemaker** — A biventricular pacemaker, also known as cardiac resynchronization therapy (CRT), stimulates both the right and left ventricles. By pacing both ventricles, the pacemaker can resynchronize a heart whose opposing walls do not contract in synchrony (a problem that occurs in 25% to 50% of heart failure patients). CRT devices have been shown to reduce mortality and improve quality of life in patients with an ejection fraction of 35% or less or in patients with heart failure symptoms.

■ **Implantable cardioverter-defibrillators (ICDs)** — These devices have the ability to pace for bradycardia, and overdrive pace for tachycardia (antitachycardia pacing) and shock therapy (cardioversion and defibrillation). They are used in the treatment of patients at risk for sudden cardiac death.

Once the pacemaker is implanted, the following information is helpful to share with the patient:

1. **Periodic pacemaker checkups** — The pacemaker is periodically checked to ensure the device is operational and performing appropriately. This can be done in the physician's office or over the phone (remote monitoring). Most pacemakers are programmable, enabling the physician to adjust pacing therapy.

2. **Pacemaker safety** — Built-in filters protect pacemakers from electrical interference from most devices encountered in daily life, including microwave ovens. Security devices at airports should not cause any interference to the normal operation of the pacemaker; however, they may detect the metal in the pacemaker. In this situation, the pacemaker wearer can present an ID card indicating they have a pacemaker. Cell phones do not seem to damage or affect how the pacemaker works. Any activity that involves intense magnetic fields (such as arc welding) should be avoided. Medical tests involving the use of magnetic resonance imaging (MRI) are usually ruled out for patients with pacemakers.

3. **Pacemaker replacement** — The life of a pacemaker is affected by the type of pacemaker and how it is programmed to pace the heart. Today's pacemakers usually contain lithium-iodine batteries, which are designed to last many years. Pacemakers have a built-in indicator to signal when the battery is approaching depletion. Most reflect battery depletion by a gradual decrease in the pacing rate. The pacemaker is designed to operate for several months to allow adequate time to schedule a replacement procedure. Because the batteries are permanently sealed inside the pacemaker, the entire pacemaker is replaced when the battery runs down. Device replacement is usually a simpler procedure than the original insertion as it does not normally require leads to be replaced.

Permanent pacemaker identification codes

A universal coding system is used to describe the function of single- and dual-chamber pacemakers (Table 10-1). The code is comprised of five positions. Various letters are used for each position to describe a pacemaker function or characteristic. Only one letter is used per position:

■ **First position** — Identifies the chamber paced.

■ **Second position** — Identifies the chamber where intrinsic electrical activity is sensed.

■ **Third position** — Indicates how the pacemaker will respond when it senses intrinsic electrical activity.

■ **Fourth position** — Identifies programmable functions, the capability for transmitting and receiving data (communication), and the availability of rate responsiveness.

■ **Fifth position** — Identifies antitachycardia functions:

1. Antitachycardia pacing (overdrive pacing) — this function paces the heart faster than the intrinsic rate to convert the tachycardia

2. Shock (synchronized cardioversion and defibrillation)

3. Dual — performs both a pacing function and a shock function.

Table 10-1.
Five-letter pacemaker identification code

First letter	Second letter	Third letter	Fourth letter	Fifth letter
Chamber paced	*Chamber sensed*	*Response to sensing*	*Programmable functions*	*Antitachycardia functions*
O = None	O = None	O = None	O = None	O = None
A = Atrium	A = Atrium	I = Inhibits pacing	P = Simple programmable	P = Antitachycardia pacing
V = Ventricle	V = Ventricle	T = Triggers pacing	M = Multiprogrammable	S = Shock
D = Dual (A and V)	D = Dual (A and V)	D = Dual (I and T)	C = Communication	D = Dual (P and S)
			R = Rate responsive	

Pacemaker terms

Pacemaker firing

A pacemaker produces a programmed current (stimulus) at a set rate to the myocardium. This energy travels from the pacemaker generator through the lead wires to the myocardial muscle. This is known as pacemaker firing and produces a pacemaker spike (a vertical line) on the ECG tracing.

Basic pacemaker operation consists of a closed-loop circuit in which electrical current flows between two metal poles (one negative, the other positive). The stimulating pulse is delivered through the negative electrode. Pacemaker systems may be either unipolar or bipolar. Unipolar pacing has one pole (electrode) within the heart, with the other pole being the metal case of the pulse generator. Pacemaker systems utilizing unipolar pacing involve a large electrical circuit. The circuit travels between the electrode on the distal tip of the pacing lead in contact with the myocar-dium (the negative pole) to the pacemaker generator located in soft tissue (the positive pole). Because of the greater distance between the two poles, the ECG tracing will show a large, easily visible pacing spike (Figure 10-7, example A). Pacemaker systems utilizing bipolar pacing involve a small electrical circuit. The current travels between the electrode on the distal tip of the pacing lead (negative pole) to the proximal electrode located a few millimeters above the distal tip (the positive pole). Because of the smaller distance between the two poles, the ECG tracing will show a small spike (Figure 10- 7, example B) or may not be visible in some leads on an ECG (Figure 10-7, example C).

Capture

The term *capture* refers to the successful stimulation of the myocardium by a pacemaker stimulus, resulting in depolarization. Capture is evidenced on the ECG by a pacemaker spike followed by either an atrial complex (P wave),

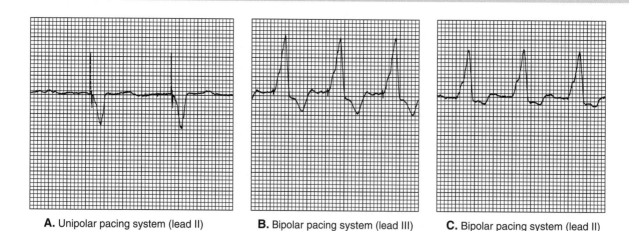

A. Unipolar pacing system (lead II)   **B.** Bipolar pacing system (lead III)   **C.** Bipolar pacing system (lead II)

Figure 10-7. Unipolar and bipolar pacing spikes. (A) Large pacing spikes are seen with a unipolar pacing system. (B) Small pacing spikes are seen with a bipolar pacing system. (C) The electrical circuit is so small in a bipolar system that some leads may not show a pacing spike.

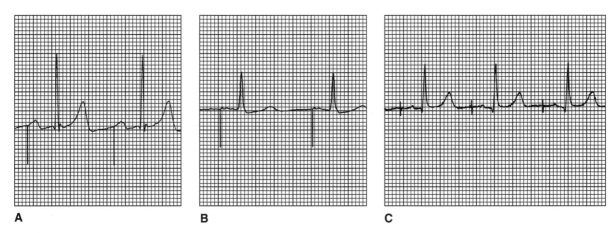

Figure 10-8. Examples of atrial capture.
(A) Atrial capture with normal-looking P waves conducted with long PR interval.
(B) Atrial capture with abnormal-looking P waves.
(C) Atrial capture with small, pointed P waves not immediately following the atrial spike.

a ventricular complex (QRS), or both, depending on the chambers being paced. Capture beats are normal.

Atrial depolarization from a pacing stimulus results in a pacing spike followed by atrial activity (P wave). The morphology of the P waves produced may resemble that of sinus beats and be normal looking, or may be abnormal in appearance and so small that they are difficult to see. The P waves may not immediately follow the atrial pacing spike. The P waves may also be associated with a long PR interval. Examples are shown in Figure 10-8.

Normal ventricular depolarization is simultaneous (both ventricles depolarize at the same time), resulting in a narrow QRS complex of 0.10 second or less in duration. Ventricular depolarization from a pacing stimulus is sequential (one ventricle depolarizes, then the other), prolonging the duration of depolarization, resulting in a wide QRS complex of 0.12 second or greater. The wide QRS complex immediately follows the pacing spike (Figure 10-9, example A). An exception to the wide QRS rule is the biventricular pacemaker. This pacemaker simultaneously paces the right and left ventricle,

resulting in normal depolarization and a narrow QRS complex.

Sensing

Sensing is the ability of the pacemaker to detect intrinsic electrical impulses (the patient's own electrical activity) or electrical impulses produced by a pacemaker (paced activity). If the pacemaker detects electrical activity, it is inhibited from delivering a stimulus. If the pacemaker does not detect electrical activity, it is triggered to initiate an electrical stimulus.

Intrinsic beat

An intrinsic beat (also called native beat) is produced by the patient's natural electrical system (Figure 10-9, example B). Intrinsic beats are normal.

Automatic interval (pacing interval)

The automatic interval refers to the heart rate at which the pacemaker is set. This interval is measured from one pacing spike to the next consecutive pacing spike. For

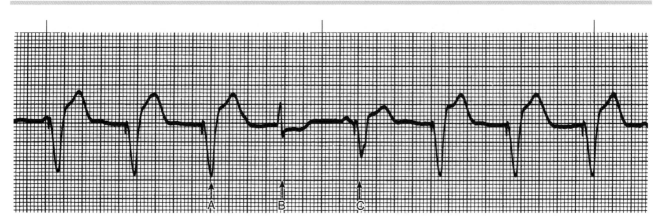

Figure 10-9. (A) Ventricular capture beat, (B) native beat, (C) fusion beat.

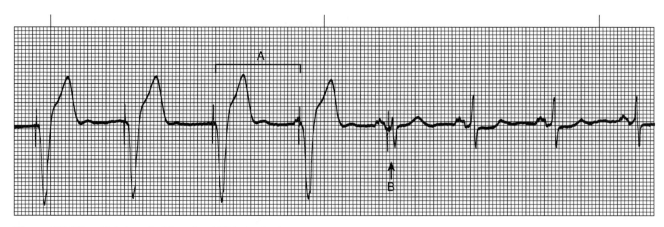

Figure 10-10.   (A) Automatic interval and (B) fusion beat.

atrial pacing, measure from one atrial pacing spike to the next consecutive atrial pacing spike. This is called the A-A interval, analogous to the P-P interval of intrinsic waveforms. For ventricular pacing, measure from one ventricular pacing spike to the next consecutive ventricular pacing spike (Figure 10-10, example A). This is called the V-V interval, analogous to the R-R interval of intrinsic waveforms.

Fusion beat

A fusion beat occurs when the pacemaker fires an electrical stimulus at the same time the patient's own electrical impulse fires an electrical stimulus. This results in part of the ventricle being depolarized by the pacemaker and part by the patient's own intrinsic impulse. The fusion beat is evidenced on the ECG by a pacemaker spike that occurs at the programmed rate (occurs on time), followed by a QRS that is different in height or width from the paced beats and the patient's intrinsic beats (Figures 10-9 and 10-10).

The fusion beat has characteristics of both pacemaker and patient forces, although one usually dominates the other. In Figure 10-9, example C, the fusion beat has more characteristics of the patient's paced beats than his intrinsic beats. In Figure 10-10, example B, the fusion beat has more characteristics of the patient's intrinsic beats than his paced beats. Fusion beats are normal and are usually seen only with ventricular pacing.

Pseudofusion beat

A pseudofusion beat occurs when the pacemaker fires an electrical stimulus after the patient's spontaneous impulse has already started depolarizing the ventricle. The pacing stimulus has no effect since the ventricle is already being depolarized. The pseudofusion beat is evidenced on the monitor by a pacemaker spike occurring at the programmed rate (occurs on time), along with a native QRS complex. The intrinsic QRS is not altered in height or width (Figure 10-11). Pseudofusion beats are normal and are usually seen only with ventricular pacing.

Pacemaker rhythm

Stimulation of the atria for one beat is called an atrial paced beat. Continuous stimulation of the atria (all P waves

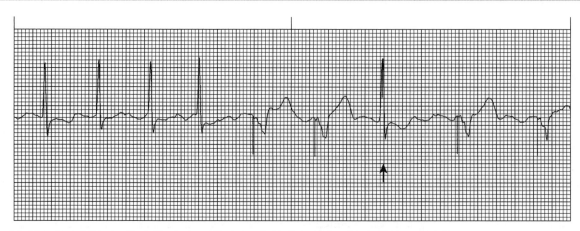

Figure 10-11.   Pseudoinfusion beat. The pacing spike is located in the middle of the QRS in complex 7.

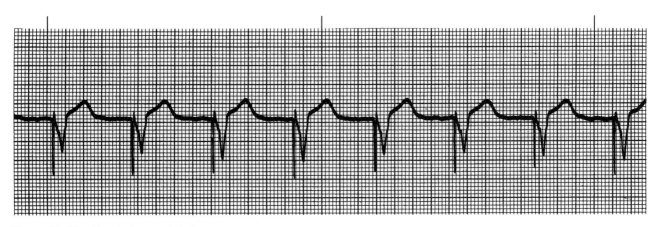

Figure 10-12.   Ventricular paced rhythm.

are pacemaker induced) is called an atrial paced rhythm. Stimulation of the ventricle for one beat is called a ventricular paced beat. Continuous stimulation of the ventricle (all QRS complexes are pacemaker induced) is called a ventricular paced rhythm (Figure 10-12). Stimulation of the atria and the ventricle for one beat is called an AV paced beat. Continuous stimulation of the atria and ventricles (all P waves and QRS complexes are pacemaker induced) is called an AV paced rhythm.

Pacemaker malfunctions

Basic functions of all pacemakers include the ability to fire (stimulus release), to sense electrical activity (intrinsic and paced), and to capture (depolarize the chambers being paced). Most malfunctions can be traced to problems with the generator (parameter settings, battery failure), the lead (problems at the interface between the catheter tip and the endocardium, fracture in the lead or its insulating surface), or to a disconnection in the system.

This section includes a description of pacemaker malfunctions, common causes, and interventions. It is directed primarily toward temporary transvenous ventricular

demand pacemakers since nurses can interact more directly with them than with permanent pacemakers. The same concepts apply to permanent pacemakers, but correction of malfunctions requires the use of a pacemaker programmer or an actual surgical procedure to reposition the pacing lead or replace the generator.

Failure to fire

With failure to fire, the pacemaker does not discharge a stimulus to the myocardium. Failure to fire will be evidenced on the ECG by an absence of a pacemaker spike where expected (Figure 10-13). Failure to fire is abnormal.

Causes and interventions for failure to fire:
1. **Battery depletion** — Replace the battery.
2. **Disconnection in the system** — Check the connections between the generator, bridging cable, and lead; reconnect or tighten connections.
3. **Fracture of lead or lead insulation** — Do an overpenetrated chest X-ray to detect fractures; have the physician replace the lead.
4. **Electromagnetic interference (EMI)** — Exposure of a pacing unit to such sources as electrocautery devices or

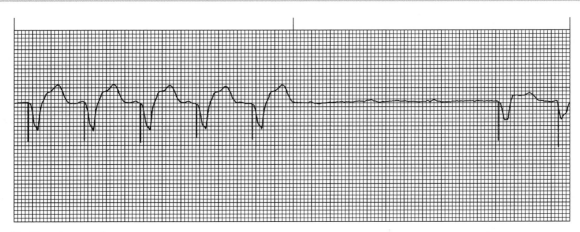

Figure 10-13.   Failure to fire.

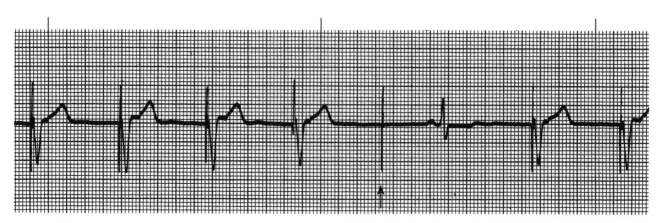

Figure 10-14.   Loss of capture.

MRI may result in inhibition of the pacing stimulus. Avoid exposure.

5. **Pacemaker is turned off** — Make sure the pacemaker is turned on; the generator should be secured away from the patient.

Failure to capture

With failure to capture, the pacemaker delivers a pacing stimulus, but electrical stimulation of the myocardium (depolarization) does not occur. This is evidenced on the ECG by pacemaker spikes that occur at the programmed rate, but are not followed by a P wave (for atrial pacing) or a QRS (for ventricular pacing). Figure 10-14 shows loss of capture with ventricular pacing. Loss of capture is abnormal.

Causes and interventions for failure to capture

1. **mA output is too low** — Increase the mA on the generator by turning the mA dial clockwise to a higher number (Figure 10-5). Over a period of days, inflammation or fibrin formation at the catheter tip may raise the stimulation threshold, requiring a higher mA output.

2. **Lead is out of position or lying in infarcted tissue** — The electrode tip must be in contact with the endocardium for the electrical stimulus to cause depolarization. Infarcted tissue does not respond to a stimulus. Do an overpenetrated chest X-ray to determine the catheter position. If the catheter is out of position, a temporary maneuver is to turn the patient on his left side (gravity may allow the catheter to contact the endocardium). A physician will have to reposition the lead.

3. **Electrolyte imbalance** — Electrolyte imbalances can alter the ability of the heart to respond to a pacing stimulus. Check serum electrolyte levels and replace if needed.

Sensing failure

Sensing failure occurs when the pacemaker either does not sense myocardial electrical activity or the pacemaker oversenses the wrong signals. Sensing failure falls into two categories: undersensing and oversensing.

Undersensing

The most common cause of sensing failure is undersensing. The pacemaker does not sense (does not "see") myocardial electrical activity (either intrinsic or paced) and fires earlier than it should. Undersensing is recognized on the ECG by a pacing spike that occurs earlier than expected. It can occur with capture (Figure 10-15, examples B and C) or without (Figure 10-15, example A).

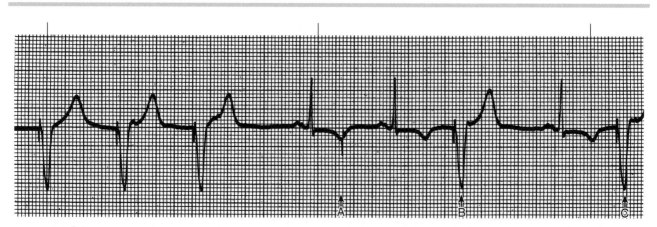

Figure 10-15.   Undersensing.

Causes and interventions for undersensing

1. **Sensitivity set too low** — Increase sensitivity by turning sensitivity dial clockwise to a lower number.

2. **Pacing catheter out of position or lying in infarcted tissue** — The electrode tip must be in contact with the endocardium to sense appropriately. Infarcted tissue does not have the ability to sense. Do an overpenetrated chest X-ray to determine catheter position. If the catheter is out of position, a temporary maneuver is to turn the patient on his left side, which may allow migration of the catheter into a better position. A physician will have to reposition the lead.

3. **Pacemaker set on asynchronous (fixed rate) mode** — With asynchronous pacing, the sensing circuit is off. Turn the sensitivity dial to synchronous (demand) pacing mode.

Oversensing

The pacemaker is too sensitive ("sees" too much) and is sensing the wrong signals (large P waves, large T waves, muscle movement), causing the pacemaker to fire later than it should. Oversensing is recognized on the ECG by a paced beat that occurs later than expected. (Figure 10-16).

Causes and interventions for oversensing

1. **Sensitivity set too high** — Decrease sensitivity by turning the sensitivity dial counterclockwise to higher number.

Analyzing pacemaker strips (ventricular demand type)

When analyzing pacemaker rhythm strips, you will again need to use either calipers or an index card. The following steps should be helpful.

■ **Step one** — Place an index card above two consecutively paced beats. Mark the automatic interval. "Left mark" and "right mark" mentioned in the steps below refer to marks on the index card. The automatic interval measurement will assist you in determining if the pacemaker fired on time, too early, too late, or not at all.

■ **Step two** — Starting on the left side of the strip, analyze each pacing spike you see. The patient's intrinsic beats

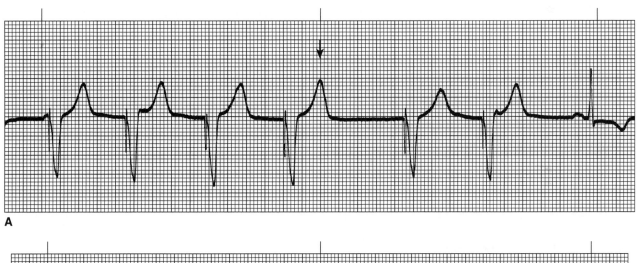

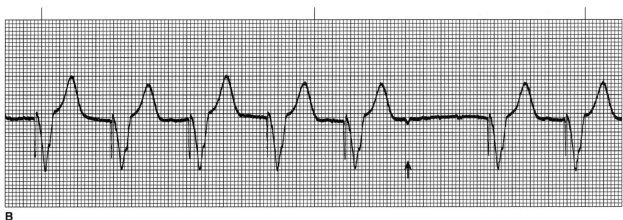

Figure 10-16.   Oversensing.
Example A: Pacemaker is sensing a large T wave.
Example B: Pacemaker is sensing a low waveform artifact. *Note*: Using the automatic interval marks on index card, place right mark on spike of late paced beat. The left mark will match whatever pacemaker is sensing.

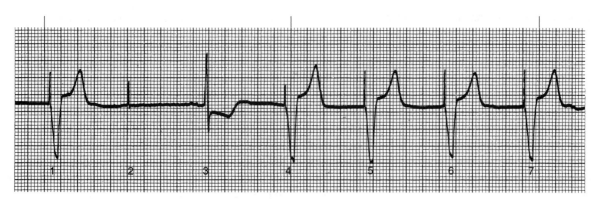

Figure 10-17. Pacemaker analysis strip #1.

■ The automatic interval can be measured from #4 to #5. Mark automatic interval on index card. Left mark and right mark in steps below refer to marks on index card.

■ #2 can be analyzed by placing left mark on spike of paced beat just before it; #2 matches right mark; #2 occurs on time, but does not cause ventricular depolarization (no QRS), so it indicates failure to capture.

■ #3 is a native beat and doesn't need analyzing.

■ #4 can be analyzed by placing left mark on R wave of native QRS just before it; #4 matches right mark; #4 occurs on time and causes ventricular depolarization (QRS present), indicating ventricular capture beat.

■ #5, #6, and #7 can be analyzed by placing left mark on spikes of the paced beats immediately preceding each beat to be analyzed; all occur on time and cause ventricular depolarization, indicating ventricular capture beats.

Interpretation: Ventricular paced rhythm with one intrinsic beat and one episode of failure to capture (abnormal pacemaker function).

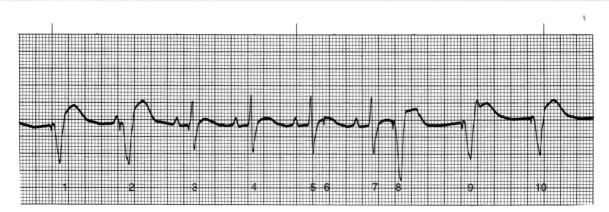

Figure 10-18. Pacemaker analysis strip #2.

■ The automatic interval can be measured from #1 to #2. Mark automatic interval on index card. Left mark and right mark in steps below refer to marks on index card.

■ #2 can be analyzed by placing left mark on spike of paced beat immediately before it; #2 matches right mark; #2 occurs on time and causes ventricular depolarization, indicating ventricular capture beat.

■ #3 has a tiny spike at the beginning of the R wave so it needs analyzing; place left mark on spike of paced beat just before it; #3 matches right mark and is different in height or width from the native and paced beats, so this represents a fusion beat.

■ #4 and #5 are native beats and do not need analyzing.

■ #6 can be analyzed by placing left mark on R wave of native beat just before it; #6 occurs earlier than right mark; #6 indicates that the pacemaker did not sense the preceding beat and represents an undersensing problem.

■ #7 is a native beat and does not need analyzing.

■ #8 can be analyzed by placing left mark on R wave of native beat just before it; #8 occurs earlier than right mark; #8 indicates that the pacemaker did not sense the preceding beat and represents an undersensing problem. *Note*: #6 represents an undersensing problem without capture, while #8 represents an undersensing problem with capture. #6 occurs during the refractory period when capture is unable to occur.

■ #9 can be analyzed by placing left mark on spike of paced beat just before it; #9 matches right mark; #9 occurs on time and causes ventricular depolarization, indicating a ventricular capture beat.

■ #10 can be analyzed by placing left mark on spike of paced beat just before it; #10 matches right mark; #10 occurs on time and causes ventricular depolarization, indicating a ventricular capture beat.

Interpretation: Ventricular paced rhythm with one fusion beat, three intrinsic beats, and two episodes of undersensing (abnormal pacemaker function).

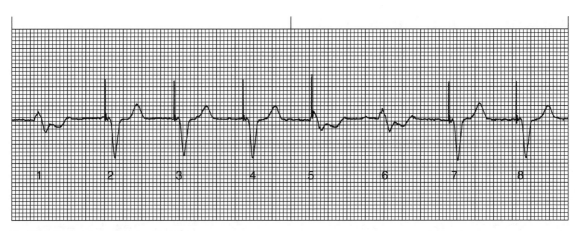

Figure 10-19.   Pacemaker analysis strip #3.

■ The automatic interval can be measured from #2 to #3. Mark automatic interval on index card. Left mark and right mark in steps below refer to marks on index card.

■ #1 is a native beat and doesn't need analyzing.

■ #2 can be analyzed by placing left mark on R wave of native QRS just before it; #2 matches right mark; #2 occurs on time and causes ventricular depolarization, indicating ventricular capture beat.

■ #3 can be analyzed by placing left mark on spike of paced beat just before it; #3 matches right mark; #3 occurs on time and causes ventricular depolarization, indicating ventricular capture beat.

■ #4 can be analyzed by placing left mark on spike of paced beat just before it; #4 matches right mark; #4 occurs on time and causes ventricular depolarization, indicating ventricular capture beat.

■ #5 can be analyzed by placing left mark on spike of paced beat just before it; #5 matches right mark; #5 shows a pacing spike which occurs at the same time as the native beat, but does not alter its height or width, indicating a pseudoinfusion beat.

■ #6 is a native beat and doesn't need analyzing.

■ #7 can be analyzed by placing left mark on R wave of native QRS just before it; #7 matches right mark; #7 occurs on time and causes ventricular depolarization, indicating ventricular capture beat.

■ #8 can be analyzed by placing left mark on spike of paced beat just before it; #8 matches right mark; #8 occurs on time and causes ventricular depolarization, indicating ventricular capture beat.

Interpretation: Ventricular paced rhythm with one pseudofusion beat and two intrinsic beats (normal pacemaker function).

do not need analyzing, but you need to be able to identify them from the paced beats.

■ **Step three** — Identify the pacing spike to be analyzed (only analyze one spike at a time). Using the marked index card, place the left mark on the spike of the paced beat or R wave of the native beat immediately preceding the pacing spike being analyzed.

■ **Step four** — Observe the relationship of the right mark with the spike being analyzed to determine the answer:

Spike occurs on time (spike matches right mark)	*Spike occurs too early* (spike earlier than right mark)
■ Ventricular capture beat (normal) ■ Fusion beat (normal) ■ Pseudofusion beat (normal) ■ Failure to capture (abnormal)	■ Undersensing (abnormal)
Spike doesn't occur	*Spike occurs too late* (spike later than right mark)
■ Failure to fire (abnormal)	■ Oversensing (abnormal)

Figures 10-17 through 10-19 have been analyzed for you.

Rhythm strip practice: Pacemakers

Follow the four basic steps for analyzing pacemaker rhythm strips. Analyze and interpret each pacing strip as shown in Figures 10-17 through 10-19. All pacemaker strips are lead II, a positive lead, unless otherwise noted. Check your answers with the answer keys in the appendix.

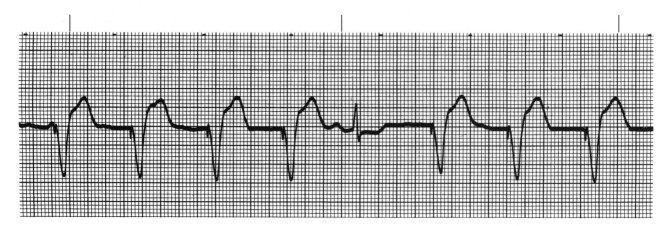

Strip 10-1. Analysis:_____

Interpretation: _____

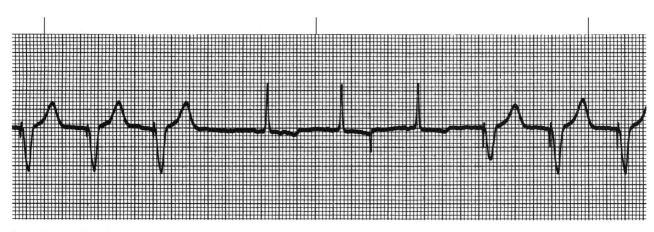

Strip 10-2. Analysis:_____

Interpretation: _____

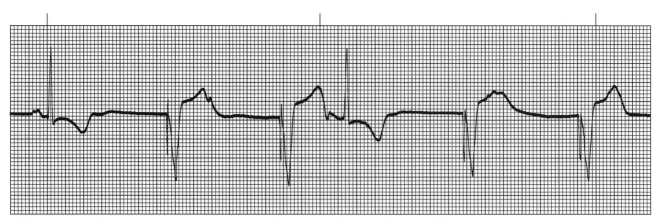

Strip 10-3. Analysis:_____

Interpretation: _____

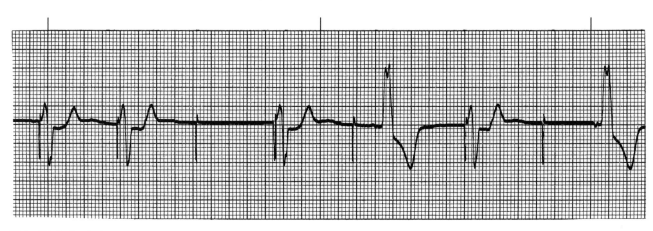

Strip 10-4. Analysis:_____

Interpretation: _____

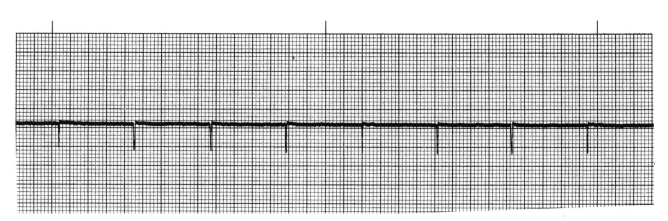

Strip 10-5. Analysis:_____

Interpretation: _____

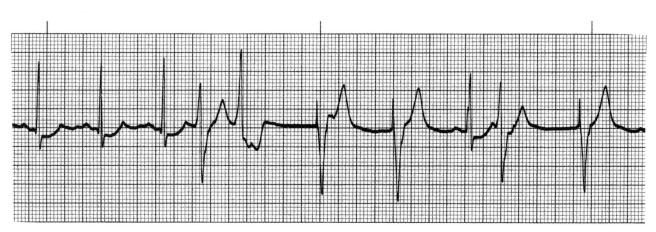

Strip 10-6. Analysis:_____

Interpretation: _____

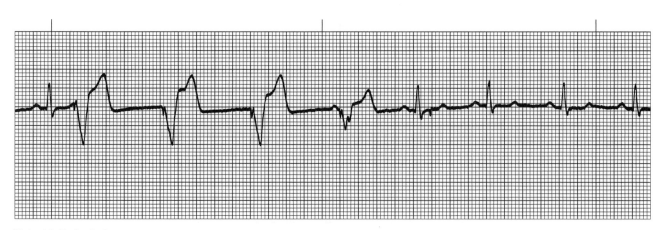

Strip 10-7. Analysis:_____

Interpretation:_____

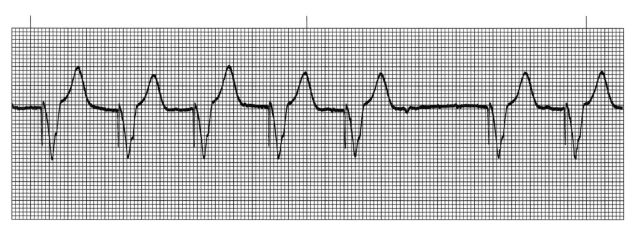

Strip 10-8. Analysis:_____

Interpretation:_____

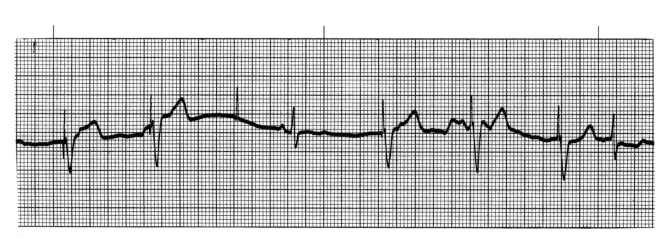

Strip 10-9. Analysis:_____

Interpretation:_____

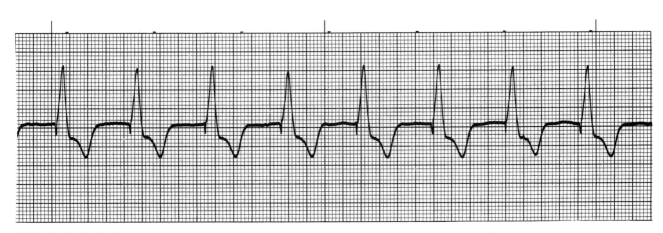

Strip 10-10. Analysis:_____

Interpretation: _____

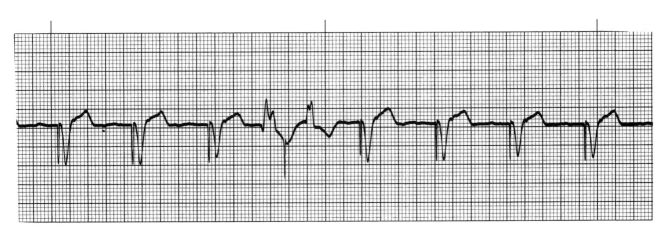

Strip 10-11. Analysis:_____

Interpretation: _____

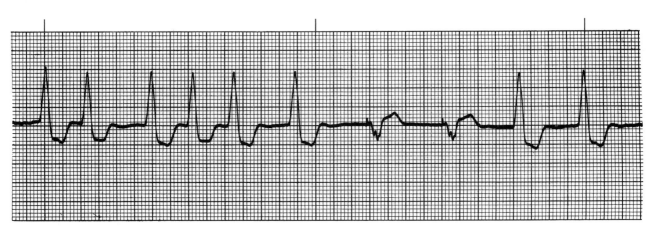

Strip 10-12. Analysis:_____

Interpretation: _____

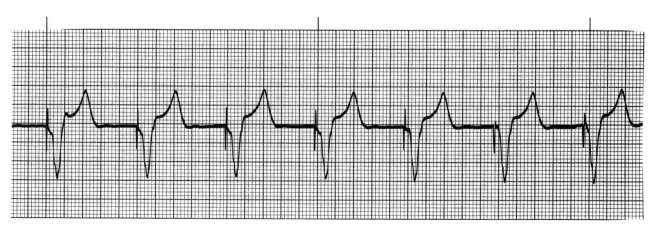

Strip 10-13. Analysis:_____

Interpretation: _____

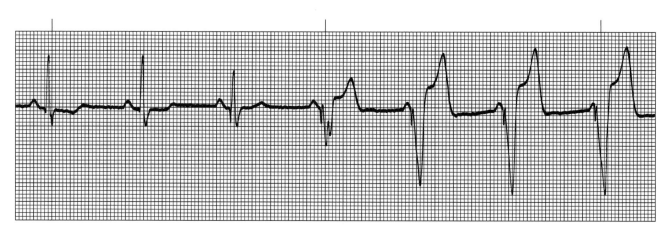

Strip 10-14. Analysis:_____

Interpretation: _____

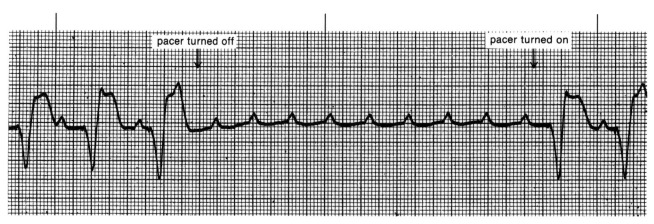

pacer turned off

pacer turned on

Strip 10-15. Analysis:_____

Interpretation: _____

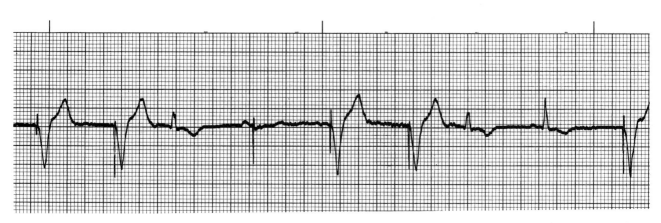

Strip 10-16. Analysis:_____

Interpretation: _____

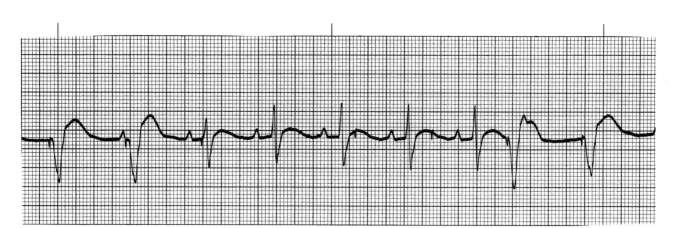

Strip 10-17. Analysis:_____

Interpretation: _____

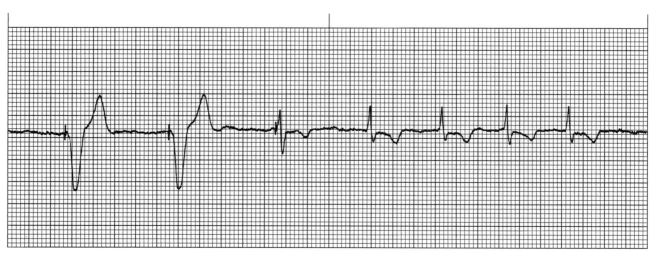

Strip 10-18. Analysis:_____

Interpretation: _____

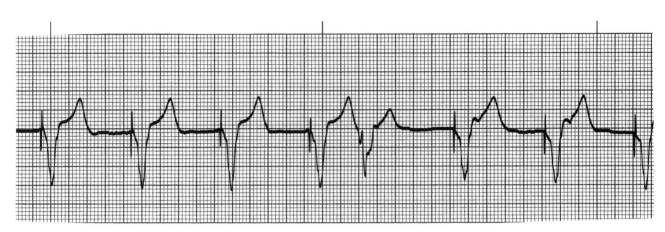

Strip 10-19. Analysis:_____

Interpretation: _____

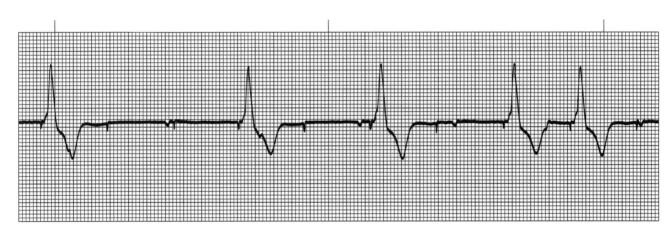

Strip 10-20. Analysis:_____

Interpretation: _____

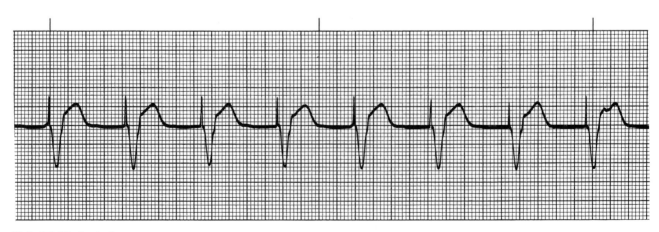

Strip 10-21. Analysis:_____

Interpretation: _____

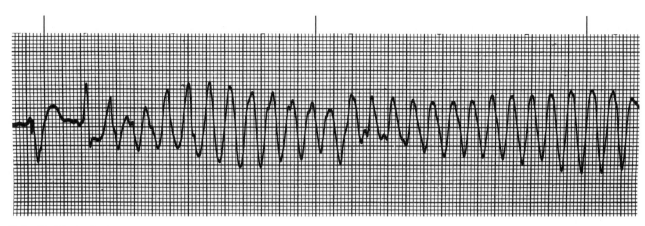

Strip 10-22. Analysis:_____

Interpretation: _____

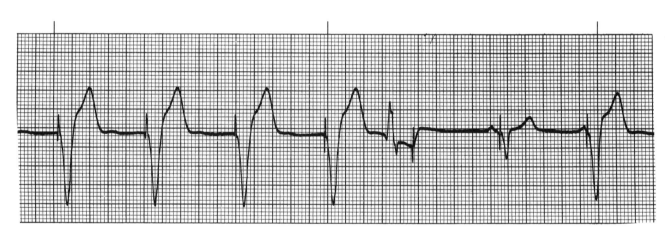

Strip 10-23. Analysis:_____

Interpretation: _____

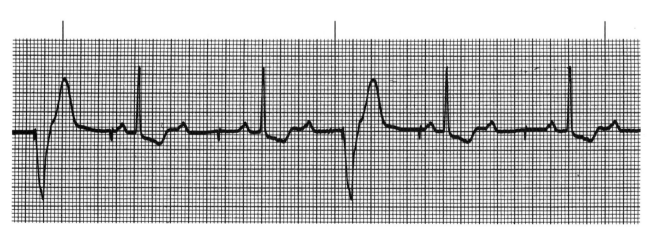

Strip 10-24. Analysis:_____

Interpretation: _____

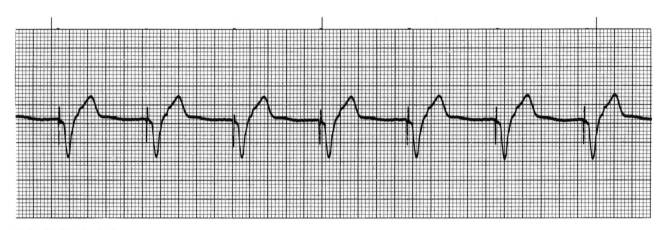

Strip 10-25. Analysis:_____

Interpretation: _____

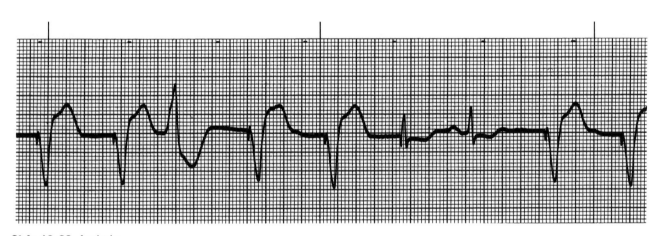

Strip 10-26. Analysis:_____

Interpretation: _____

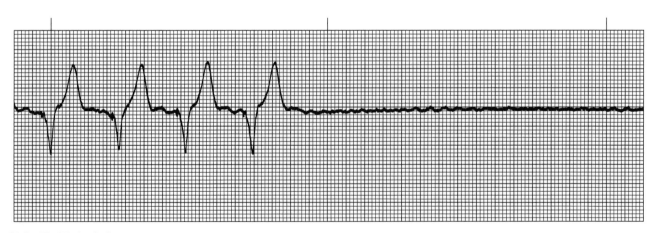

Strip 10-27. Analysis:_____

Interpretation: _____

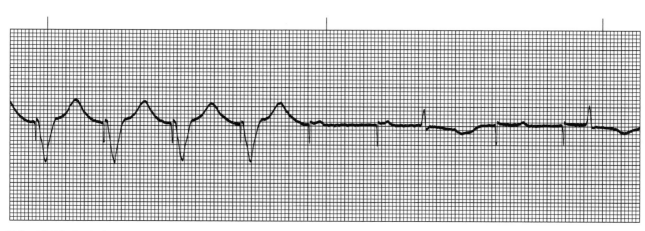

Strip 10-28. Analysis:_____

Interpretation: _____

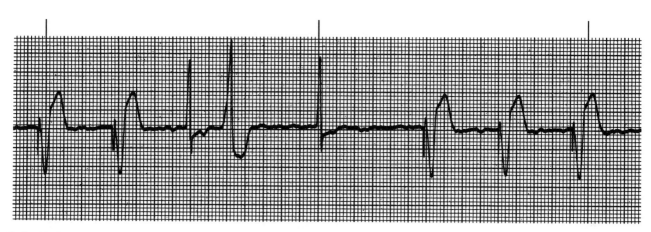

Strip 10-29. Analysis:_____

Interpretation: _____

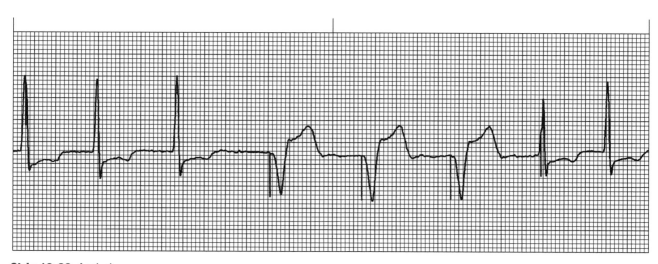

Strip 10-30. Analysis:_____

Interpretation: _____

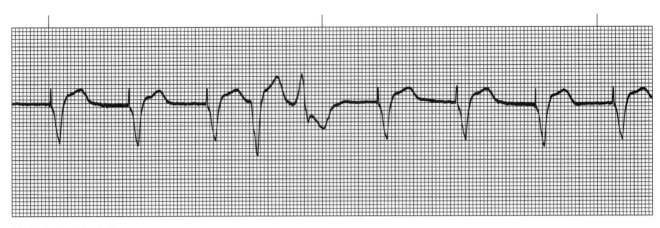

Strip 10-31. Analysis:_____

Interpretation: _____

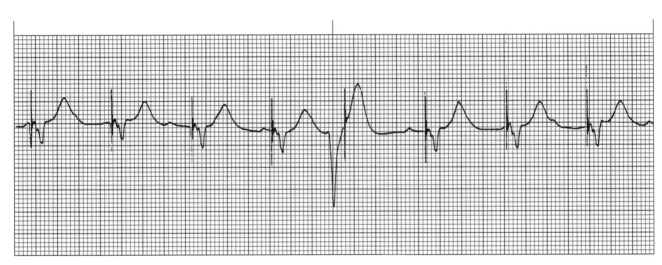

Strip 10-32. Analysis:_____

Interpretation: _____

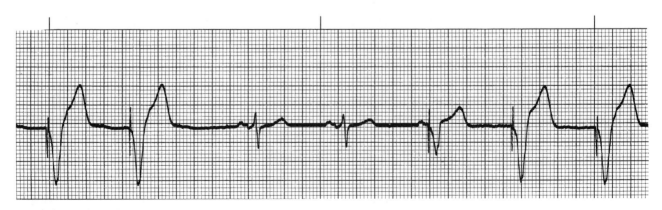

Strip 10-33. Analysis:_____

Interpretation: _____

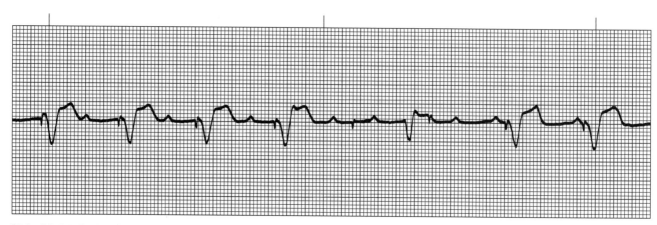

Strip 10-34. Analysis:_____

Interpretation:_____

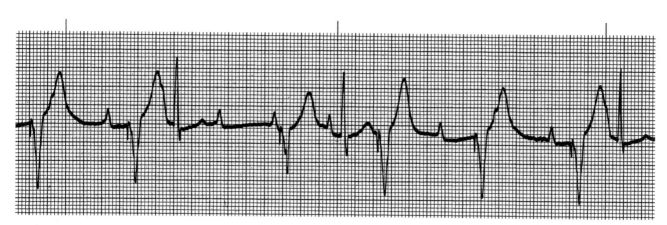

Strip 10-35. Analysis:_____

Interpretation:_____

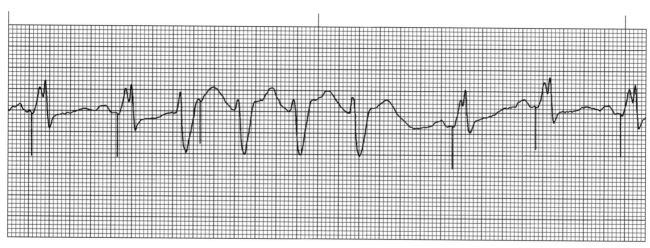

Strip 10-36. Analysis:_____

Interpretation:_____

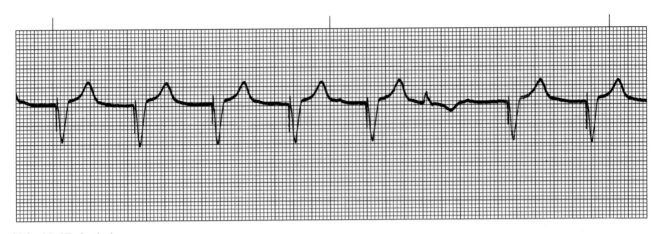

Strip 10-37. Analysis:_____

Interpretation: _____

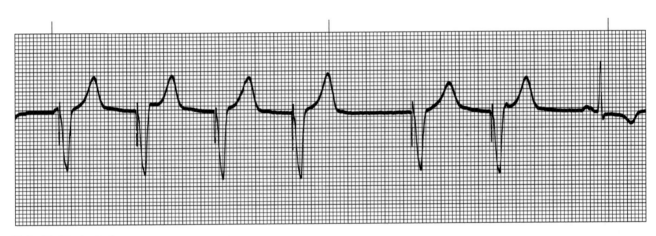

Strip 10-38. Analysis:_____

Interpretation: _____

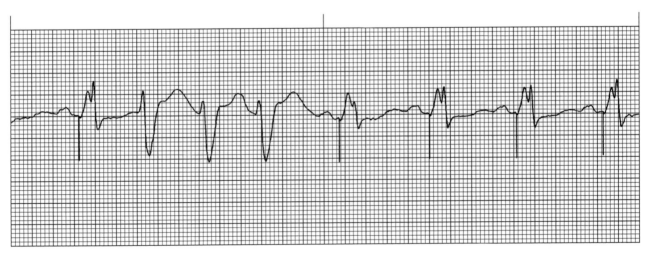

Strip 10-39. Analysis:_____

Interpretation: _____

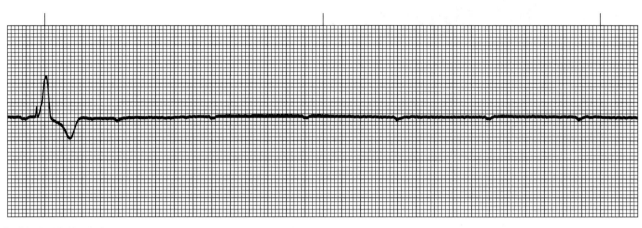

Strip 10-40. Analysis:_____

Interpretation: _____

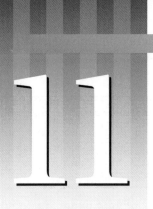

11 Posttest

Posttest: All rhythm groups
For arrhythmia strips

Follow the five basic steps in analyzing a rhythm strip. Interpret the rhythm by comparing this data with the ECG characteristics for each rhythm.

For pacemaker strips

Follow the four basic steps for analyzing pacemaker rhythm strips. Analyze and interpret each pacing strip as shown in Figures 10-17 through 10-19.

All strips are lead II, a positive lead, unless otherwise noted. Check your answers with the answer key in the appendix.

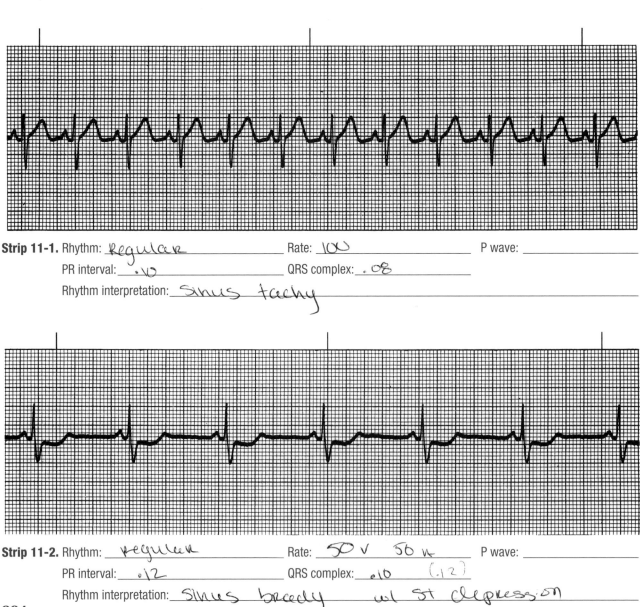

Strip 11-1. Rhythm: _Regular_ Rate: _100_ P wave: _____

PR interval: _.10_ QRS complex: _.08_

Rhythm interpretation: _Sinus tachy_

Strip 11-2. Rhythm: _Regular_ Rate: _50 v 50 A_ P wave: _____

PR interval: _.12_ QRS complex: _.10 (.12)_

Rhythm interpretation: _Sinus brady w/ ST depression_

284

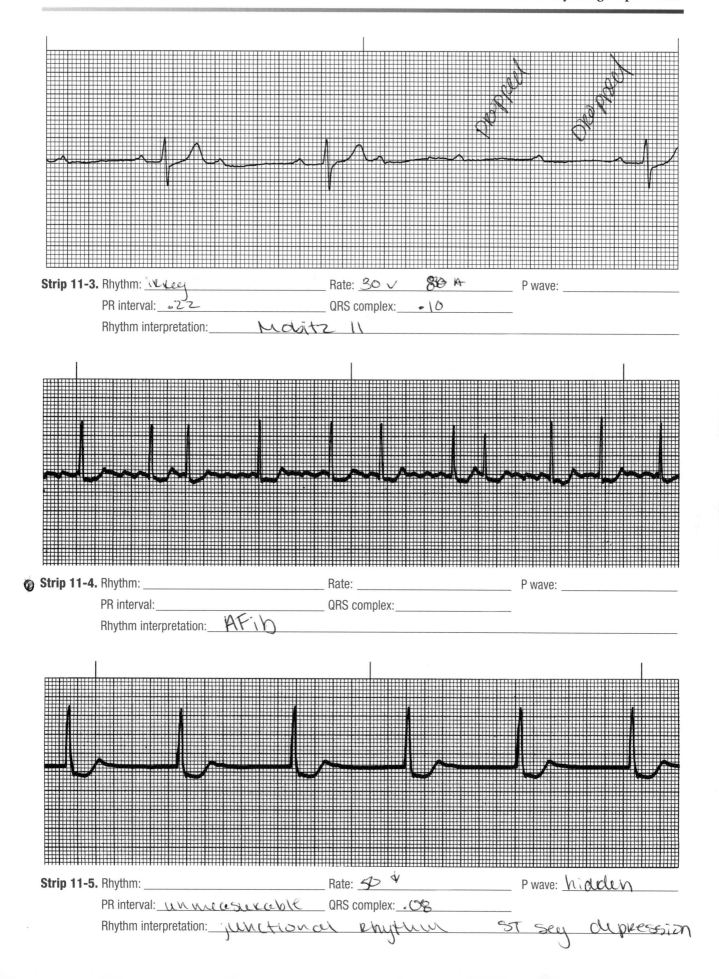

Strip 11-3. Rhythm: _irreg_   Rate: _30 ∨_   _80 A_   P wave: _____

PR interval: _.22_   QRS complex: _.10_

Rhythm interpretation: _____ Mobitz II _____

Strip 11-4. Rhythm: _____ Rate: _____ P wave: _____

PR interval: _____ QRS complex: _____

Rhythm interpretation: _AFib_

Strip 11-5. Rhythm: _____ Rate: _40 ∨_   P wave: _hidden_

PR interval: _unmeasurable_ QRS complex: _.08_

Rhythm interpretation: _junctional rhythm_   _ST seg depression_

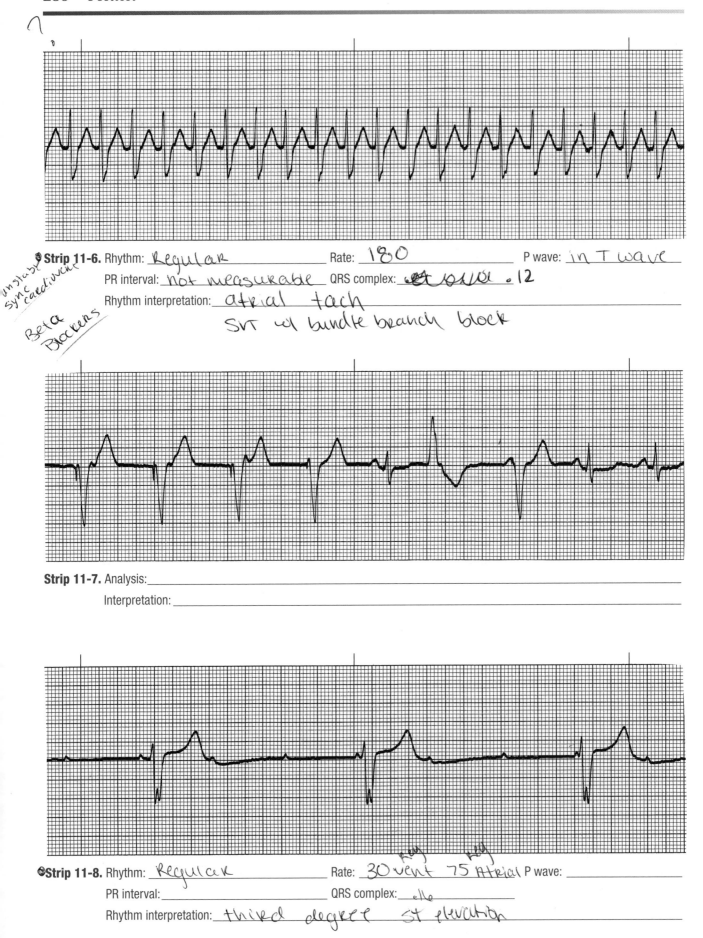

Strip 11-6. Rhythm: _Regular_ Rate: _180_ P wave: _in T wave_

PR interval: _not measurable_ QRS complex: _at least .12_

Rhythm interpretation: _atrial tach_

SVT w/ bundle branch block

unstable sync cardivian

Beta Blockers

Strip 11-7. Analysis: _____

Interpretation: _____

Strip 11-8. Rhythm: _Regular_ Rate: _30 vent 75 Atrial_ P wave: _____

PR interval: _____ QRS complex: _.16_

Rhythm interpretation: _third degree ST elevation_

anti

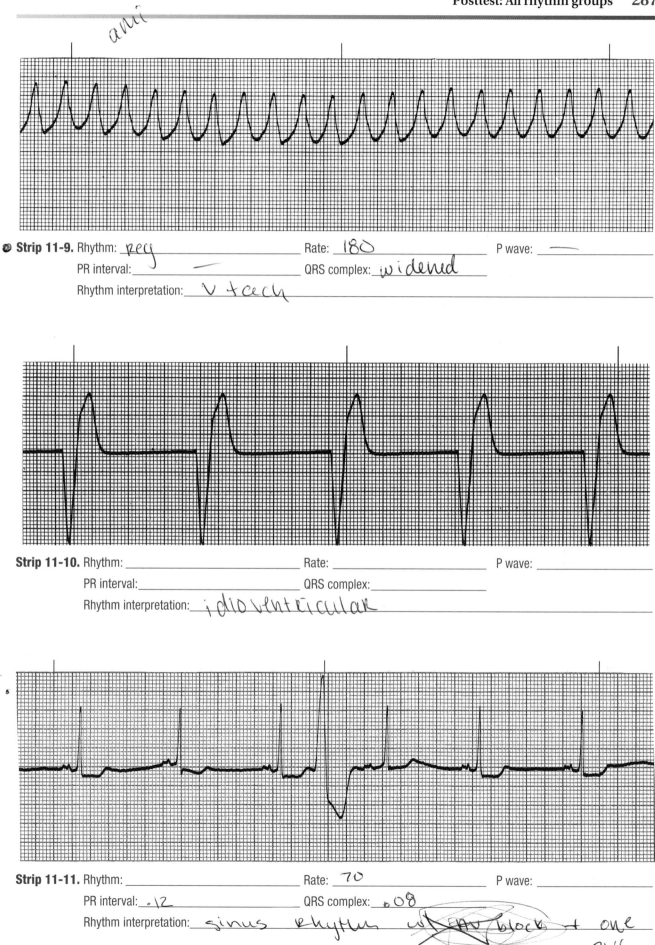

Strip 11-9. Rhythm: _reg_____ Rate: _180_____ P wave: _____

PR interval: _____—_____ QRS complex: _widened_____

Rhythm interpretation: _V tech_____

Strip 11-10. Rhythm: _____ Rate: _____ P wave: _____

PR interval: _____ QRS complex: _____

Rhythm interpretation: _idioventricular_____

Strip 11-11. Rhythm: _____ Rate: _70_____ P wave: _____

PR interval: _.12_____ QRS complex: _.08_____

Rhythm interpretation: _sinus rhythm w/ AV block + one_____
PVC

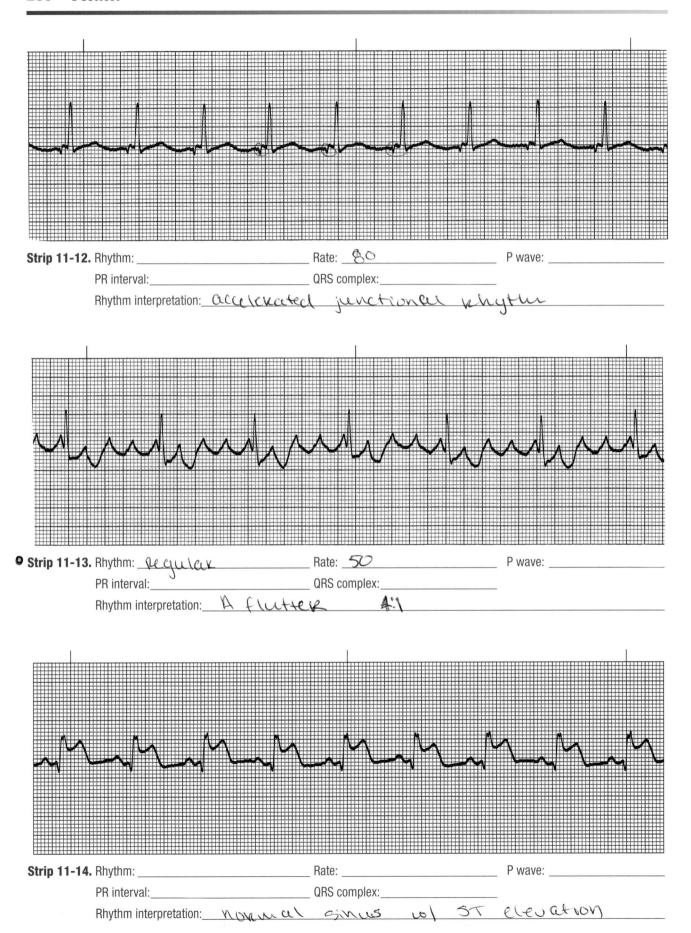

Strip 11-12. Rhythm: _____ Rate: _80_____ P wave: _____

PR interval: _____ QRS complex: _____

Rhythm interpretation: _accelerated junctional rhythm_____

Strip 11-13. Rhythm: _Regular_____ Rate: _50_____ P wave: _____

PR interval: _____ QRS complex: _____

Rhythm interpretation: _A flutter   4:1_____

Strip 11-14. Rhythm: _____ Rate: _____ P wave: _____

PR interval: _____ QRS complex: _____

Rhythm interpretation: _normal sinus w/ ST elevation_____

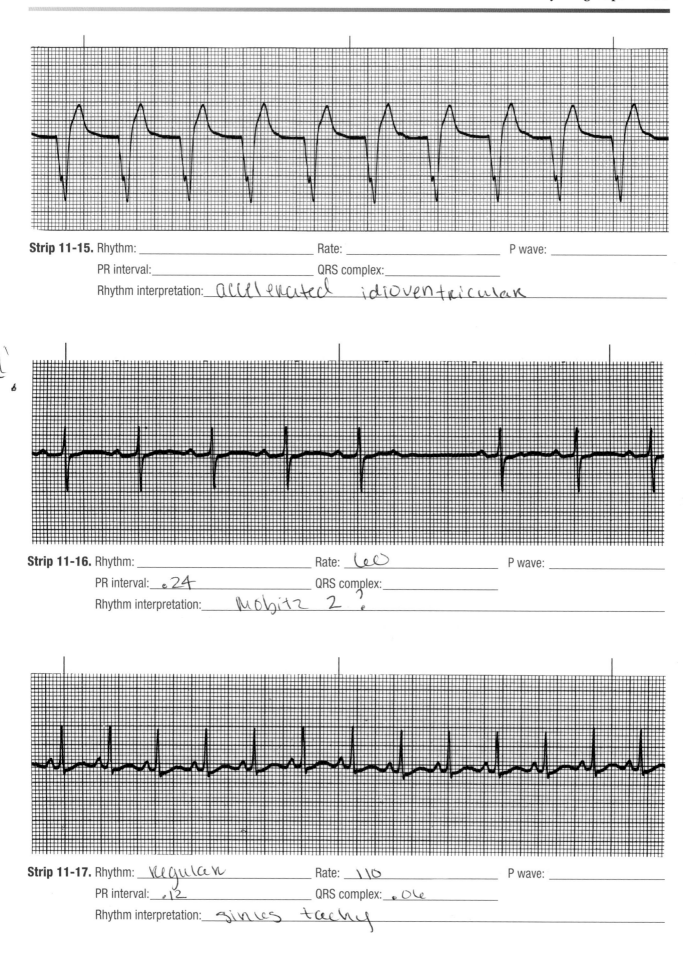

Strip 11-15. Rhythm: _____ Rate: _____ P wave: _____

PR interval: _____ QRS complex: _____

Rhythm interpretation: _accellerated idioventricular_____

Strip 11-16. Rhythm: _____ Rate: _60__ P wave: _____

PR interval: _.24_____ QRS complex: _____

Rhythm interpretation: _Mobitz 2 ?_____

Strip 11-17. Rhythm: _regular_____ Rate: _110__ P wave: _____

PR interval: _.12_____ QRS complex: _.06__

Rhythm interpretation: _sinus tachy_____

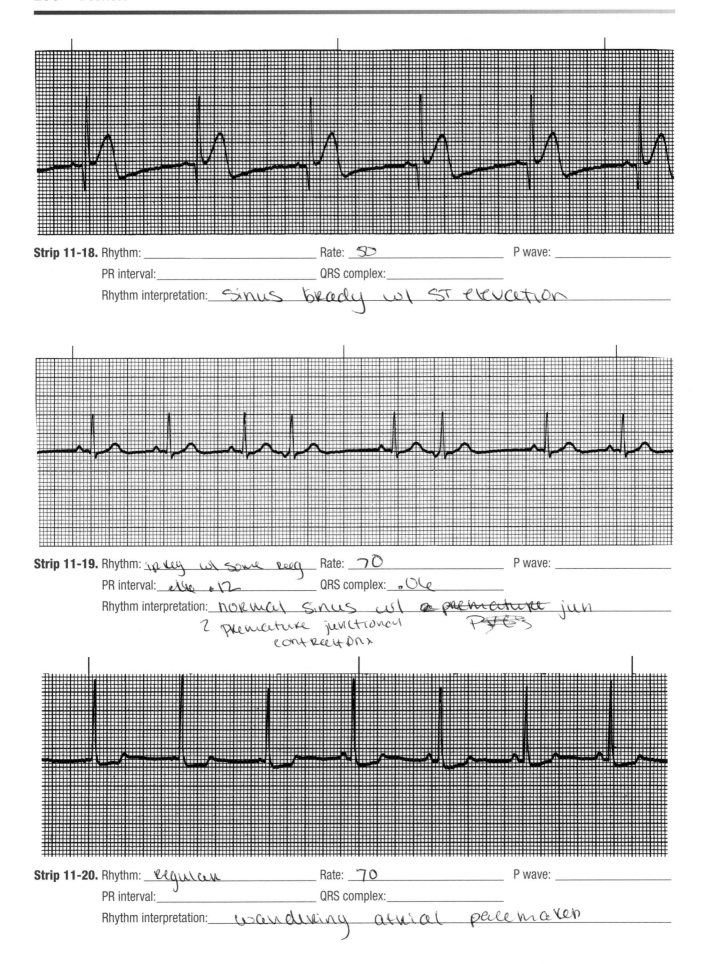

Strip 11-18. Rhythm: _____ Rate: _SD_____ P wave: _____

PR interval: _____ QRS complex: _____

Rhythm interpretation: _Sinus brady w/ ST elevation_____

Strip 11-19. Rhythm: _irreg w/ some reg_ Rate: _70_____ P wave: _____

PR interval: _else .12_____ QRS complex: _.06_____

Rhythm interpretation: _normal sinus w/ a premature jun_

2 premature junctional   PJC's

contractions

Strip 11-20. Rhythm: _regular_____ Rate: _70_____ P wave: _____

PR interval: _____ QRS complex: _____

Rhythm interpretation: _wandering atrial pacemaker_____

chaotic

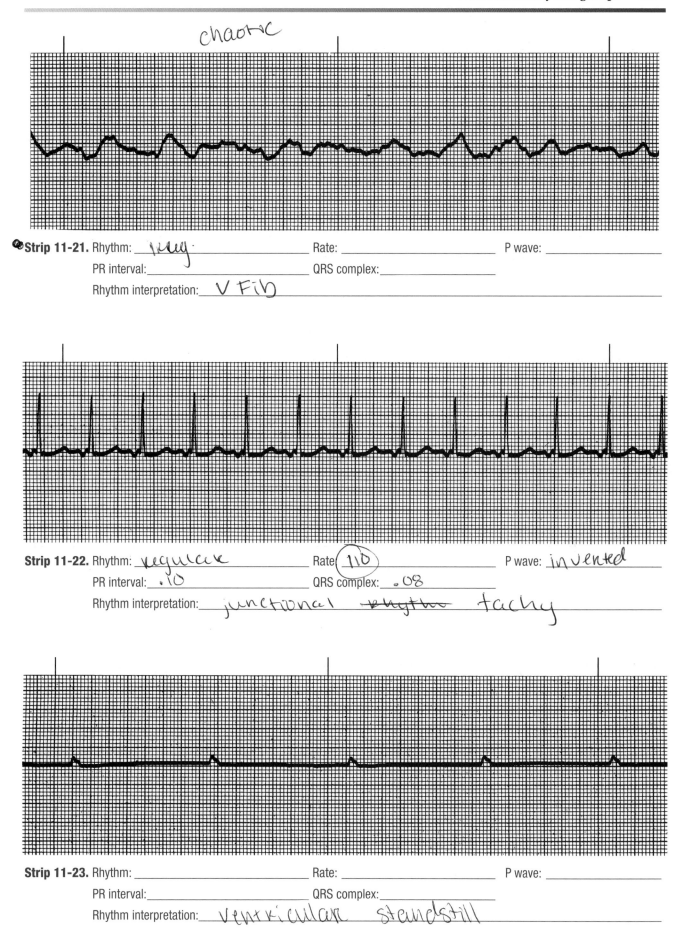

Strip 11-21. Rhythm: _irreg_ _____ Rate: _____ P wave: _____
PR interval: _____ QRS complex: _____
Rhythm interpretation: _V Fib_ _____

Strip 11-22. Rhythm: _regular_ _____ Rate: (_110_) _____ P wave: _inverted_
PR interval: _.10_ _____ QRS complex: _.08_ _____
Rhythm interpretation: _junctional_ ~~rhythm~~ _tachy_ _____

Strip 11-23. Rhythm: _____ Rate: _____ P wave: _____
PR interval: _____ QRS complex: _____
Rhythm interpretation: _ventricular standstill_ _____

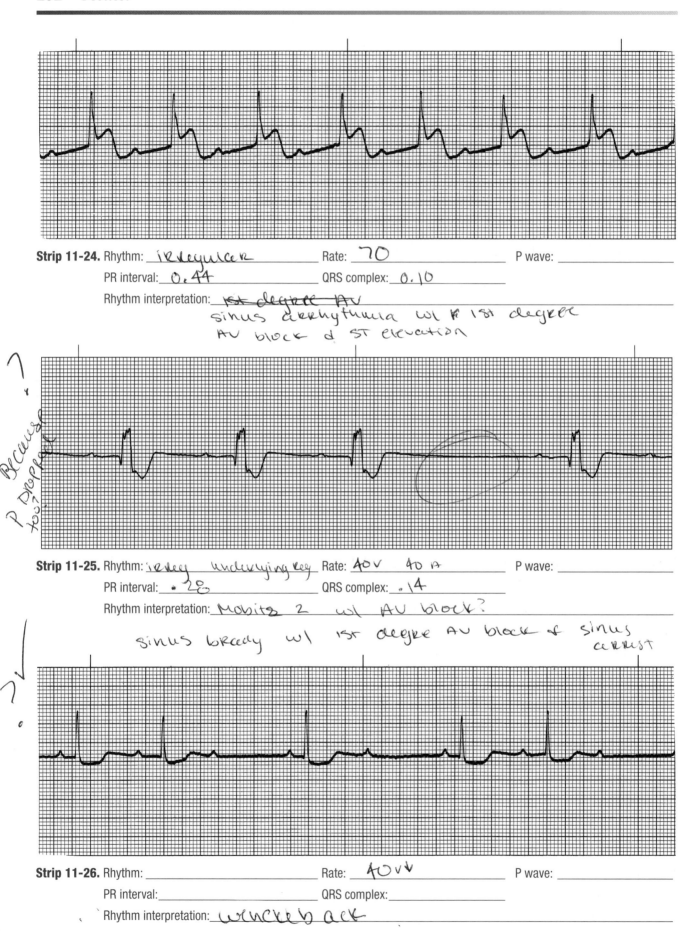

Strip 11-24. Rhythm: _irregular_   Rate: _70_   P wave: _____

PR interval: _0.44_   QRS complex: _0.10_

Rhythm interpretation: _~~1st degree AV~~_
sinus arrhythmia w/ ~~R~~ 1st degree
AV block & ST elevation

Because ↗
P Dropped ↗
too ?

Strip 11-25. Rhythm: _irreg   underlying reg_   Rate: _40 v   40 A_   P wave: _____

PR interval: _.28_   QRS complex: _.14_

Rhythm interpretation: _Mobitz 2   w/ AV block?_
sinus brady w/ 1st degree AV block & sinus
arrest

? ↗

Strip 11-26. Rhythm: _____   Rate: _40 v v_   P wave: _____

PR interval: _____   QRS complex: _____

Rhythm interpretation: _ventric act_

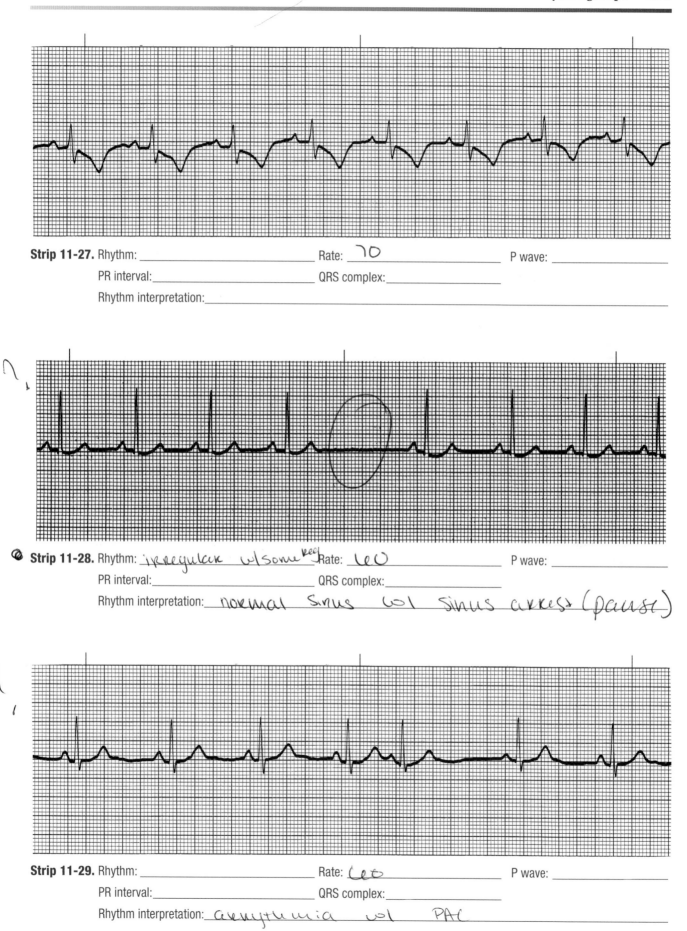

Strip 11-27. Rhythm: _____ Rate: _70_____ P wave: _____

PR interval:_____ QRS complex:_____

Rhythm interpretation:_____

Strip 11-28. Rhythm: _irregular w/some beat_ Rate: _60_____ P wave: _____

PR interval:_____ QRS complex:_____

Rhythm interpretation: _normal sinus w/ sinus arrest (pause)_

Strip 11-29. Rhythm: _____ Rate: _60_____ P wave: _____

PR interval:_____ QRS complex:_____

Rhythm interpretation: _arrhythmia w/ PAC_

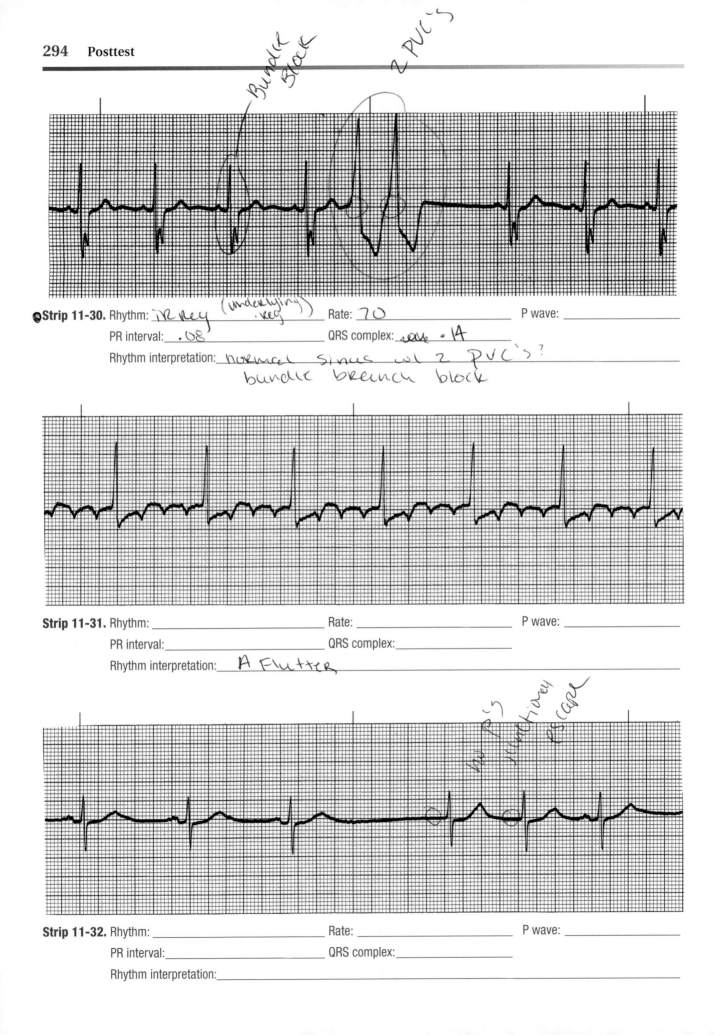

Bundle Block

2 PVC's

Strip 11-30. Rhythm: _NR Reg (underlying reg)_ Rate: _70_ P wave: _____

PR interval: _.08_ QRS complex: _.14_

Rhythm interpretation: _normal sinus w/ 2 PVC's?_
bundle branch block

Strip 11-31. Rhythm: _____ Rate: _____ P wave: _____

PR interval: _____ QRS complex: _____

Rhythm interpretation: _A Flutter_

Strip 11-32. Rhythm: _____ Rate: _____ P wave: _____

PR interval: _____ QRS complex: _____

Rhythm interpretation: _____

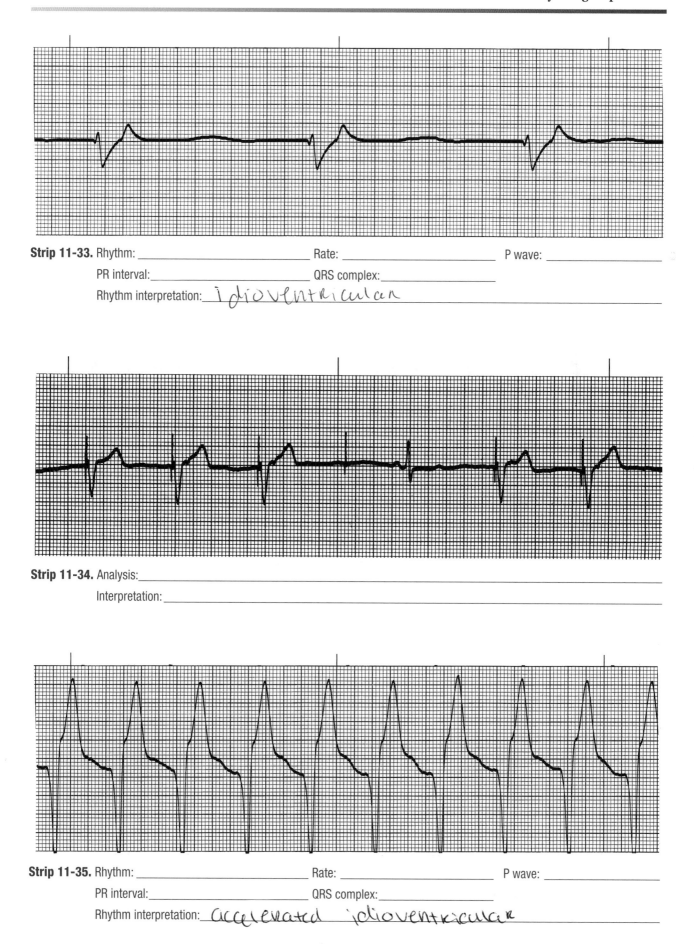

Strip 11-33. Rhythm: _____ Rate: _____ P wave: _____

PR interval:_____ QRS complex:_____

Rhythm interpretation: _idioventricular_____

Strip 11-34. Analysis:_____

Interpretation: _____

Strip 11-35. Rhythm: _____ Rate: _____ P wave: _____

PR interval:_____ QRS complex:_____

Rhythm interpretation: _accelerated idioventricular_____

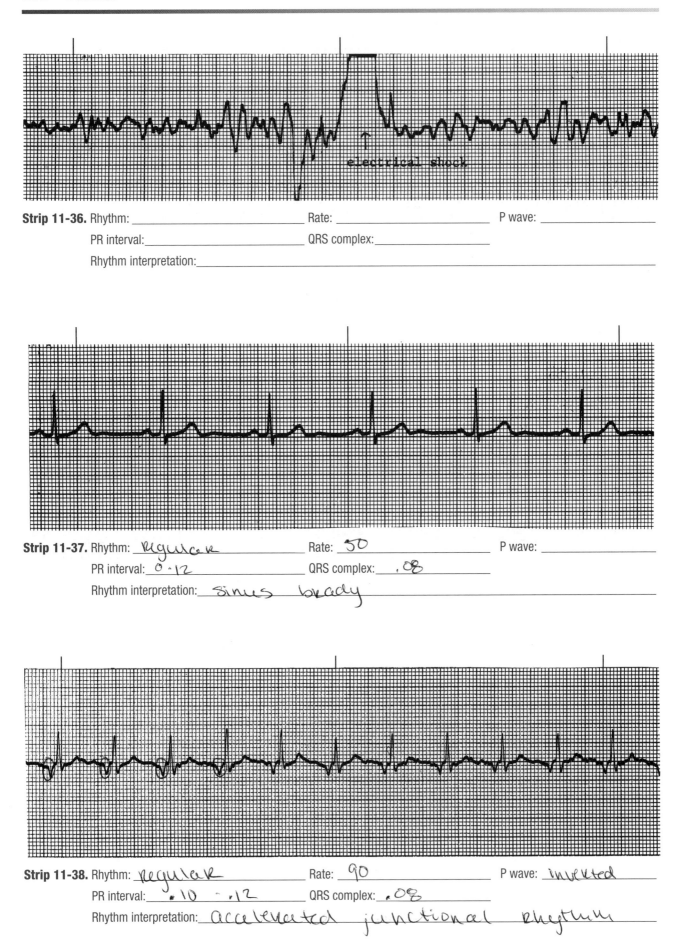

Strip 11-36. Rhythm: _____ Rate: _____ P wave: _____

PR interval: _____ QRS complex: _____

Rhythm interpretation: _____

Strip 11-37. Rhythm: _regular_ Rate: _50_ P wave: _____

PR interval: _0·12_ QRS complex: _.08_

Rhythm interpretation: _sinus brady_

Strip 11-38. Rhythm: _regular_ Rate: _90_ P wave: _inverted_

PR interval: _.10 - .12_ QRS complex: _.08_

Rhythm interpretation: _accelerated junctional rhythm_

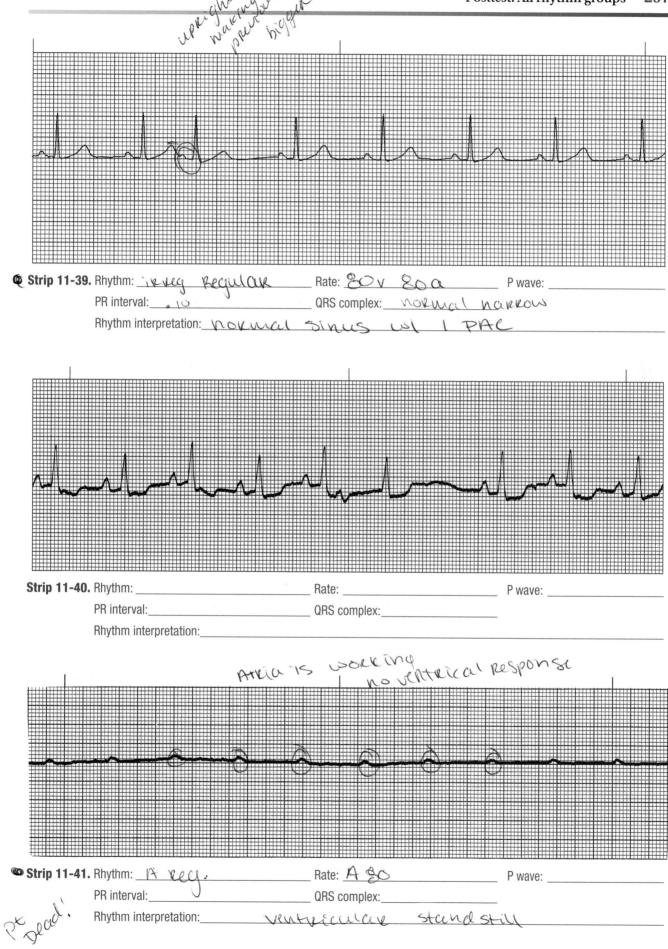

upright P
wanting's T
previous's
bigger

Q Strip 11-39. Rhythm: _irreg Regular_   Rate: _80v 80a_   P wave: _____

PR interval: _.10_   QRS complex: _normal narrow_

Rhythm interpretation: _normal Sinus w/ 1 PAC_

Strip 11-40. Rhythm: _____   Rate: _____   P wave: _____

PR interval: _____   QRS complex: _____

Rhythm interpretation: _____

Atria is working
no ventrical response

Strip 11-41. Rhythm: _A reg._   Rate: _A 80_   P wave: _____

PR interval: _____   QRS complex: _____

Rhythm interpretation: _ventricular standstill_

Pt Dead!

pacemaker

Strip 11-42. Rhythm: _____   Rate: _60_   P wave: _____

PR interval: _____   QRS complex: _____

Rhythm interpretation: _normal sinus with PAC & N._
bundle block   (PVC's)

Strip 11-43. Rhythm: __   Rate: _130_   P wave: _____

PR interval: _.12_   QRS complex: _.08_

Rhythm interpretation: _sinus tachy w/ 2 PAC's_

Strip 11-44. Rhythm: _____   Rate: _70_   P wave: _____

PR interval: _.18_   QRS complex: _.10_

Rhythm interpretation: _normal sinus rhythm w/ sinus arrest_
t wave inversion st depression

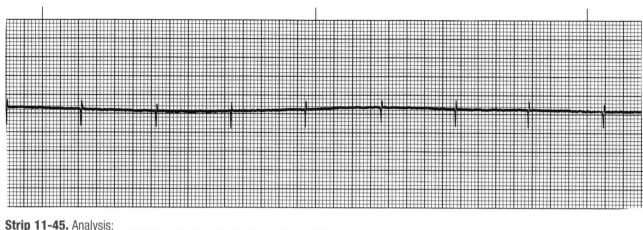

Strip 11-45. Analysis:_____

Interpretation: _____

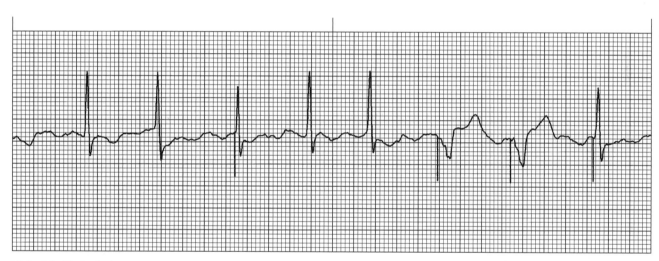

Strip 11-46. Analysis:_____

Interpretation: _____

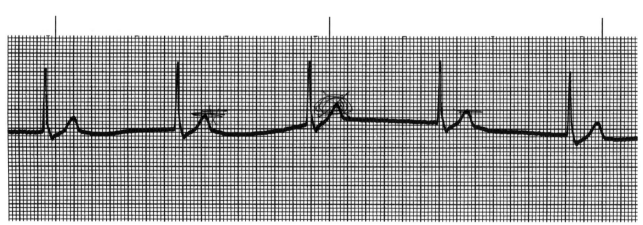

Strip 11-47. Rhythm: _regular_____ Rate: _40_ ↓_____ P wave: _hidden in T_

PR interval:_____—_____ QRS complex: _.08_____

Rhythm interpretation: _junctional rhythm_____

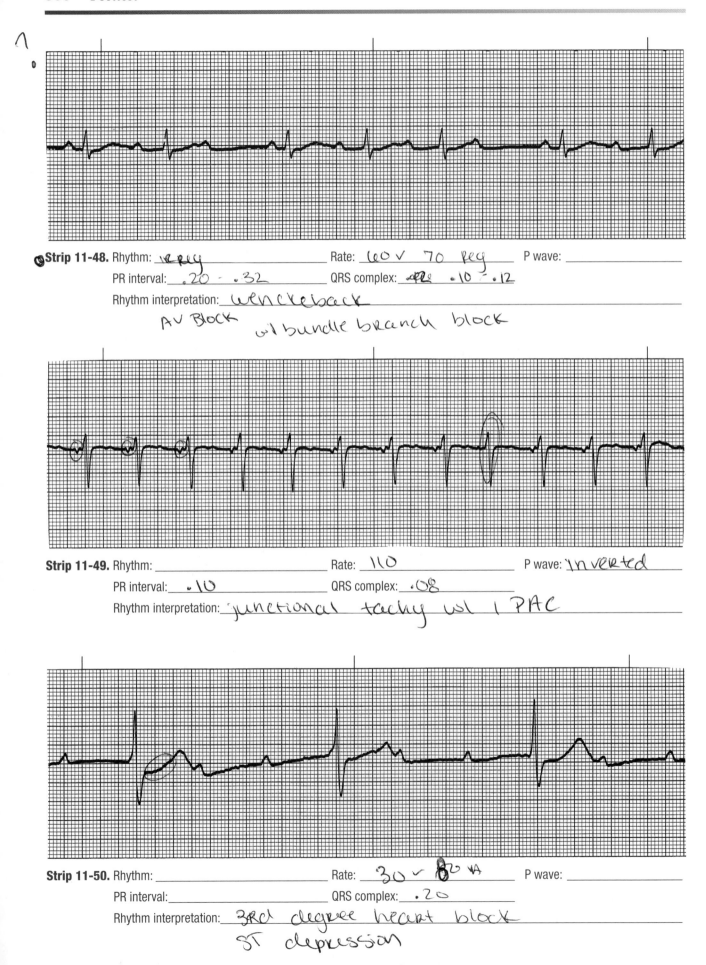

Strip 11-48. Rhythm: _reg_ _____ Rate: _160 ∨ 70 reg_ ___ P wave: _____

PR interval: _.20 - .32_ _____ QRS complex: _wide .10 ≈ .12_ ___

Rhythm interpretation: _Wenckeback_ _____

AV Block   w/ bundle branch block

Strip 11-49. Rhythm: _____ Rate: _110_ ____ P wave: _Inverted_ ___

PR interval: _.10_ _____ QRS complex: _.08_ _____

Rhythm interpretation: _junctional tachy w/ 1 PAC_ _____

Strip 11-50. Rhythm: _____ Rate: _30 ∨ 80 VA_ __ P wave: _____

PR interval: _____ QRS complex: _.20_ _____

Rhythm interpretation: _3rd degree heart block_ _____

ST depression

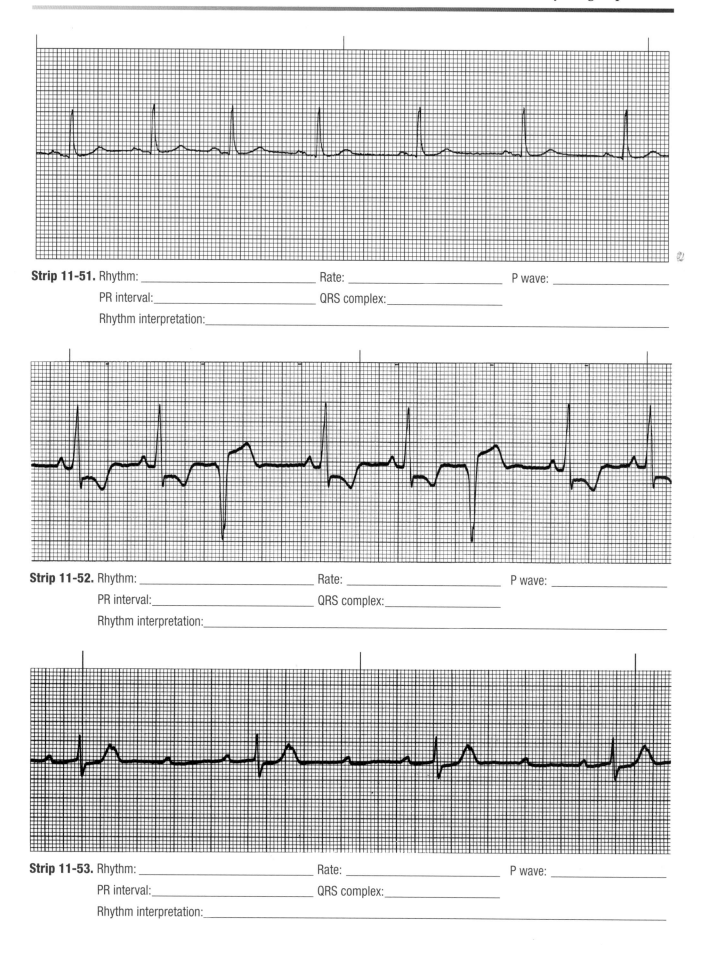

Strip 11-51. Rhythm: _____ Rate: _____ P wave: _____

PR interval: _____ QRS complex: _____

Rhythm interpretation: _____

Strip 11-52. Rhythm: _____ Rate: _____ P wave: _____

PR interval: _____ QRS complex: _____

Rhythm interpretation: _____

Strip 11-53. Rhythm: _____ Rate: _____ P wave: _____

PR interval: _____ QRS complex: _____

Rhythm interpretation: _____

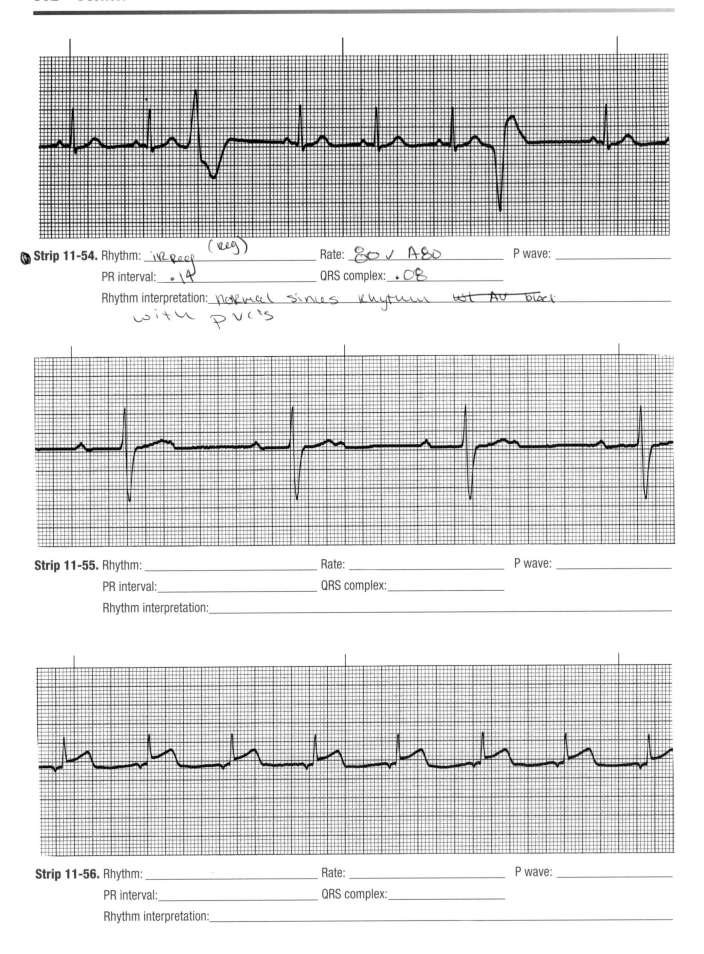

Strip 11-54. Rhythm: _irregular (reg)_ Rate: _80 √ A80_ P wave: _____

PR interval: _.14_ QRS complex: _.08_

Rhythm interpretation: _normal sinus rhythm tot AV block_
with pvc's

Strip 11-55. Rhythm: _____ Rate: _____ P wave: _____

PR interval: _____ QRS complex: _____

Rhythm interpretation: _____

Strip 11-56. Rhythm: _____ Rate: _____ P wave: _____

PR interval: _____ QRS complex: _____

Rhythm interpretation: _____

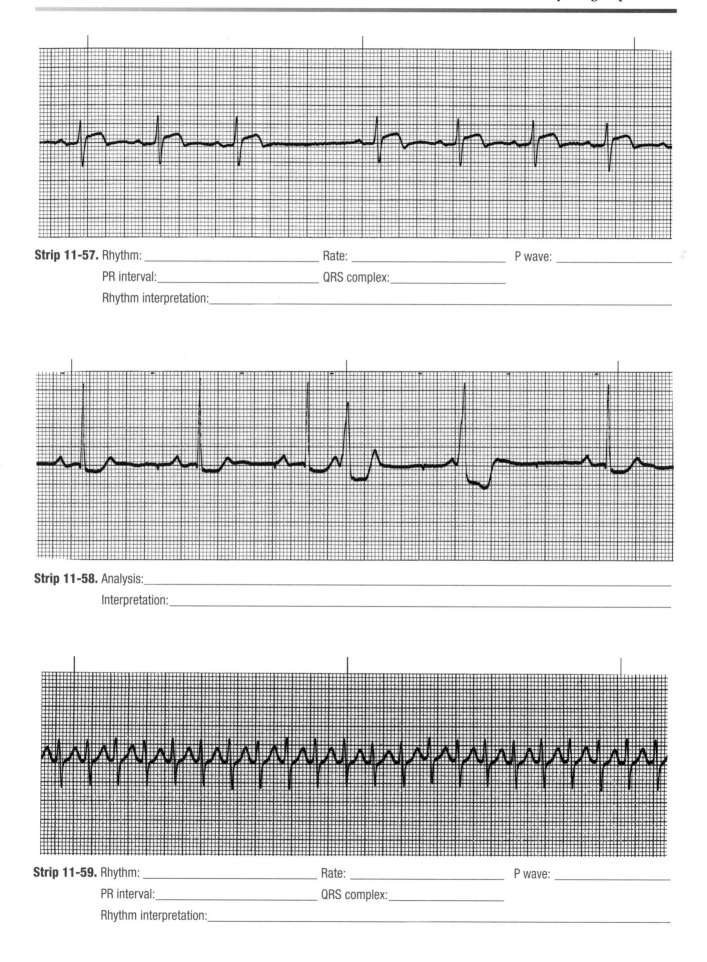

Strip 11-57. Rhythm: _____ Rate: _____ P wave: _____

PR interval:_____ QRS complex:_____

Rhythm interpretation:_____

Strip 11-58. Analysis:_____

Interpretation:_____

Strip 11-59. Rhythm: _____ Rate: _____ P wave: _____

PR interval:_____ QRS complex:_____

Rhythm interpretation:_____

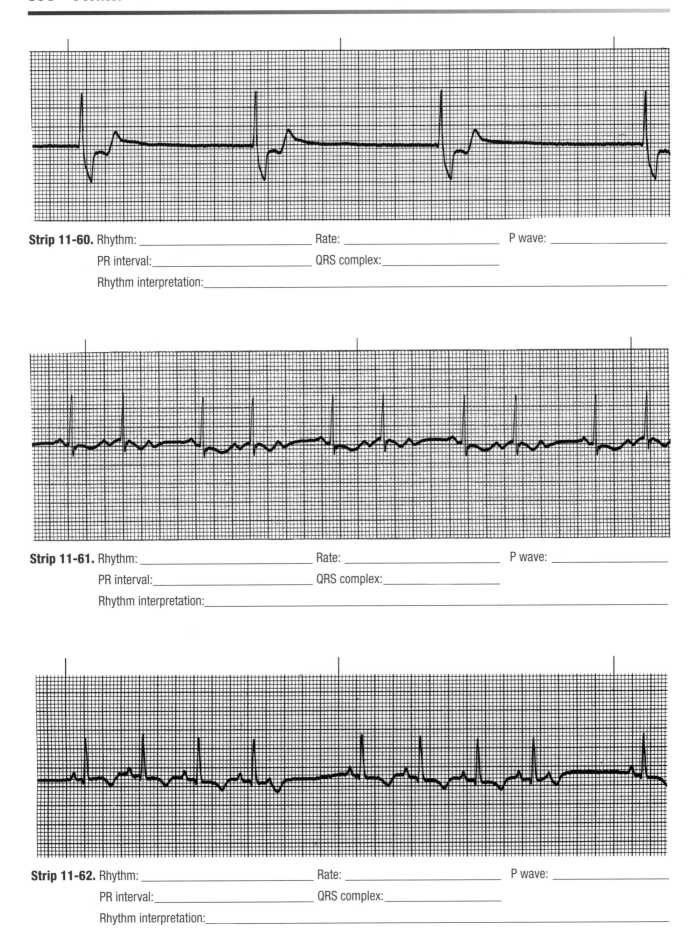

Strip 11-60. Rhythm: _____ Rate: _____ P wave: _____

PR interval: _____ QRS complex: _____

Rhythm interpretation: _____

Strip 11-61. Rhythm: _____ Rate: _____ P wave: _____

PR interval: _____ QRS complex: _____

Rhythm interpretation: _____

Strip 11-62. Rhythm: _____ Rate: _____ P wave: _____

PR interval: _____ QRS complex: _____

Rhythm interpretation: _____

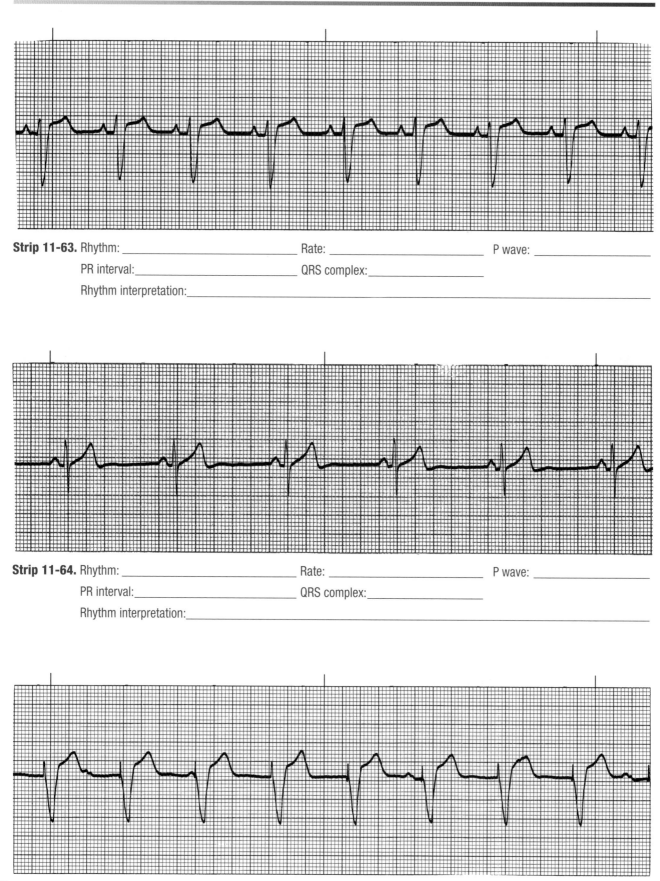

Strip 11-63. Rhythm: _____ Rate: _____ P wave: _____

PR interval:_____ QRS complex:_____

Rhythm interpretation:_____

Strip 11-64. Rhythm: _____ Rate: _____ P wave: _____

PR interval:_____ QRS complex:_____

Rhythm interpretation:_____

Strip 11-65. Analysis:_____

Interpretation: ventricular paced Rhythm

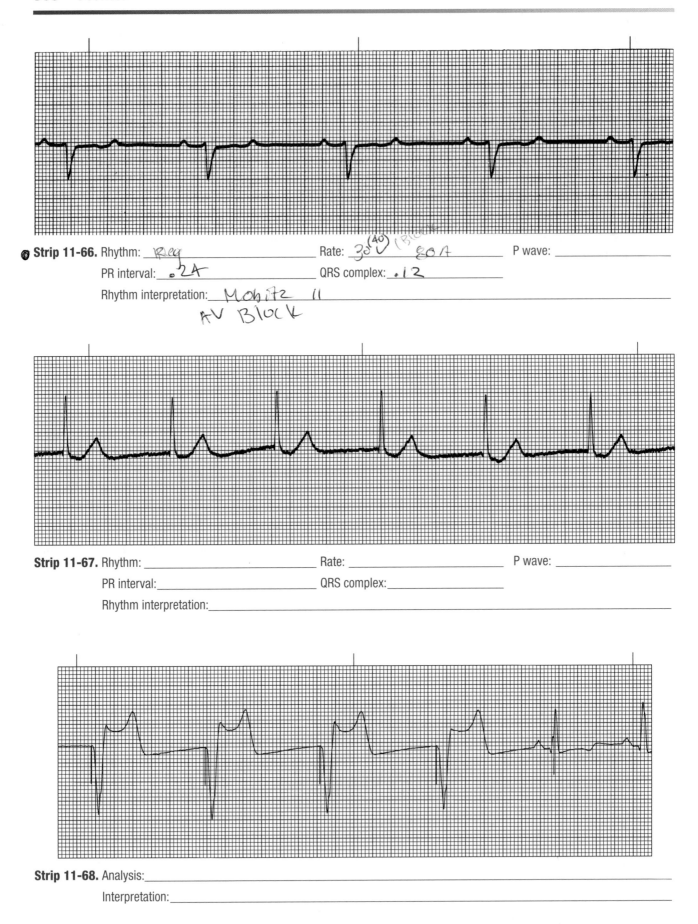

Strip 11-66. Rhythm: _Reg_   Rate: _3°0_ (40) (Block _80A_   P wave: _____

PR interval: _.24_   QRS complex: _.12_

Rhythm interpretation: _Mobitz 11_ _AV Block_

Strip 11-67. Rhythm: _____ Rate: _____ P wave: _____

PR interval: _____ QRS complex: _____

Rhythm interpretation: _____

Strip 11-68. Analysis: _____

Interpretation: _____

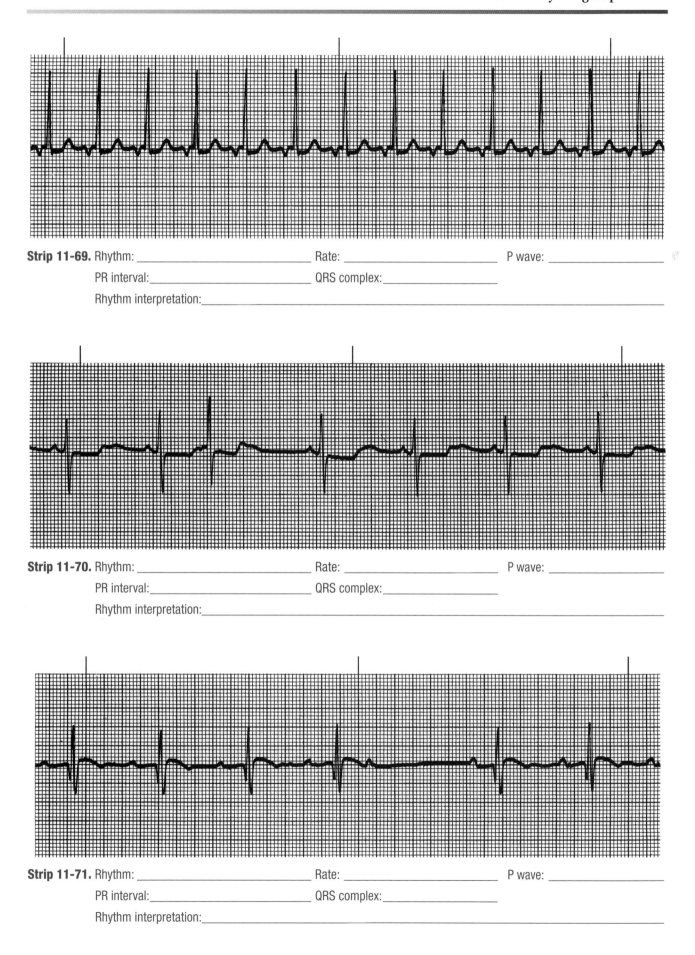

Strip 11-69. Rhythm: _____ Rate: _____ P wave: _____

PR interval:_____ QRS complex:_____

Rhythm interpretation:_____

Strip 11-70. Rhythm: _____ Rate: _____ P wave: _____

PR interval:_____ QRS complex:_____

Rhythm interpretation:_____

Strip 11-71. Rhythm: _____ Rate: _____ P wave: _____

PR interval:_____ QRS complex:_____

Rhythm interpretation:_____

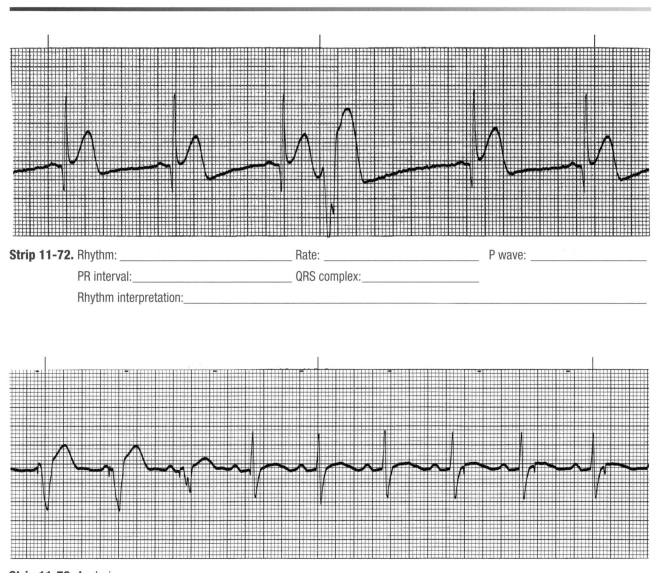

Strip 11-72. Rhythm: _____ Rate: _____ P wave: _____

PR interval:_____ QRS complex:_____

Rhythm interpretation:_____

Strip 11-73. Analysis:_____

Interpretation: _____

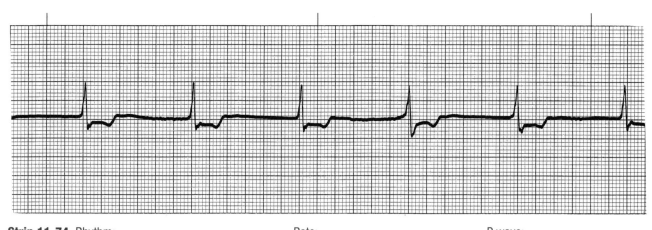

Strip 11-74. Rhythm: _____ Rate: _____ P wave: _____

PR interval:_____ QRS complex:_____

Rhythm interpretation:_____

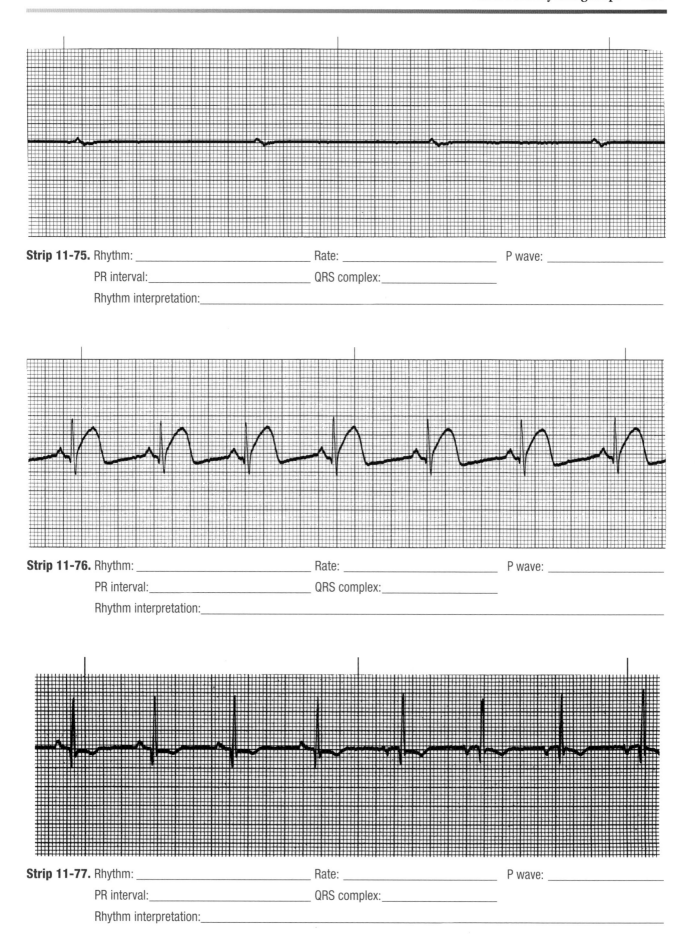

Strip 11-75. Rhythm: _____ Rate: _____ P wave: _____

PR interval:_____ QRS complex:_____

Rhythm interpretation:_____

Strip 11-76. Rhythm: _____ Rate: _____ P wave: _____

PR interval:_____ QRS complex:_____

Rhythm interpretation:_____

Strip 11-77. Rhythm: _____ Rate: _____ P wave: _____

PR interval:_____ QRS complex:_____

Rhythm interpretation:_____

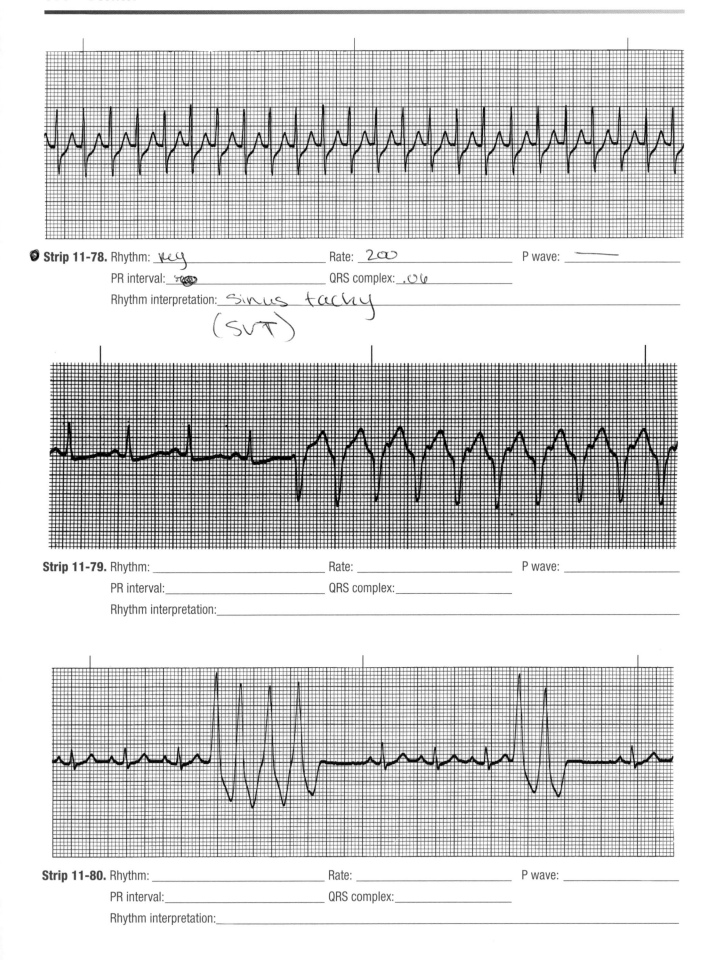

Strip 11-78. Rhythm: _reg_   Rate: _200_   P wave: _____

PR interval: _____   QRS complex: _.06_

Rhythm interpretation: _sinus tachy_

(SVT)

Strip 11-79. Rhythm: _____ Rate: _____ P wave: _____

PR interval: _____ QRS complex: _____

Rhythm interpretation: _____

Strip 11-80. Rhythm: _____ Rate: _____ P wave: _____

PR interval: _____ QRS complex: _____

Rhythm interpretation: _____

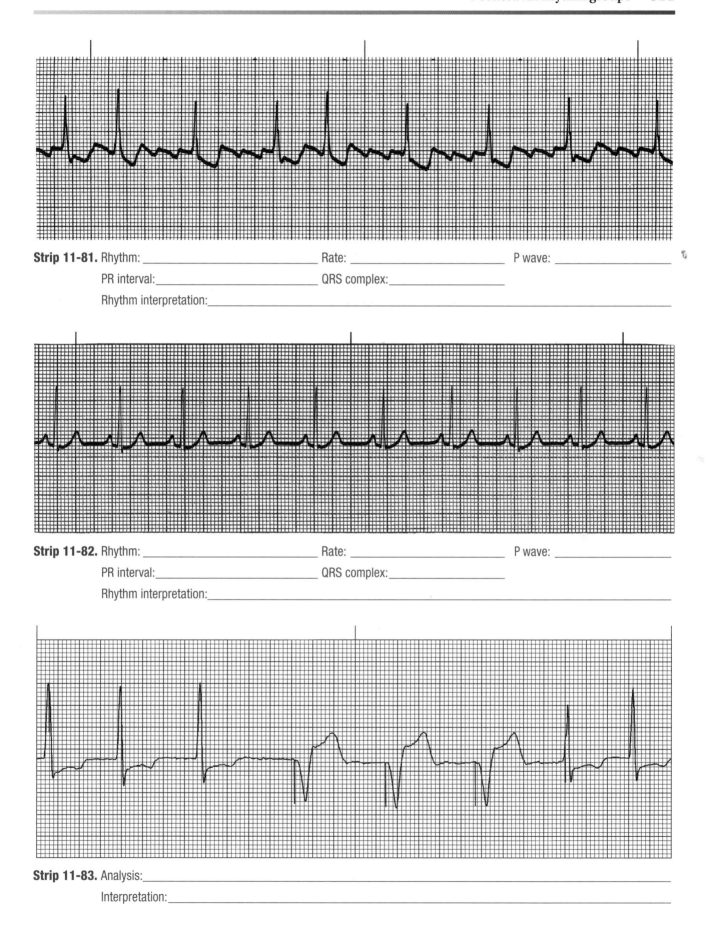

Strip 11-81. Rhythm: _____ Rate: _____ P wave: _____

PR interval:_____ QRS complex:_____

Rhythm interpretation:_____

Strip 11-82. Rhythm: _____ Rate: _____ P wave: _____

PR interval:_____ QRS complex:_____

Rhythm interpretation:_____

Strip 11-83. Analysis:_____

Interpretation: _____

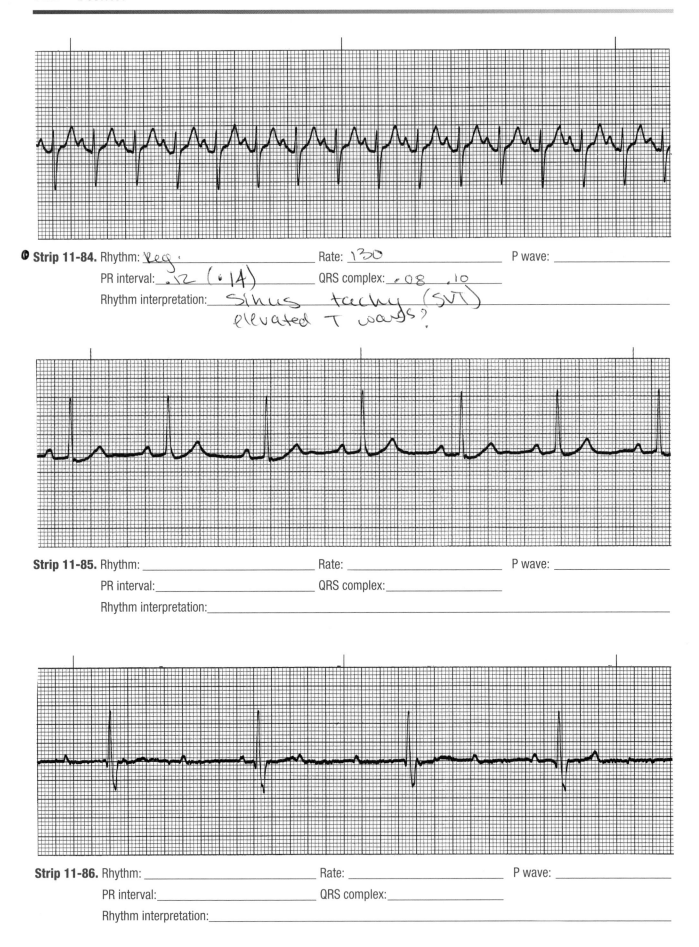

Strip 11-84. Rhythm: _Reg._   Rate: _130_   P wave: _____

PR interval: _.12 (.14)_   QRS complex: _.08 .10_

Rhythm interpretation: _Sinus tachy (SVT)_
elevated T waves?

Strip 11-85. Rhythm: _____ Rate: _____ P wave: _____

PR interval: _____ QRS complex: _____

Rhythm interpretation: _____

Strip 11-86. Rhythm: _____ Rate: _____ P wave: _____

PR interval: _____ QRS complex: _____

Rhythm interpretation: _____

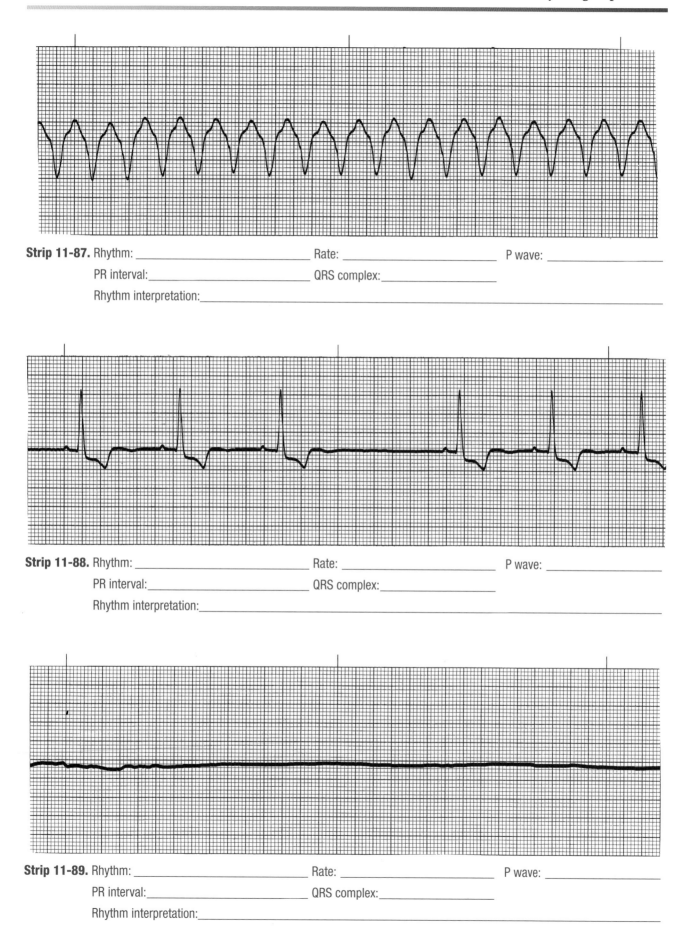

Strip 11-87. Rhythm: _____ Rate: _____ P wave: _____

PR interval: _____ QRS complex: _____

Rhythm interpretation: _____

Strip 11-88. Rhythm: _____ Rate: _____ P wave: _____

PR interval: _____ QRS complex: _____

Rhythm interpretation: _____

Strip 11-89. Rhythm: _____ Rate: _____ P wave: _____

PR interval: _____ QRS complex: _____

Rhythm interpretation: _____

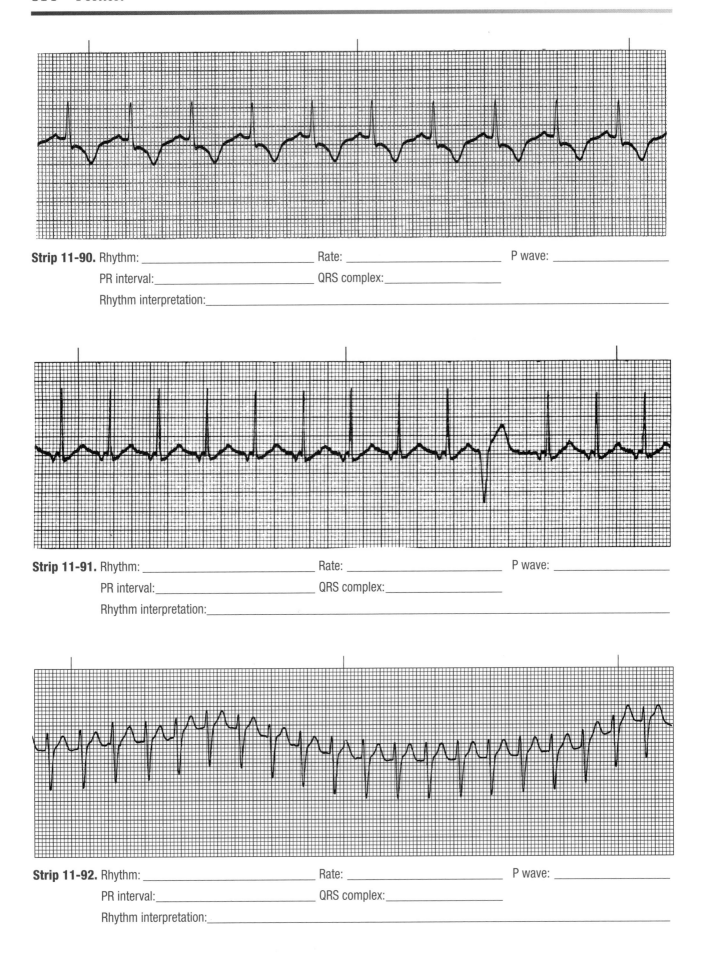

Strip 11-90. Rhythm: _____ Rate: _____ P wave: _____

PR interval:_____ QRS complex:_____

Rhythm interpretation:_____

Strip 11-91. Rhythm: _____ Rate: _____ P wave: _____

PR interval:_____ QRS complex:_____

Rhythm interpretation:_____

Strip 11-92. Rhythm: _____ Rate: _____ P wave: _____

PR interval:_____ QRS complex:_____

Rhythm interpretation:_____

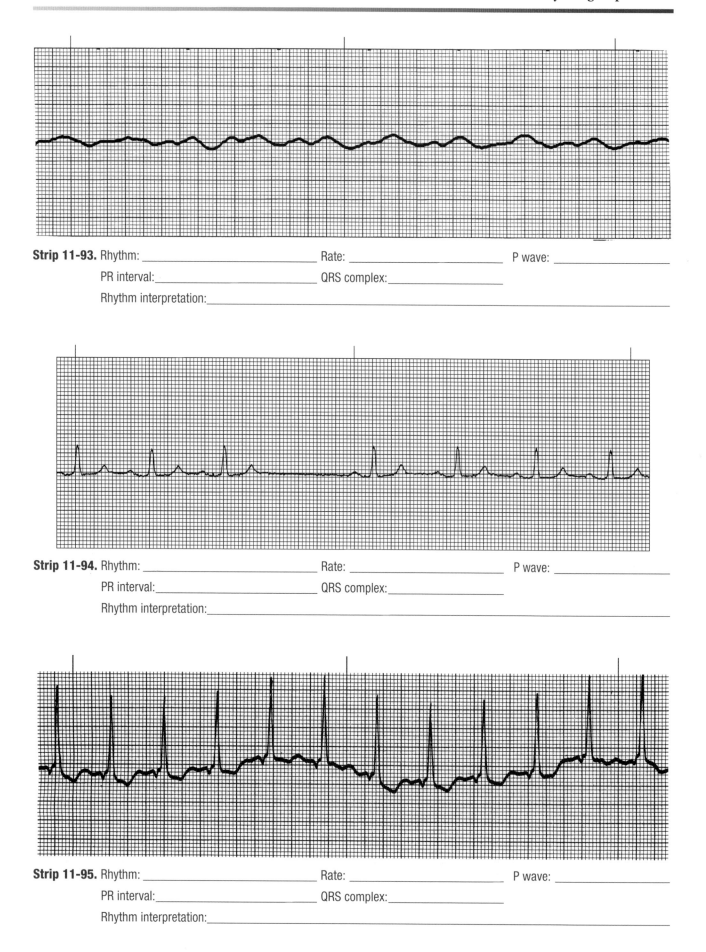

Strip 11-93. Rhythm: _____ Rate: _____ P wave: _____

PR interval:_____ QRS complex:_____

Rhythm interpretation:_____

Strip 11-94. Rhythm: _____ Rate: _____ P wave: _____

PR interval:_____ QRS complex:_____

Rhythm interpretation:_____

Strip 11-95. Rhythm: _____ Rate: _____ P wave: _____

PR interval:_____ QRS complex:_____

Rhythm interpretation:_____

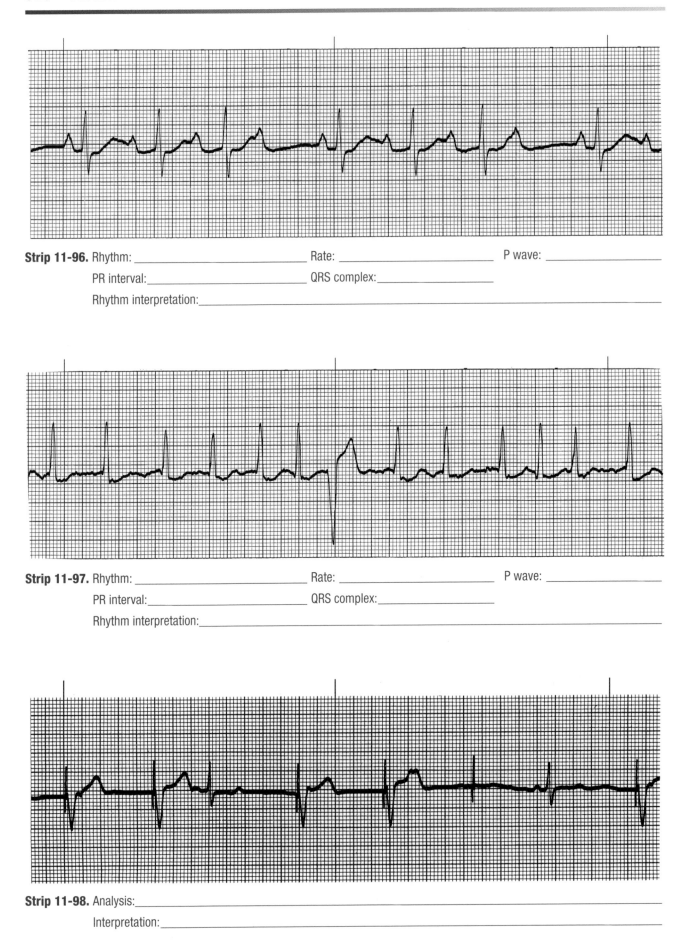

Strip 11-96. Rhythm: _____ Rate: _____ P wave: _____

PR interval:_____ QRS complex:_____

Rhythm interpretation:_____

Strip 11-97. Rhythm: _____ Rate: _____ P wave: _____

PR interval:_____ QRS complex:_____

Rhythm interpretation:_____

Strip 11-98. Analysis:_____

Interpretation:_____

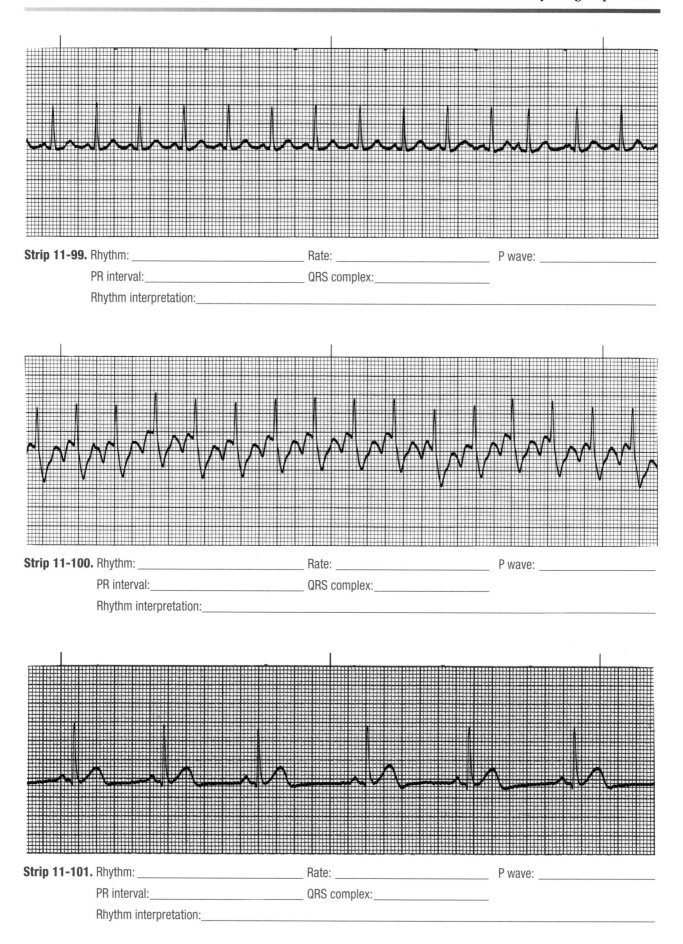

Strip 11-99. Rhythm: _____ Rate: _____ P wave: _____

PR interval:_____ QRS complex:_____

Rhythm interpretation:_____

Strip 11-100. Rhythm: _____ Rate: _____ P wave: _____

PR interval:_____ QRS complex:_____

Rhythm interpretation:_____

Strip 11-101. Rhythm: _____ Rate: _____ P wave: _____

PR interval:_____ QRS complex:_____

Rhythm interpretation:_____

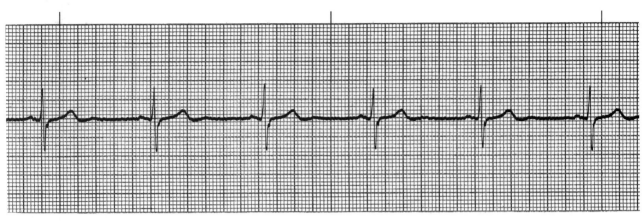

Strip 11-102. Rhythm: _____ Rate: _____ P wave: _____

PR interval:_____ QRS complex:_____

Rhythm interpretation:_____

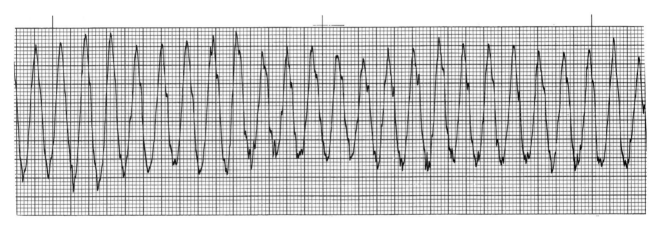

Strip 11-103. Rhythm: _____ Rate: _____ P wave: _____

PR interval:_____ QRS complex:_____

Rhythm interpretation:_____

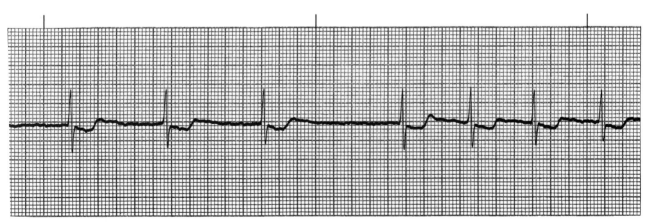

Strip 11-104. Rhythm: _____ Rate: _____ P wave: _____

PR interval:_____ QRS complex:_____

Rhythm interpretation:_____

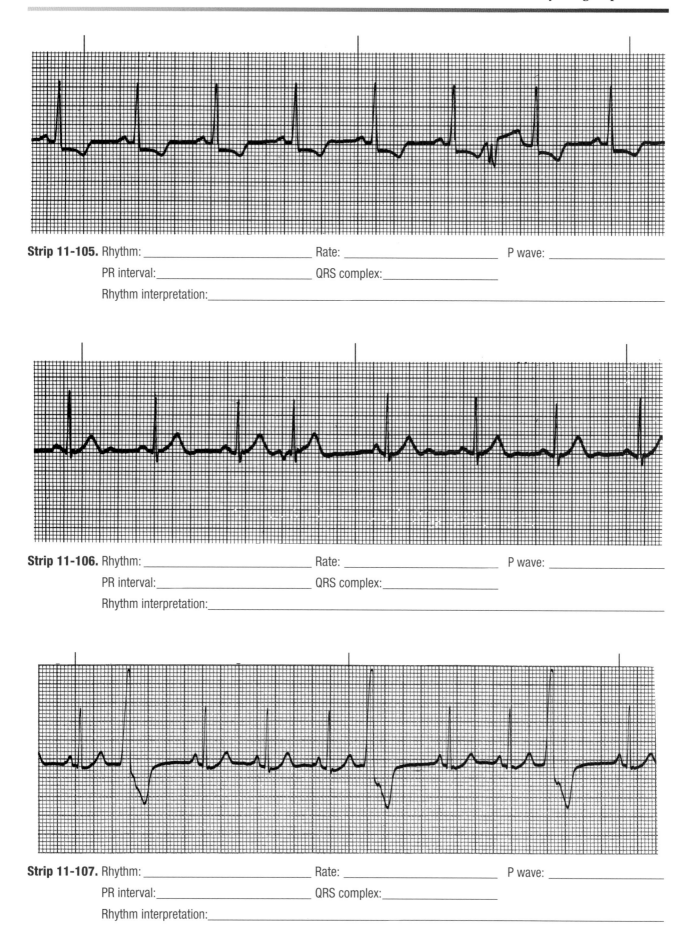

Strip 11-105. Rhythm: _____ Rate: _____ P wave: _____

PR interval:_____ QRS complex:_____

Rhythm interpretation:_____

Strip 11-106. Rhythm: _____ Rate: _____ P wave: _____

PR interval:_____ QRS complex:_____

Rhythm interpretation:_____

Strip 11-107. Rhythm: _____ Rate: _____ P wave: _____

PR interval:_____ QRS complex:_____

Rhythm interpretation:_____

Answer key to Chapter 3

Answer key to Chapters 5 through 11

Glossary

Index

Answer key to Chapter 3

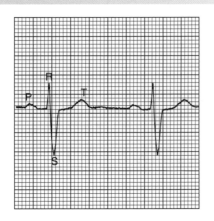

Strip 3-1.

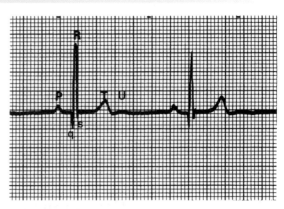

Strip 3-2.

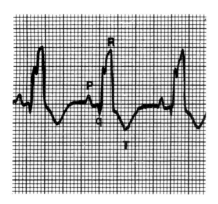

Strip 3-3.

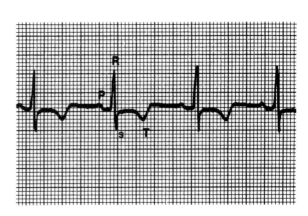

Strip 3-4.

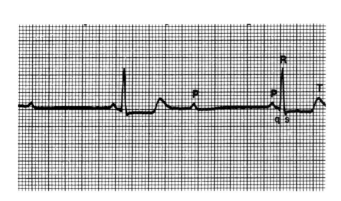

Strip 3-5.

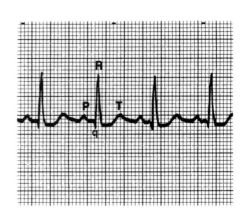

Strip 3-6.

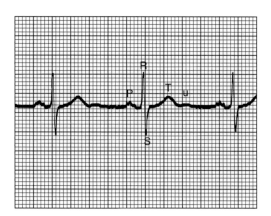

Strip 3-7.

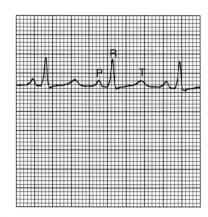

Strip 3-8.

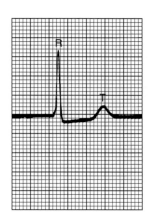

Strip 3-9.

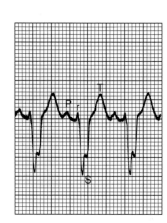

Strip 3-10.

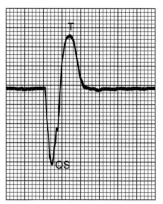

Strip 3-11.

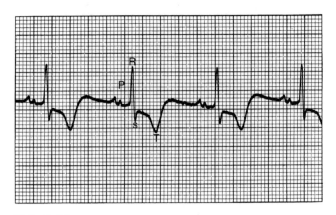

Strip 3-12.

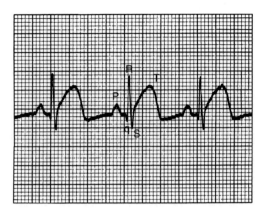

Strip 3-13.

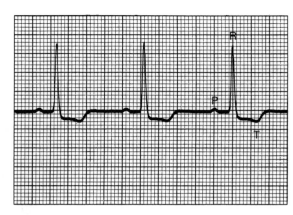

Strip 3-14.

Answer key to Chapters 5 through 11

Strip 5-1
Rhythm: Regular
Rate: 79 beats/minute
P waves: Sinus
PR interval: 0.14 to 0.16 second
QRS complex: 0.06 to 0.08 second
Comment: An inverted T wave is present.

Strip 5-2
Rhythm: Regular
Rate: 45 beats/minute
P waves: Sinus
PR interval: 0.14 to 0.16 second
QRS complex: 0.08 second
Comment: A small U wave is seen after the T wave.

Strip 5-3
Rhythm: Regular
Rate: 88 beats/minute
P waves: Sinus
PR interval: 0.20 second
QRS complex: 0.08 to 0.10 second
Comment: A depressed ST segment and biphasic T wave are present.

Strip 5-4
Rhythm: Irregular
Rate: 50 beats/minute
P waves: Sinus
PR interval: 0.16 to 0.18 second
QRS complex: 0.04 second

Strip 5-5
Rhythm: Regular
Rate: 50 beats/minute
P waves: Sinus
PR interval: 0.18 to 0.20 second
QRS complex: 0.06 to 0.08 second
Comment: An elevated ST segment is present.

Strip 5-6
Rhythm: Regular
Rate: 136 beats/minute
P waves: Sinus
PR interval: 0.14 to 0.16 second
QRS complex: 0.06 to 0.08 second

Strip 5-7
Rhythm: Regular
Rate: 68 beats/minute
P waves: Sinus
PR interval: 0.16 to 0.18 second
QRS complex: 0.12 to 0.14 second
Comment: A U wave is present.

Strip 5-8
Rhythm: Irregular
Rate: 50 beats/minute
P waves: Sinus
PR interval: 0.12 to 0.14 second
QRS complex: 0.06 to 0.08 second
Comment: An elevated ST segment and inverted T wave are present.

Strip 5-9
Rhythm: Regular
Rate: 94 beats/minute
P waves: Sinus
PR interval: 0.14 to 0.16 second
QRS complex: 0.06 to 0.08 second
Comment: A depressed ST segment is present

Strip 5-10
Rhythm: Regular
Rate: 58 beats/minute
P waves: Sinus
PR interval: 0.16 to 0.18 second
QRS complex: 0.14 to 0.16 second

Strip 5-11
Rhythm: Regular
Rate: 56 beats/minute
P waves: Sinus
PR interval: 0.24 to 0.26 second
QRS complex: 0.04 to 0.06 second

Strip 6-1
Rhythm: Regular
Rate: 54 beats/minute
P waves: Sinus
PR interval: 0.18 to 0.20 second
QRS complex: 0.08 second
Rhythm interpretation: Sinus bradycardia

Strip 6-2
Rhythm: Regular
Rate: 68 beats/minute
P waves: Sinus
PR interval: 0.16 to 0.18 second
QRS complex: 0.06 to 0.08 second
Rhythm interpretation: Normal sinus rhythm; ST-segment depression and T-wave inversion are present.

Strip 6-3
Rhythm: Regular
Rate: 79 beats/minute
P waves: Sinus
PR interval: 0.14 to 0.16 second
QRS complex: 0.06 to 0.08 second
Rhythm interpretation: Normal sinus rhythm

Strip 6-4
Rhythm: Regular
Rate: 107 beats/minute
P waves: Sinus
PR interval: 0.12 to 0.16 second
QRS complex: 0.06 to 0.08 second
Rhythm interpretation: Sinus tachycardia; ST-segment depression and T-wave inversion are present.

Strip 6-5
Rhythm: Regular
Rate: 58 beats/minute
P waves: Sinus
PR interval: 0.16 to 0.18 second
QRS complex: 0.06 to 0.08 second
Rhythm interpretation: Sinus bradycardia; a U wave is present.

Strip 6-6
Rhythm: Regular (basic rhythm); irregular during pause
Rate: 100 beats/minute (basic rhythm)
P waves: Sinus (basic rhythm); absent during pause
PR interval: 0.16 to 0.20 second
QRS complex: 0.08 to 0.10 second (basic rhythm)
Rhythm interpretation: Normal sinus rhythm with sinus block; ST-segment depression and T-wave inversion are present.

Strip 6-7
Rhythm: Regular
Rate: 54 beats/minute
P waves: Sinus (notched P waves
usually indicate left atrial
hypertrophy)
PR interval: 0.14 to 0.16 second
QRS complex: 0.06 to 0.08 second
Rhythm interpretation: Sinus
bradycardia; a U wave is present.

Strip 6-8
Rhythm: Irregular
Rate: 50 beats/minute
P waves: Sinus
PR interval: 0.20 second
QRS complex: 0.06 to 0.08 second
Rhythm interpretation: Sinus
arrhythmia with a bradycardic rate;
a U wave is present.

Strip 6-9
Rhythm: Regular (basic rhythm);
irregular during pause
Rate: 58 beats/minute (basic rhythm)
P waves: Sinus (basic rhythm);
absent during pause
PR interval: 0.14 to 0.18 second
(basic rhythm); absent during
pause
QRS complex: 0.08 to 0.10 second
(basic rhythm); absent during
pause
Rhythm interpretation: Sinus
bradycardia with sinus arrest;
a depressed ST segment and an
inverted T wave are present.

Strip 6-10
Rhythm: Regular
Rate: 125 beats/minute
P waves: Sinus
PR interval: 0.12 to 0.14 second
QRS complex: 0.06 to 0.08 second
Rhythm interpretation: Sinus
tachycardia

Strip 6-11
Rhythm: Regular
Rate: 63 beats/minute
P waves: Sinus
PR interval: 0.18 to 0.20 second
QRS complex: 0.08 second
Rhythm interpretation: Normal sinus
rhythm; a U wave is present.

Strip 6-12
Rhythm: Regular
Rate: 47 beats/minute
P waves: Sinus
PR interval: 0.18 to 0.20 second
QRS complex: 0.08 second
Rhythm interpretation: Sinus
bradycardia; an elevated ST segment
is present.

Strip 6-13
Rhythm: Irregular
Rate: 80 beats/minute
P waves: Sinus
PR interval: 0.12 to 0.14 second
QRS complex: 0.08 second
Rhythm interpretation: Sinus
arrhythmia

Strip 6-14
Rhythm: Regular
Rate: 63 beats/minute
P waves: Sinus
PR interval: 0.18 to 0.20 second
QRS complex: 0.08 to 0.10 second
Rhythm interpretation: Normal sinus
rhythm; ST-segment depression and
T-wave inversion are present.

Strip 6-15
Rhythm: Regular (basic rhythm);
irregular during pause
Rate: 84 beats/minute (basic
rhythm); slows to 56 beats/minute
after a pause (temporary rate
suppression may occur after a pause
in the basic rhythm)
P waves: Sinus (basic rhythm);
absent during pause
PR interval: 0.16 to 0.18 second
(basic rhythm); absent during pause
QRS complex: 0.08 to 0.10 second
(basic rhythm); absent during pause
Rhythm interpretation: Normal
sinus rhythm with sinus arrest;
rate suppression is present after the
pause.

Strip 6-16
Rhythm: Regular
Rate: 150 beats/minute
P waves: Sinus
PR interval: 0.12 to 0.16 second
QRS complex: 0.04 to 0.06 second
Rhythm interpretation: Sinus
tachycardia

Strip 6-17
Rhythm: Regular
Rate: 52 beats/minute
P waves: Sinus
PR interval: 0.16 to 0.18 second
QRS complex: 0.08 to 0.10 second
Rhythm interpretation: Sinus
bradycardia

Strip 6-18
Rhythm: Irregular
Rate: 60 beats/minute
P waves: Sinus
PR interval: 0.16 to 0.18 second
QRS complex: 0.08 to 0.10 second
Rhythm interpretation: Sinus
arrhythmia

Strip 6-19
Rhythm: Regular
Rate: 79 beats/minute
P waves: Sinus
PR interval: 0.16 to 0.20 second
QRS complex: 0.06 second
Rhythm interpretation: Normal sinus
rhythm

Strip 6-20
Rhythm: Regular (basic rhythm);
irregular during pause
Rate: 88 beats/minute (basic rhythm)
P waves: Sinus (basic rhythm);
absent during pause
PR interval: 0.14 to 0.16 second
(basic rhythm)
QRS complex: 0.08 second (basic
rhythm)
Rhythm interpretation: Normal sinus
rhythm with sinus block; a U wave is
present.

Strip 6-21
Rhythm: Regular
Rate: 150 beats/minute
P waves: Sinus
PR interval: 0.12 second
QRS complex: 0.06 second
Rhythm interpretation: Sinus
tachycardia

Strip 6-22
Rhythm: Regular
Rate: 60 beats/minute
P waves: Sinus
PR interval: 0.12 second
QRS complex: 0.08 second
Rhythm interpretation: Normal
sinus rhythm; T-wave inversion is
present.

Strip 6-23
Rhythm: Irregular
Rate: 60 beats/minute
P waves: Sinus
PR interval: 0.16 second
QRS complex: 0.08 second
Rhythm interpretation: Sinus
arrhythmia

Strip 6-24
Rhythm: Regular (basic rhythm);
irregular during pause
Rate: 60 beats/minute (basic
rhythm); slows to 47 beats/minute
after a pause (temporary rate
suppression can occur after a pause
in the basic rhythm)
P waves: Sinus (basic rhythm);
absent during pause
PR interval: 0.16 to 0.18 second
(basic rhythm); absent during
pause
QRS complex: 0.06 to 0.08 second
(basic rhythm); absent during
pause
Rhythm interpretation: Normal sinus
rhythm with sinus arrest

Strip 6-25
Rhythm: Regular
Rate: 125 beats/minute
P waves: Sinus
PR interval: 0.12 to 0.14 second
QRS complex: 0.04 to 0.06 second
Rhythm interpretation: Sinus
tachycardia

Strip 6-26
Rhythm: Regular
Rate: 35 beats/minute
P waves: Sinus
PR interval: 0.14 to 0.16 second
QRS complex: 0.10 second
Rhythm interpretation: Marked sinus
bradycardia

Strip 6-27
Rhythm: Regular (basic rhythm);
irregular during pause
Rate: 72 beats/minute (basic
rhythm)
P waves: Sinus (basic rhythm);
absent during pause
PR interval: 0.14 to 0.16 second
(basic rhythm); absent during
pause
QRS complex: 0.08 to 0.10 second
(basic rhythm); absent during
pause
Rhythm interpretation: Normal sinus
rhythm with sinus block

Strip 6-28
Rhythm: Irregular
Rate: 60 beats/minute
P waves: Sinus
PR interval: 0.12 to 0.14 second
QRS complex: 0.10 second
Rhythm interpretation: Sinus
arrhythmia; a U wave is present.

Strip 6-29
Rhythm: Regular
Rate: 65 beats/minute
P waves: Sinus
PR interval: 0.20 second
QRS complex: 0.08 to 0.10 second
Rhythm interpretation: Normal sinus
rhythm; ST-segment depression and
T-wave inversion are present.

Strip 6-30
Rhythm: Regular (basic rhythm);
irregular during pause
Rate: 68 beats/minute (basic rhythm);
slows to 63 beats/minute after a
pause (temporary rate suppression
can occur after a pause in the basic
rhythm; after several cycles the rate
returns to the basic rate)
P waves: Sinus (basic rhythm);
absent during pause
PR interval: 0.16 second (basic
rhythm); absent during pause
QRS complex: 0.06 to 0.08 second
(basic rhythm); absent during
pause
Rhythm interpretation: Normal sinus
rhythm with sinus arrest; a U wave is
present.

Strip 6-31
Rhythm: Regular
Rate: 48 beats/minute
P waves: Sinus
PR interval: 0.16 to 0.18 second
QRS complex: 0.06 to 0.08 second
Rhythm interpretation: Sinus
bradycardia

Strip 6-32
Rhythm: Irregular
Rate: 60 beats/minute
P waves: Sinus
PR interval: 0.14 to 0.16 second
QRS complex: 0.06 to 0.08 second
Rhythm interpretation: Sinus
arrhythmia

Strip 6-33
Rhythm: Regular
Rate: 115 beats/minute
P waves: Sinus
PR interval: 0.16 to 0.18 second
QRS complex: 0.06 to 0.08 second
Rhythm interpretation: Sinus
tachycardia

Strip 6-34
Rhythm: Regular
Rate: 88 beats/minute
P waves: Sinus
PR interval: 0.18 to 0.20 second
QRS complex: 0.08 second
Rhythm interpretation: Normal sinus
rhythm; ST-segment depression is
present.

Strip 6-35
Rhythm: Irregular
Rate: 60 beats/minute
P waves: Sinus
PR interval: 0.14 to 0.16 second
QRS complex: 0.06 to 0.08 second
Rhythm interpretation: Sinus
arrhythmia

Strip 6-36
Rhythm: Regular
Rate: 41 beats/minute
P waves: Sinus
PR interval: 0.16 to 0.18 second
QRS complex: 0.06 to 0.08 second
Rhythm interpretation: Sinus
bradycardia; ST-segment depression
is present.

Strip 6-37
Rhythm: Regular (basic rhythm);
irregular during pause
Rate: 88 beats/minute (basic rhythm)
P waves: Sinus
PR interval: 0.20 second
QRS complex: 0.06 to 0.08 second
Rhythm interpretation: Normal
sinus rhythm with sinus arrest;
ST-segment depression is present.

Strip 6-38
Rhythm: Regular
Rate: 107 beats/minute
P waves: Sinus
PR interval: 0.16 to 0.18 second
QRS complex: 0.06 to 0.08 second
Rhythm interpretation: Sinus
tachycardia

Strip 6-39
Rhythm: Regular
Rate: 107 beats/minute
P waves: Sinus
PR interval: 0.16 to 0.18 second
QRS complex: 0.06 to 0.08 second
Rhythm interpretation: Sinus
tachycardia; ST-segment elevation is
present.

Strip 6-40
Rhythm: Regular
Rate: 54 beats/minute
P waves: Sinus (notched P waves
usually indicate left atrial hypertrophy)
PR interval: 0.16 to 0.20 second
QRS complex: 0.06 to 0.08 second
Rhythm interpretation: Sinus
bradycardia

Strip 6-41
Rhythm: Regular
Rate: 84 beats/minute
P waves: Sinus
PR interval: 0.16 second
QRS complex: 0.06 to 0.08 second
Rhythm interpretation: Normal sinus
rhythm

Strip 6-42
Rhythm: Irregular
Rate: 60 beats/minute
P waves: Sinus
PR interval: 0.14 to 0.16 second
QRS complex: 0.06 to 0.08 second
Rhythm interpretation: Sinus
arrhythmia

Strip 6-43
Rhythm: Regular (basic rhythm);
irregular during pause
Rate: 63 beats/minute (basic
rhythm)
P waves: Sinus (basic rhythm);
absent during pause
PR interval: 0.18 to 0.20 second
(basic rhythm); absent during
pause
QRS complex: 0.04 to 0.06 second
(basic rhythm); absent during
pause
Rhythm interpretation: Normal
sinus rhythm with sinus arrest;
ST-segment depression is present.

Strip 6-44
Rhythm: Irregular
Rate: 60 beats/minute
P waves: Sinus
PR interval: 0.12 to 0.14 second
QRS complex: 0.08 to 0.10 second
Rhythm interpretation: Sinus
arrhythmia; ST-segment elevation is
present.

Strip 6-45
Rhythm: Regular
Rate: 27 beats/minute
P waves: Sinus
PR interval: 0.14 to 0.16 second
QRS complex: 0.08 to 0.10 second
Rhythm interpretation: Sinus
bradycardia with extremely slow
rate; ST-segment depression is
present.

Strip 6-46
Rhythm: Irregular
Rate: 50 beats/minute
P waves: Sinus
PR interval: 0.12 to 0.14 second
QRS complex: 0.06 to 0.08 second
Rhythm interpretation: Sinus
arrhythmia with a bradycardic rate

Strip 6-47
Rhythm: Regular
Rate: 136 beats/minute
P waves: Sinus
PR interval: 0.12 to 0.14 second
QRS complex: 0.06 to 0.08 second
Rhythm interpretation: Sinus
tachycardia

Strip 6-48
Rhythm: Irregular
Rate: 70 beats/minute
P waves: Sinus
PR interval: 0.16 to 0.20 second
QRS complex: 0.04 to 0.06 second
Rhythm interpretation: Sinus
arrhythmia; a U wave is present.

Strip 6-49
Rhythm: Regular
Rate: 52 beats/minute
P waves: Sinus
PR interval: 0.12 second
QRS complex: 0.08 second
Rhythm interpretation: Sinus
bradycardia

Strip 6-50
Rhythm: Regular
Rate: 60 beats/minute
P waves: Sinus
PR interval: 0.16 to 0.18 second
QRS complex: 0.08 second
Rhythm interpretation: Normal sinus
rhythm; an elevated ST segment is
present.

Strip 6-51
Rhythm: Regular
Rate: 107 beats/minute
P waves: Sinus
PR interval: 0.12 to 0.14 second
QRS complex: 0.06 to 0.08 second
Rhythm interpretation: Sinus
tachycardia

Strip 6-52
Rhythm: Regular (basic rhythm);
irregular during pause
Rate: 60 beats/minute (basic
rhythm); slows to 31 beats/minute
after a pause (temporary rate
suppression is common after a pause
in the basic rhythm)
P waves: Sinus
PR interval: 0.16 to 0.20 second
QRS complex: 0.06 to 0.08 second
Rhythm interpretation: Normal
sinus rhythm with sinus arrest;
ST-segment depression and T-wave
inversion are present.

Strip 6-53
Rhythm: Irregular
Rate: 80 beats/minute
P waves: Sinus
PR interval: 0.12 to 0.14 second
QRS complex: 0.06 to 0.08 second
Rhythm interpretation: Sinus
arrhythmia

Strip 6-54
Rhythm: Regular (basic rhythm);
irregular during pause
Rate: 94 beats/minute (basic
rhythm); rate slows to 54 beats/
minute after a pause (temporary rate
suppression can occur after a pause
in the basic rhythm)
P waves: Sinus (basic rhythm);
absent during pause
PR interval: 0.16 to 0.18 second
(basic rhythm); absent during
pause
QRS complex: 0.08 to 0.10 second
Rhythm interpretation: Normal sinus
rhythm with sinus block

Strip 6-55
Rhythm: Regular
Rate: 65 beats/minute
P waves: Sinus
PR interval: 0.16 to 0.18 second
QRS complex: 0.06 second
Rhythm interpretation: Normal sinus
rhythm

Strip 6-56
Rhythm: Regular
Rate: 125 beats/minute
P waves: Sinus
PR interval: 0.16 second
QRS complex: 0.08 second
Rhythm interpretation: Sinus
tachycardia; ST-segment depression
is present.

Strip 6-57
Rhythm: Irregular
Rate: 40 beats/minute
P waves: Sinus
PR interval: 0.16 to 0.18 second
QRS complex: 0.08 second
Rhythm interpretation: Sinus
arrhythmia with a bradycardic rate; a
U wave is present.

Strip 6-58
Rhythm: Regular
Rate: 72 beats/minute
P waves: Sinus
PR interval: 0.16 to 0.20 second
QRS complex: 0.06 to 0.08 second
Rhythm interpretation: Normal sinus
rhythm; ST-segment depression and
T-wave inversion are present.

Strip 6-59
Rhythm: Regular
Rate: 50 beats/minute
P waves: Sinus
PR interval: 0.20 second
QRS complex: 0.06 to 0.08 second
Rhythm interpretation: Sinus
bradycardia; ST-segment depression
and T-wave inversion are present.

Strip 6-60
Rhythm: Regular (basic rhythm);
irregular during pause
Rate: 88 beats/minute (basic rhythm)
P waves: Sinus (basic rhythm);
absent during pause
PR interval: 0.14 to 0.20 second
(basic rhythm); absent during pause
QRS complex: 0.08 to 0.10 second
(basic rhythm); absent during
pause
Rhythm interpretation: Normal
sinus rhythm with sinus block;
ST-segment depression is present.

Strip 6-61
Rhythm: Regular
Rate: 72 beats/minute
P waves: Sinus
PR interval: 0.12 to 0.14 second
QRS complex: 0.06 to 0.08 second
Rhythm interpretation: Normal
sinus rhythm; an inverted T wave is
present.

Strip 6-62
Rhythm: Regular
Rate: 125 beats/minute
P waves: Sinus
PR interval: 0.12 second
QRS complex: 0.04 second
Rhythm interpretation: Sinus
tachycardia; ST-segment depression
is present.

Strip 6-63
Rhythm: Regular
Rate: 44 beats/minute
P waves: Sinus
PR interval: 0.18 to 0.20 second
QRS complex: 0.06 to 0.08 second
Rhythm interpretation: Sinus
bradycardia; a U wave is present.

Strip 6-64
Rhythm: Regular
Rate: 79 beats/minute
P waves: Sinus
PR interval: 0.14 to 0.16 second
QRS complex: 0.04 to 0.06 second
Rhythm interpretation: Normal sinus
rhythm; T-wave inversion is present.

Strip 6-65
Rhythm: Regular
Rate: 107 beats/minute
P waves: Sinus
PR interval: 0.18 to 0.20 second
QRS complex: 0.08 to 0.10 second
Rhythm interpretation: Sinus
tachycardia; an elevated ST segment
is present.

Strip 6-66
Rhythm: Regular
Rate: 136 beats/minute
P waves: Sinus
PR interval: 0.16 to 0.20 second
QRS complex: 0.08 to 0.10 second
Rhythm interpretation: Sinus
tachycardia; an elevated ST segment
is present.

Strip 6-67
Rhythm: Regular
Rate: 44 beats/minute
P waves: Sinus
PR interval: 0.14 to 0.16 second
QRS complex: 0.08 second
Rhythm interpretation: Sinus
bradycardia; a U wave is present.

Strip 6-68
Rhythm: Regular
Rate: 88 beats/minute
P waves: Sinus
PR interval: 0.18 to 0.20 second
QRS complex: 0.06 to 0.08 second
Rhythm interpretation: Normal sinus
rhythm; a depressed ST segment is
present.

Strip 6-69
Rhythm: Regular
Rate: 136 beats/minute
P waves: Sinus
PR interval: 0.14 to 0.16 second
QRS complex: 0.08 second
Rhythm interpretation: Sinus
tachycardia; an elevated ST segment
is present.

Strip 6-70
Rhythm: Regular (basic rhythm);
irregular during pause
Rate: 56 beats/minute (basic rhythm);
slows to 50 beats/minute after a
pause (temporary rate suppression
can occur after a pause in the basic
rhythm; after several cycles the rate
returns to the basic rate)
P waves: Sinus (basic rhythm);
absent during pause
PR interval: 0.14 to 0.16 second
(basic rhythm); absent during pause
QRS complex: 0.08 to 0.10 second
(basic rhythm); absent during pause
Rhythm interpretation: Sinus
bradycardia with sinus arrest

Strip 6-71
Rhythm: Regular
Rate: 115 beats/minute
P waves: Sinus
PR interval: 0.14 to 0.16 second
QRS complex: 0.08 to 0.10 second
Rhythm interpretation: Sinus
tachycardia; ST-segment depression
is present.

Strip 6-72
Rhythm: Regular
Rate: 79 beats/minute
P waves: Sinus
PR interval: 0.14 to 0.16 second
QRS complex: 0.06 to 0.08 second
Rhythm interpretation: Normal sinus
rhythm; a depressed ST segment and
a biphasic T wave are present.

Strip 6-73
Rhythm: Regular
Rate: 54 beats/minute
P waves: Sinus
PR interval: 0.14 to 0.16 second
QRS complex: 0.06 to 0.08 second
Rhythm interpretation: Sinus
bradycardia; an elevated ST segment
is present.

Strip 6-74
Rhythm: Regular
Rate: 94 beats/minute
P waves: Sinus
PR interval: 0.16 second
QRS complex: 0.08 to 0.10 second
Rhythm interpretation: Normal
sinus rhythm; ST-segment
depression and a biphasic T wave
are present.

Strip 6-75
Rhythm: Regular
Rate: 94 beats/minute
P waves: Sinus
PR interval: 0.16 to 0.20 second
QRS complex: 0.06 to 0.08 second
Rhythm interpretation: Normal sinus
rhythm

Strip 6-76
Rhythm: Regular
Rate: 125 beats/minute
P waves: Sinus
PR interval: 0.12 second
QRS complex: 0.06 to 0.08 second
Rhythm interpretation: Sinus
tachycardia

Strip 6-77
Rhythm: Regular
Rate: 79 beats/minute
P waves: Sinus
PR interval: 0.18 to 0.20 second
QRS complex: 0.06 to 0.08 second
Rhythm interpretation: Normal sinus
rhythm; an elevated ST segment is
present.

Strip 6-78
Rhythm: Regular
Rate: 58 beats/minute
P waves: Sinus
PR interval: 0.16 to 0.18 second
QRS complex: 0.06 to 0.08 second
Rhythm interpretation: Sinus
bradycardia; an elevated ST segment
and a U wave are present.

Strip 6-79
Rhythm: Regular (basic rhythm);
irregular during pause
Rate: 107 beats/minute (basic
rhythm); slows to 94 beats/
minute for one cycle after a pause
(temporary rate suppression can
occur after a pause in the basic
rhythm)
P waves: Sinus in basic rhythm;
absent during pause
PR interval: 0.16 to 0.20 second
(basic rhythm); absent during
pause
QRS complex: 0.10 second (basic
rhythm); absent during pause
Rhythm interpretation: Sinus
tachycardia with sinus block;
baseline artifact is present.

Strip 6-80
Rhythm: Regular
Rate: 84 beats/minute
P waves: Sinus
PR interval: 0.16 second
QRS complex: 0.06 second
Rhythm interpretation: Normal
sinus rhythm; T-wave inversion is
present.

Strip 6-81
Rhythm: Regular
Rate: 56 beats/minute
P waves: Sinus
PR interval: 0.16 to 0.18 second
QRS complex: 0.06 to 0.08 second
Rhythm interpretation: Sinus
bradycardia; T-wave inversion is
present.

Strip 6-82
Rhythm: Regular
Rate: 125 beats/minute
P waves: Sinus
PR interval: 0.16 to 0.18 second
QRS complex: 0.04 to 0.06 second
Rhythm interpretation: Sinus
tachycardia

Strip 6-83
Rhythm: Irregular (basic rhythm)
Rate: 60 beats/minute (basic rhythm)
P waves: Sinus (basic rhythm);
absent during pause
PR interval: 0.14 to 0.16 second
(basic rhythm); absent during
pause
QRS complex: 0.04 second (basic
rhythm); absent during pause
Rhythm interpretation: Sinus
arrhythmia with sinus pause (with
an irregular basic rhythm it's
impossible to distinguish sinus arrest
from sinus block, so the rhythm is
interpreted using the broad term
sinus pause).

Strip 6-84
Rhythm: Regular
Rate: 79 beats/minute
P waves: Sinus
PR interval: 0.12 second
QRS complex: 0.06 to 0.08 second
Rhythm interpretation: Normal sinus
rhythm; an elevated ST segment is
present.

Strip 6-85
Rhythm: Regular
Rate: 136 beats/minute
P waves: Sinus
PR interval: 0.14 to 0.16 second
QRS complex: 0.06 to 0.08 second
Rhythm interpretation: Sinus
tachycardia

Strip 6-86
Rhythm: Regular
Rate: 54 beats/minute
P waves: Sinus
PR interval: 0.16 second
QRS complex: 0.06 to 0.08 second
Rhythm interpretation: Sinus
bradycardia

Strip 6-87
Rhythm: Regular (basic rhythm);
irregular during pause
Rate: 84 beats/minute (basic rhythm);
slows to 75 beats/minute for one
cycle after the pause (temporary rate
suppression is common after a pause
in the basic rhythm)
P waves: Sinus (basic rhythm);
absent during pause
PR interval: 0.16 to 0.18 second
(basic rhythm); absent during pause
QRS complex: 0.06 to 0.08 second
(basic rhythm); absent during pause
Rhythm interpretation: Normal sinus
rhythm with sinus arrest

Strip 6-88
Rhythm: Regular
Rate: 100 beats/minute
P waves: Sinus
PR interval: 0.12 to 0.14 second
QRS complex: 0.08 to 0.10 second
Rhythm interpretation: Normal sinus
rhythm; an elevated ST segment is
present.

Strip 6-89
Rhythm: Regular
Rate: 54 beats/minute
P waves: Sinus
PR interval: 0.18 to 0.20 second
QRS complex: 0.06 to 0.08 second
Rhythm interpretation: Sinus
bradycardia; an elevated ST segment
and T-wave inversion are present.

Strip 6-90
Rhythm: Regular (basic rhythm);
irregular during pause
Rate: 72 beats/minute (basic rhythm);
slows to 68 beats/minute for two
cycles after a pause (temporary rate
suppression can occur after a pause in
the basic rhythm)
P waves: Sinus (basic rhythm);
absent during pause
PR interval: 0.12 to 0.14 second
(basic rhythm); absent during pause
QRS complex: 0.06 to 0.08 second
(basic rhythm); absent during pause
Rhythm interpretation: Normal sinus
rhythm with sinus arrest; T-wave
inversion is present.

Strip 6-91
Rhythm: Regular
Rate: 65 beats/minute
P waves: Sinus
PR interval: 0.14 to 0.16 second
QRS complex: 0.06 to 0.08 second
Rhythm interpretation: Normal sinus
rhythm; a U wave is present.

Strip 6-92
Rhythm: Regular
Rate: 63 beats/minute
P waves: Sinus
PR interval: 0.18 to 0.20 second
QRS complex: 0.08 to 0.10 second
Rhythm interpretation: Normal sinus
rhythm; ST-segment depression and
T-wave inversion are present.

Strip 6-93
Rhythm: Regular (basic rhythm);
irregular during pause
Rate: 79 beats/minute (basic
rhythm); slows to 72 beats/minute
after a pause (temporary rate
suppression can occur after a pause
in the basic rhythm)
P waves: Sinus (basic rhythm);
absent during pause
PR interval: 0.20 second (basic
rhythm); absent during pause
QRS complex: 0.08 to 0.10 second
(basic rhythm); absent during pause
Rhythm interpretation: Normal
sinus rhythm with sinus arrest;
ST-segment depression and T-wave
inversion are present.

Strip 6-94
Rhythm: Regular
Rate: 150 beats/minute
P waves: Sinus
PR interval: 0.12 second
QRS complex: 0.04 to 0.06 second
Rhythm interpretation: Sinus
tachycardia

Strip 6-95
Rhythm: Regular
Rate: 136 beats/minute
P waves: Sinus
PR interval: 0.12 second
QRS complex: 0.06 to 0.08 second
Rhythm interpretation: Sinus
tachycardia

Strip 6-96
Rhythm: Irregular
Rate: 50 beats/minute
P waves: Sinus
PR interval: 0.14 to 0.16 second
QRS complex: 0.08 second
Rhythm interpretation: Sinus
arrhythmia with a bradycardic rate

Strip 6-97
Rhythm: Irregular
Rate: 40 beats/minute
P waves: Sinus
PR interval: 0.18 to 0.20 second
QRS complex: 0.06 to 0.08 second
Rhythm interpretation: Sinus
arrhythmia with a bradycardic
rate and sinus pause. (With
an irregular basic rhythm it's
impossible to distinguish sinus arrest
from sinus block, so the rhythm is
interpreted using the broad term
sinus pause.)

Strip 6-98
Rhythm: Regular
Rate: 136 beats/minute
P waves: Sinus
PR interval: 0.14 to 0.16 second
QRS complex: 0.08 to 0.10 second
Rhythm interpretation: Sinus
tachycardia; ST-segment elevation is
present.

Strip 6-99
Rhythm: Irregular
Rate: 50 beats/minute
P waves: Sinus
PR interval: 0.14 to 0.16 second
QRS complex: 0.08 to 0.10 second
Rhythm interpretation: Sinus
arrhythmia with a bradycardic rate

Strip 7-1
Rhythm: Irregular
Rate: 60 beats/minute (ventricular);
atrial not measurable
P waves: Fibrillation waves present
PR interval: Not measurable
QRS complex: 0.06 to 0.08 second
Rhythm interpretation: Atrial
fibrillation; ST-segment depression
is present.

Strip 7-2
Rhythm: Regular
Rate: 188 beats/minute
P waves: Hidden in T waves
PR interval: Not measurable
QRS complex: 0.06 to 0.08 second
Rhythm interpretation: Paroxysmal
atrial tachycardia

Strip 7-3
Rhythm: Regular (basic rhythm);
irregular (PACs)
Rate: 94 beats/minute (basic rhythm)
P waves: Sinus (basic rhythm);
premature and abnormal (PACs)
PR interval: 0.12 second (basic
rhythm); 0.14 second (PACs)
QRS complex: 0.08 to 0.10 second
(basic rhythm and PACs)
Rhythm interpretation: Normal
sinus rhythm with two PACs (fourth
and eighth complexes); ST-segment
depression is present.

Strip 7-4
Rhythm: Regular (off by one square)
Rate: 65 to 68 beats/minute
P waves: Vary in size, shape, and
position
PR interval: 0.12 to 0.16 second
QRS complex: 0.06 to 0.08 second
Rhythm interpretation: Wandering
atrial pacemaker

Strip 7-5
Rhythm: Regular (basic rhythm);
irregular (PAC)
Rate: 125 beats/minute (basic rhythm)
P waves: Sinus (basic rhythm); pre-
mature and pointed (PAC)
PR interval: 0.12 second (basic
rhythm)
QRS complex: 0.04 to 0.06 second
(basic rhythm)
Rhythm interpretation: Sinus tachy-
cardia with one PAC (eighth complex)

Strip 7-6
Rhythm: Regular
Rate: 167 beats/minute
P waves: Pointed, abnormal
PR interval: 0.14 to 0.16 second
QRS complex: 0.06 to 0.08 second
Rhythm interpretation: Paroxys-
mal atrial tachycardia; ST-segment
depression is present.

Strip 7-7
Rhythm: Regular (basic rhythm);
irregular (nonconducted PAC)
Rate: 88 beats/minute (basic rhythm)
P waves: Sinus (basic rhythm);
premature and abnormal
(nonconducted PAC)
PR interval: 0.16 second
QRS complex: 0.06 to 0.08 second
Rhythm interpretation: Normal sinus
rhythm with nonconducted PAC
(after the seventh QRS complex); ST-
segment depression is present.

Strip 7-8
Rhythm: Irregular
Rate: 320 beats/minute (atrial);
120 beats/minute (ventricular)
P waves: Flutter waves present
(varying ratios)
PR interval: Not measurable
QRS complex: 0.06 to 0.08 second
Rhythm interpretation: Atrial flutter
with variable AV conduction

Strip 7-9
Rhythm: Irregular
Rate: 70 beats/minute
P waves: Vary in size, shape, and
direction
PR interval: 0.12 to 0.14 second
QRS complex: 0.06 to 0.08 second
Rhythm interpretation: Wandering
atrial pacemaker

Strip 7-10
Rhythm: Irregular
Rate: 60 beats/minute (ventricular);
atrial not measurable
P waves: Fibrillatory waves present
PR interval: Not measurable
QRS complex: 0.04 to 0.06 second
Rhythm interpretation: Atrial
fibrillation

Strip 7-11
Rhythm: Regular (basic rhythm);
irregular (PAC)
Rate: 72 beats/minute (basic rhythm)
P waves: Sinus (basic rhythm);
premature and pointed (PAC)
PR interval: 0.18 to 0.20 second
(basic rhythm)
QRS complex: 0.06 to 0.08 second
(basic rhythm)
Rhythm interpretation: Normal sinus
rhythm with one PAC (sixth complex)

Strip 7-12
Rhythm: Regular
Rate: 237 beats/minute (atrial);
79 beats/minute (ventricular)
P waves: Three flutter waves to each
QRS complex
PR interval: Not necessary to
measure
QRS complex: 0.04 second
Rhythm interpretation: Atrial flutter
with 3:1 AV conduction

Strip 7-13
Rhythm: Regular (basic rhythm);
irregular (PAC)
Rate: 107 beats/minute (basic
rhythm)
P waves: Sinus (basic rhythm);
premature and pointed P wave
without a QRS complex after the fifth
QRS complex
PR interval: 0.18 to 0.20 second
QRS complex: 0.04 to 0.06 second
Rhythm interpretation: Sinus
tachycardia with one nonconducted
PAC (after the fifth QRS complex)

Strip 7-14
Rhythm: Irregular
Rate: 110 beats/minute (ventricular);
atrial not measurable
P waves: Fibrillatory waves present
PR interval: Not measurable
QRS complex: 0.06 to 0.08 second
Rhythm interpretation: Atrial
fibrillation; some flutter waves are
noted.

Strip 7-15
Rhythm: Regular (both rhythms)
Rate: 167 beats/minute (first
rhythm); 100 beats/minute (second
rhythm)
P waves: Obscured in T waves
(first rhythm); sinus (second
rhythm)
PR interval: Not measurable (first
rhythm); 0.16 to 0.18 second (second
rhythm)
QRS complex: 0.08 second (both
rhythms)
Rhythm interpretation: Paroxysmal
atrial tachycardia converting to
normal sinus rhythm

Strip 7-16
Rhythm: Regular
Rate: 300 beats/minute (atrial);
100 beats/minute (ventricular)
P waves: Three flutter waves before
each QRS complex
PR interval: Not measurable
QRS complex: 0.08 second
Rhythm interpretation: Atrial flutter
with 3:1 AV conduction

Strip 7-17
Rhythm: Irregular
Rate: 40 beats/minute
P waves: Fibrillatory waves
PR interval: Not measurable
QRS complex: 0.08 second
Rhythm interpretation: Atrial
fibrillation

Strip 7-18
Rhythm: Irregular
Rate: 320 beats/minute (atrial);
90 beats/minute (ventricular)
P waves: Flutter waves (varying ratios)
PR interval: Not discernible
QRS complex: 0.04 to 0.06 second
Rhythm interpretation: Atrial flutter
with variable AV conduction

Strip 7-19
Rhythm: Regular (basic rhythm);
irregular (PACs and nonconducted
PACs)
Rate: 84 beats/minute (basic rhythm)
P waves: Sinus (basic rhythm);
premature and abnormal (PACs and
nonconducted PACs)
PR interval: 0.16 second (basic
rhythm)
QRS complex: 0.06 to 0.08 second
(basic rhythm and PACs)
Rhythm interpretation: Normal
sinus rhythm with two PACs (third
and ninth complexes) and two
nonconducted PACs (after the fourth
and fifth complexes)

Strip 7-20
Rhythm: Regular
Rate: 167 beats/minute
P waves: Pointed and abnormal
PR interval: 0.16 to 0.18 second
QRS complex: 0.06 to 0.08 second
Rhythm interpretation: Paroxysmal
atrial tachycardia

Strip 7-21
Rhythm: Regular (basic rhythm);
irregular (nonconducted PAC)
Rate: 75 beats/minute (basic
rhythm); slows to 72 beats/
minute for two cycles after a
pause (temporary rate suppression
is common after a pause in the
underlying rhythm)
P waves: Sinus (basic rhythm);
premature and pointed without QRS
complex after the third QRS complex
PR interval: 0.16 second
QRS complex: 0.08 second
Rhythm interpretation: Normal sinus
rhythm with one nonconducted
PAC (after the third QRS complex);
a U wave is present.

Strip 7-22
Rhythm: Regular
Rate: 260 beats/minute (atrial);
65 beats/minute (ventricular)
P waves: Four flutter waves to each
QRS complex
PR interval: Not measurable
QRS complex: 0.08 second
Rhythm interpretation: Atrial flutter
with 4:1 AV conduction

Strip 7-23
Rhythm: Regular (basic rhythm);
irregular with pause
Rate: 79 beats/minute (basic rhythm)
P waves: Sinus (basic rhythm);
premature and abnormal without
QRS complex after the fourth QRS
complex
PR interval: 0.16 to 0.18 second
(basic rhythm)
QRS complex: 0.06 to 0.08 second
(basic rhythm)
Rhythm interpretation: Normal sinus
rhythm with one nonconducted
PAC (after the fourth QRS complex);
ST-segment depression and T-wave
inversion are present.

Strip 7-24
Rhythm: Irregular
Rate: 100 beats/minute
P waves: Fibrillatory waves present
PR interval: Not measurable
QRS complex: 0.06 to 0.08 second
Rhythm interpretation: Atrial
fibrillation

Strip 7-25
Rhythm: Regular
Rate: 84 beats/minute
P waves: Vary in size, shape, and position
PR interval: 0.12 to 0.14 second
QRS complex: 0.06 to 0.08 second
Rhythm interpretation: Wandering atrial pacemaker; T-wave inversion is present.

Strip 7-26
Rhythm: Regular (basic rhythm); irregular (PAC)
Rate: 68 beats/minute (basic rhythm)
P waves: Sinus (basic rhythm); premature and inverted (PAC)
PR interval: 0.12 to 0.14 second (basic rhythm); 0.12 second (PAC)
QRS complex: 0.06 to 0.08 second (basic rhythm); 0.08 second (PAC)
Rhythm interpretation: Normal sinus rhythm with one PAC (fourth complex); a U wave is present.

Strip 7-27
Rhythm: Regular
Rate: 232 beats/minute (atrial); 58 beats/minute (ventricular)
P waves: Four flutter waves to each QRS complex
PR interval: Not measurable
QRS complex: 0.06 to 0.08 second
Rhythm interpretation: Atrial flutter with 4:1 AV conduction

Strip 7-28
Rhythm: Regular (basic rhythm); irregular (PACs)
Rate: 42 beats/minute (basic rhythm; measured between the fifth and sixth complexes)
P waves: Sinus (basic rhythm); premature and abnormal (PACs)
PR interval: 0.12 to 0.14 second (basic rhythm); 0.16 second (PACs)
QRS complex: 0.08 to 0.10 second
Rhythm interpretation: Sinus bradycardia with four PACs (second, fourth, seventh, and ninth complexes)

Strip 7-29
Rhythm: Regular
Rate: 150 beats/minute
P waves: Obscured in preceding T wave
PR interval: Not measurable
QRS complex: 0.08 second
Rhythm interpretation: Paroxysmal atrial tachycardia

Strip 7-30
Rhythm: Regular
Rate: 272 beats/minute (atrial); 136 beats/minute (ventricular)
P waves: Two flutter waves to each QRS complex
PR interval: Not measurable
QRS complex: 0.06 second
Rhythm interpretation: Atrial flutter with 2:1 AV conduction

Strip 7-31
Rhythm: Regular (basic rhythm); irregular (PACs and atrial fibrillation)
Rate: 68 beats/minute (basic rhythm); 140 beats/minute (atrial fibrillation)
P waves: Sinus (basic rhythm); premature and abnormal (PACs); fibrillation waves (atrial fibrillation)
PR interval: 0.12 to 0.14 second (basic rhythm)
QRS complex: 0.08 to 0.10 second
Rhythm interpretation: Normal sinus rhythm with two PACs (second and fifth complexes); last PAC initiates atrial fibrillation; ST-segment depression is present.

Strip 7-32
Rhythm: Regular (basic rhythm); irregular (nonconducted PAC)
Rate: 94 beats/minute (basic rhythm); slows to 84 beats/minute for one cycle after a pause (temporary rate suppression can occur after a pause in the basic rhythm)
P waves: Sinus (basic rhythm); premature, abnormal P wave without a QRS complex hidden in T wave after the seventh QRS complex
PR interval: 0.16 to 0.18 second
QRS complex: 0.06 to 0.08 second
Rhythm interpretation: Normal sinus rhythm with one nonconducted PAC (after the seventh QRS complex)

Strip 7-33
Rhythm: Regular (basic rhythm); irregular (PAC)
Rate: 47 beats/minute (basic rhythm)
P waves: Sinus (basic rhythm); premature and pointed (PAC)
PR interval: 0.18 to 0.20 second
QRS complex: 0.08 second
Rhythm interpretation: Sinus bradycardia with one PAC (fifth complex); a U wave is present.

Strip 7-34
Rhythm: Irregular
Rate: 50 beats/minute (ventricular); atrial not measurable
P waves: Fibrillatory waves present
PR interval: Not measurable
QRS complex: 0.06 to 0.08 second
Rhythm interpretation: Atrial fibrillation; ST-segment depression and T-wave inversion are present.

Strip 7-35
Rhythm: Regular
Rate: 188 beats/minute
P waves: Obscured in T waves
PR interval: Unmeasurable
QRS complex: 0.04 to 0.08 second
Rhythm interpretation: Paroxysmal atrial tachycardia; ST-segment depression is present.

Strip 7-36
Rhythm: Irregular
Rate: 50 beats/minute
P waves: Vary in size, shape, or direction across strip
PR interval: 0.12 to 0.16 second
QRS complex: 0.04 to 0.06 second
Rhythm interpretation: Wandering atrial pacemaker

Strip 7-37
Rhythm: Irregular
Rate: 260 beats/minute (atrial); 70 beats/minute (ventricular)
P waves: Flutter waves (varying ratios)
PR interval: Not measurable
QRS complex: 0.08 second
Rhythm interpretation: Atrial flutter with variable AV conduction

Strip 7-38
Rhythm: Regular
Rate: 150 beats/minute
P waves: Obscured in T waves
(T-P waves)
PR interval: Not measurable
QRS complex: 0.06 to 0.08 second
Rhythm interpretation: Paroxysmal
atrial tachycardia

Strip 7-39
Rhythm: Regular (basic rhythm);
irregular (PAC)
Rate: 136 beats/minute (basic
rhythm)
P waves: Sinus (basic rhythm);
premature and pointed (PAC)
PR interval: 0.16 to 0.18 second
(basic rhythm); 0.18 second (PAC)
QRS complex: 0.06 to 0.08 second
(basic rhythm); 0.06 second (PAC)
Rhythm interpretation: Sinus
tachycardia with one PAC (eleventh
complex)

Strip 7-40
Rhythm: Irregular
Rate: 130 beats/minute (ventricular);
atrial not measurable
P waves: Fibrillatory waves present
PR interval: Not measurable
QRS complex: 0.04 to 0.06 second
Rhythm interpretation: Atrial
fibrillation (uncontrolled rate)

Strip 7-41
Rhythm: Regular (basic rhythm);
irregular (nonconducted PAC)
Rate: 79 beats/minute (basic
rhythm)
P waves: Sinus (basic rhythm);
premature, abnormal P wave hidden
in the T wave after the seventh QRS
complex
PR interval: 0.20 second
QRS complex: 0.08 to 0.10 second
Rhythm interpretation: Normal sinus
rhythm with one nonconducted
PAC (hidden in the T wave after the
seventh QRS complex); a U wave is
present.

Strip 7-42
Rhythm: Regular (basic rhythm);
irregular with premature atrial
contraction (PAC)
Rate: 84 beats/minute (basic
rhythm)
P waves: Sinus (basic rhythm);
abnormal, pointed (PAC)
PR interval: 0.12 to 0.14 second
(basic rhythm); 0.28 second (PAC)
QRS complex: 0.06 to 0.08 second
(basic rhythm); 0.06 second (PAC)
Rhythm interpretation: Normal sinus
rhythm with one PAC (conducted
with long PR interval)

Strip 7-43
Rhythm: Regular
Rate: 68 beats/minute
P waves: Vary in size, shape, and
position
PR interval: 0.12 second
QRS complex: 0.06 to 0.08 second
Rhythm interpretation: Wander-
ing atrial pacemaker; ST-segment
depression is present.

Strip 7-44
Rhythm: Regular
Rate: 272 beats/minute (atrial);
136 beats/minute (ventricular)
P waves: Two flutter waves to each
QRS complex
PR interval: Not measurable
QRS complex: 0.06 to 0.08 second
Rhythm interpretation: Atrial flutter
with 2:1 AV conduction

Strip 7-45
Rhythm: Regular
Rate: 188 beats/minute
P waves: Hidden in T waves
PR interval: Not measurable
QRS complex: 0.04 to 0.06 second
Rhythm interpretation: Paroxysmal
atrial tachycardia; ST-segment
depression is present.

Strip 7-46
Rhythm: Regular (basic rhythm);
irregular (premature beat)
Rate: 79 beats/minute (basic rhythm)
P waves: Sinus (basic rhythm);
premature and pointed (PAC)
PR interval: 0.14 to 0.16 second
(basic rhythm); 0.12 second (PAC)
QRS complex: 0.06 to 0.08 second
Rhythm interpretation: Normal sinus
rhythm with one PAC (fifth complex)

Strip 7-47
Rhythm: Regular (basic rhythm);
irregular (PAC)
Rate: 84 beats/minute (basic rhythm)
P waves: Sinus; premature and
pointed (PAC)
PR interval: 0.14 to 0.16 (basic
rhythm); 0.16 second (PAC)
QRS complex: 0.06 to 0.08 second
(basic rhythm); 0.08 second (PAC)
Rhythm interpretation: Normal
sinus rhythm with one PAC (seventh
complex); ST-segment depression is
present.

Strip 7-48
Rhythm: Irregular
Rate: 40 beats/minute
P waves: Fibrillatory waves present
PR interval: Not measurable
QRS complex: 0.08 second
Rhythm interpretation: Atrial
fibrillation (controlled rate)

Strip 7-49
Rhythm: Irregular
Rate: 280 beats/minute (atrial);
50 beats/minute (ventricular)
P waves: Flutter waves present
(varying ratios)
PR interval: Not measurable
QRS complex: 0.06 to 0.08 second
Rhythm interpretation: Atrial flutter
with variable AV conduction

Strip 7-50
Rhythm: Irregular
Rate: 300 beats/minute (atrial);
100 beats/minute (ventricular)
P waves: Flutter waves (varying ratios)
PR interval: Not measurable
QRS complex: 0.04 to 0.06 second
Rhythm interpretation: Atrial flutter
with variable AV conduction

Strip 7-51
Rhythm: Regular
Rate: 150 beats/minute
P waves: Hidden in T waves
PR interval: Not measurable
QRS complex: 0.08 to 0.10 second
Rhythm interpretation: Paroxysmal atrial tachycardia

Strip 7-52
Rhythm: Regular (basic rhythm); irregular with PACs
Rate: 65 beats/minute (basic rhythm)
P waves: Sinus (basic rhythm); abnormal, inverted (PACs)
PR interval: 0.20 second (basic rhythm); 0.12 second (PACs)
QRS complex: 0.06 to 0.08 second (basic rhythm and PACs)
Rhythm interpretation: Normal sinus rhythm with paired PACs

Strip 7-53
Rhythm: Irregular
Rate: 70 beats/minute
P waves: Fibrillatory waves
PR interval: Not measurable
QRS complex: 0.06 to 0.08 second
Rhythm interpretation: Atrial fibrillation; ST-segment depression is present.

Strip 7-54
Rhythm: Regular (basic rhythm); irregular (PAC)
Rate: 94 beats/minute (basic rhythm)
P waves: Sinus (basic rhythm); premature and pointed (PAC)
PR interval: 0.12 to 0.16 second
QRS complex: 0.06 to 0.08 second
Rhythm interpretation: Normal sinus rhythm with one PAC (eighth complex); ST-segment depression is present.

Strip 7-55
Rhythm: Irregular (first rhythm); regular (second rhythm)
Rate: 120 beats/minute (first rhythm); 75 beats/minute (second rhythm)
P waves: Fibrillatory waves to sinus
PR interval: Not measurable (first rhythm); 0.12 to 0.14 second (second rhythm)
QRS complex: 0.04 to 0.08 second (both rhythms)
Rhythm interpretation: Atrial fibrillation to normal sinus rhythm

Strip 7-56
Rhythm: Regular (basic rhythm); irregular (PAC)
Rate: 84 beats/minute (basic rhythm)
P waves: Sinus (basic rhythm); premature and pointed (PAC)
PR interval: 0.12 to 0.14 second (basic rhythm); 0.12 second (PAC)
QRS complex: 0.06 to 0.08 second (basic rhythm); 0.08 second (PAC)
Rhythm interpretation: Normal sinus rhythm with one PAC (fifth complex); baseline artifact is present (baseline artifact shouldn't be confused with atrial fibrillation).

Strip 7-57
Rhythm: Regular
Rate: 225 beats/minute (atrial); 75 beats/minute (ventricular)
P waves: Three flutter waves to each QRS complex
PR interval: Not measurable
QRS complex: 0.06 to 0.08 second
Rhythm interpretation: Atrial flutter with 3:1 AV conduction

Strip 7-58
Rhythm: Regular (basic rhythm); irregular (nonconducted PACs)
Rate: 88 beats/minute (basic rhythm); rate slows to 72 beats/minute after a pause (temporary rate suppression is common after a pause in the basic rhythm)
P waves: Sinus (basic rhythm); premature, abnormal P wave without a QRS complex hidden in the T wave after the seventh QRS complex
PR interval: 0.12 to 0.14 second (basic rhythm)
QRS complex: 0.08 to 0.10 second
Rhythm interpretation: Normal sinus rhythm with one nonconducted PAC (after the seventh QRS complex)

Strip 7-59
Rhythm: Irregular
Rate: 70 beats/minute
P waves: Vary in size, shape, and direction
PR interval: 0.14 to 0.16 second
QRS complex: 0.06 to 0.08 second
Rhythm interpretation: Wandering atrial pacemaker; T-wave inversion is present.

Strip 7-60
Rhythm: Irregular
Rate: 50 beats/minute
P waves: Fibrillatory waves
PR interval: Not measurable
QRS complex: 0.04 to 0.06 second
Rhythm interpretation: Atrial fibrillation

Strip 7-61
Rhythm: Irregular
Rate: 210 beats/minute
P waves: Fibrillatory waves
PR interval: Not measurable
QRS complex: 0.04 to 0.06 second
Rhythm interpretation: Atrial fibrillation

Strip 7-62
Rhythm: Regular (basic rhythm); irregular (PAC)
Rate: 58 beats/minute (basic rhythm)
P waves: Sinus (basic rhythm); premature, abnormal P wave (PAC)
PR interval: 0.16 to 0.18 second (basic rhythm)
QRS complex: 0.06 to 0.08 second
Rhythm interpretation: Sinus bradycardia with one PAC (fifth complex); a U wave is present.

Strip 7-63
Rhythm: Irregular
Rate: 40 beats/minute
P waves: Fibrillatory waves
PR interval: Not measurable
QRS complex: 0.08 to 0.10 second
Rhythm interpretation: Atrial fibrillation

Strip 7-64
Rhythm: Regular
Rate: 214 beats/minute
P waves: Hidden in T waves
PR interval: Not measurable
QRS complex: 0.08 second
Rhythm interpretation: Paroxysmal atrial tachycardia

Strip 7-65
Rhythm: Regular (basic rhythm); irregular (PAC)
Rate: 52 beats/minute (basic rhythm)
P waves: Sinus (basic rhythm); premature, pointed P wave associated with PAC hidden in the T wave after the fourth QRS complex
PR interval: 0.16 to 0.18 second
QRS complex: 0.06 to 0.08 second
Rhythm interpretation: Sinus bradycardia with one PAC (fifth complex); a U wave is present.

Strip 7-66
Rhythm: Regular (basic rhythm); irregular (nonconducted PAC)
Rate: 75 beats/minute (basic rhythm)
P waves: Sinus (basic rhythm); premature, abnormal P wave hidden in the T wave after the fourth QRS complex
PR interval: 0.20 second
QRS complex: 0.06 to 0.08 second
Rhythm interpretation: Normal sinus rhythm with one nonconducted PAC (after the fourth QRS complex); a U wave is present.

Strip 7-67
Rhythm: Regular (off by two squares)
Rate: 79 beats/minute
P waves: Vary in size, shape, and direction
PR interval: 0.12 to 0.18 second
QRS complex: 0.08 to 0.10 second
Rhythm interpretation: Wandering atrial pacemaker

Strip 7-68
Rhythm: Regular
Rate: 150 beats/minute
P waves: Hidden in preceding T waves
PR interval: Not measurable
QRS complex: 0.04 to 0.06 second
Rhythm interpretation: Paroxysmal atrial tachycardia; ST-segment depression is present.

Strip 7-69
Rhythm: Irregular
Rate: 250 beats/minute (atrial); 70 beats/minute (ventricular)
P waves: Flutter waves before each QRS complex (varying ratios)
PR interval: Not measurable
QRS complex: 0.06 to 0.08 second
Rhythm interpretation: Atrial flutter with variable AV conduction

Strip 7-70
Rhythm: Irregular
Rate: 130 beats/minute (ventricular); atrial not measurable
P waves: Fibrillatory waves; some flutter waves
PR interval: Not measurable
QRS complex: 0.04 second
Rhythm interpretation: Atrial fibrillation; ST-segment depression is present.

Strip 7-71
Rhythm: Regular (basic rhythm); irregular (PACs)
Rate: 88 beats/minute (basic rhythm)
P waves: Sinus (basic rhythm); premature and abnormal (PACs)
PR interval: 0.14 to 0.16 second (basic rhythm)
QRS complex: 0.06 to 0.08 second
Rhythm interpretation: Normal sinus rhythm with paired PACs (third and fourth complexes)

Strip 7-72
Rhythm: Regular
Rate: 54 beats/minute
P waves: Varying in size and shape
PR interval: 0.12 second
QRS complex: 0.08 to 0.10 second
Rhythm interpretation: Wandering atrial pacemaker; ST-segment depression is present.

Strip 7-73
Rhythm: Regular
Rate: 272 beats/minute (atrial); 136 beats/minute (ventricular)
P waves: Two flutter waves to each QRS complex
PR interval: Not measurable
QRS complex: 0.08 second
Rhythm interpretation: Atrial flutter with 2:1 AV conduction

Strip 7-74
Rhythm: Regular (basic rhythm); irregular (PAC)
Rate: 63 beats/minute (basic rhythm)
P waves: Sinus (basic rhythm); premature and abnormal (PAC)
PR interval: 0.12 to 0.14 second (basic rhythm); 0.14 second (PAC)
QRS complex: 0.06 to 0.08 second (basic rhythm); 0.08 second (PAC)
Rhythm interpretation: Normal sinus rhythm with one PAC (fourth complex); a small U wave is present.

Strip 7-75
Rhythm: Regular
Rate: 150 beats/minute
P waves: Hidden in T waves
PR interval: Not measurable
QRS complex: 0.06 to 0.08 second
Rhythm interpretation: Paroxysmal atrial tachycardia; ST-segment depression is present.

Strip 7-76
Rhythm: Irregular
Rate: 80 beats/minute (ventricular); atrial not measurable
P waves: Fibrillatory waves present
PR interval: Not measurable
QRS complex: 0.04 second
Rhythm interpretation: Atrial fibrillation; ST-segment depression and T-wave inversion are present.

Strip 7-77
Rhythm: Regular
Rate: 88 beats/minute
P waves: Vary in size, shape, and position
PR interval: 0.12 to 0.14 second
QRS complex: 0.06 to 0.08 second
Rhythm interpretation: Wandering atrial pacemaker; T-wave inversion is present.

Strip 7-78
Rhythm: Irregular
Rate: 50 beats/minute
P waves: Vary in size, shape, and position
PR interval: 0.12 to 0.16 second
QRS complex: 0.08 second
Rhythm interpretation: Wandering atrial pacemaker; ST-segment depression is present.

Strip 7-79
Rhythm: Irregular
Rate: 280 beats/minute (atrial);
100 beats/minute (ventricular)
P waves: Flutter waves
PR interval: Not measurable
QRS complex: 0.04 to 0.06 second
Rhythm interpretation: Atrial flutter
with variable AV conduction

Strip 7-80
Rhythm: Regular (basic rhythm);
irregular (nonconducted PACs)
Rate: 107 beats/minute (basic
rhythm)
P waves: Sinus (basic rhythm);
premature and abnormal
(nonconducted PACs)
PR interval: 0.16 to 0.18 second
QRS complex: 0.06 to 0.08 second
Rhythm interpretation: Sinus
tachycardia with two nonconducted
PACs (after the third and eighth QRS
complexes)

Strip 7-81
Rhythm: Regular
Rate: 68 beats/minute
P waves: Vary in size, shape, and
direction
PR interval: 0.12 to 0.16 second
QRS complex: 0.08 second
Rhythm interpretation: Wandering
atrial pacemaker; a U wave is present.

Strip 7-82
Rhythm: Regular
Rate: 260 beats/minute (atrial);
65 beats/minute (ventricular)
P waves: Flutter waves
PR interval: Not measurable
QRS complex: 0.08 to 0.10 second
Rhythm interpretation: Atrial flutter
with 4:1 AV conduction

Strip 7-83
Rhythm: Regular
Rate: 167 beats/minute
P waves: Hidden in preceding T wave
PR interval: Not measurable
QRS complex: 0.08 to 0.10 second
Rhythm interpretation: Paroxysmal
atrial tachycardia

Strip 7-84
Rhythm: Irregular
Rate: 50 beats/minute
P waves: Fibrillatory waves
PR interval: Not measurable
QRS complex: 0.08 to 0.10 second
Rhythm interpretation: Atrial
fibrillation

Strip 7-85
Rhythm: Irregular
Rate: 40 beats/minute
P waves: Vary in size, shape, and
direction
PR interval: 0.14 to 0.16 second
QRS complex: 0.08 second
Rhythm interpretation: Wandering
atrial pacemaker

Strip 7-86
Rhythm: Regular (basic rhythm);
irregular (PACs)
Rate: 107 beats/minute (basic
rhythm)
P waves: Sinus (basic rhythm);
premature and pointed (PACs)
PR interval: 0.16 second (basic
rhythm)
QRS complex: 0.06 second
Rhythm interpretation: Sinus
tachycardia with three PACs (fourth,
ninth, and eleventh complexes)

Strip 7-87
Rhythm: Irregular
Rate: 60 beats/minute
P waves: Fibrillatory waves
PR interval: Not measurable
QRS complex: 0.04 to 0.08 second
Rhythm interpretation: Atrial
fibrillation

Strip 7-88
Rhythm: Regular (first rhythm);
irregular (second rhythm)
Rate: 79 beats/minute (first rhythm);
140 beats/minute (second rhythm)
P waves: Sinus to fibrillatory waves
PR interval: 0.12 to 0.14 second (first
rhythm); not measurable (second
rhythm)
QRS complex: 0.04 to 0.08 second
(both rhythms)
Rhythm interpretation: Normal sinus
rhythm to atrial fibrillation

Strip 7-89
Rhythm: Regular (basic rhythm);
irregular (nonconducted PAC)
Rate: 84 beats/minute (basic
rhythm)
P waves: Sinus (basic rhythm);
premature and pointed
(nonconducted PAC)
PR interval: 0.16 to 0.20 second
QRS complex: 0.06 to 0.08 second
Rhythm interpretation:
Normal sinus rhythm with one
nonconducted PAC (after the
fifth QRS complex); ST-segment
depression is present.

Strip 7-90
Rhythm: Regular (basic rhythm);
irregular (PAC)
Rate: 54 beats/minute (basic
rhythm)
P waves: Sinus (basic rhythm);
premature and abnormal (PAC)
PR interval: 0.16 to 0.18 second
QRS complex: 0.06 second
Rhythm interpretation: Sinus
bradycardia with one PAC (fourth
complex)

Strip 7-91
Rhythm: Regular (basic rhythm);
irregular (PAC)
Rate: 63 beats/minute (basic
rhythm)
P waves: Sinus (basic rhythm);
premature and abnormal (PAC)
PR interval: 0.14 to 0.16 second
QRS complex: 0.06 second
Rhythm interpretation: Normal
sinus rhythm with one PAC (fifth
complex); a U wave is present.

Strip 7-92
Rhythm: Regular
Rate: 235 beats/minute (atrial);
47 beats/minute (ventricular)
P waves: Five flutter waves to each
QRS complex
PR interval: Not discernible
QRS complex: 0.08 second
Rhythm interpretation: Atrial flutter
with 5:1 AV conduction; T-wave
inversion is present.

Strip 7-93
Rhythm: Regular
Rate: 150 beats/minute
P waves: Obscured in T waves
(T-P waves)
PR interval: Not measurable
QRS complex: 0.04 to 0.08 second
Rhythm interpretation: Paroxysmal
atrial tachycardia

Strip 7-94
Rhythm: Irregular
Rate: 50 beats/minute
P waves: Wavy
PR interval: Not measurable
QRS complex: 0.04 to 0.06 second
Rhythm interpretation: Atrial
fibrillation

Strip 7-95
Rhythm: Regular (basic rhythm);
irregular after a burst of PAT
Rate: 84 beats/minute (basic rhythm)
P waves: Sinus (basic rhythm); abnor-
mal and premature with a run of PAT
PR interval: 0.16 to 0.18 second (basic
rhythm); not measurable in PAT
QRS complex: 0.04 to 0.06 second
(basic rhythm and PAT)
Rhythm interpretation: Normal sinus
rhythm with burst of PAT (three
PACs after the fourth QRS complex)

Strip 7-96
Rhythm: Regular
Rate: 88 beats/minute
P waves: Sinus
PR interval: 0.16 to 0.18 second
QRS complex: 0.06 to 0.08 second
Rhythm interpretation: Normal sinus
rhythm

Strip 7-97
Rhythm: Regular (basic rhythm)
but off by one square; irregular with
PACs
Rate: 84 to 88 beats/minute (basic
rhythm)
P waves: Sinus (basic rhythm);
abnormal, pointed (PACs)
PR interval: 0.14 to 0.16 (basic
rhythm and PACs)
QRS complex: 0.08 second (basic
rhythm and PACs)
Rhythm interpretation: Normal sinus
rhythm with PACs every fourth beat
(quadrigeminal pattern)

Strip 7-98
Rhythm: Regular
Rate: 150 beats/minute
P waves: Sinus
PR interval: 0.14 to 0.16 second
QRS complex: 0.04 to 0.06 second
Rhythm interpretation: Sinus
tachycardia

Strip 7-99
Rhythm: Regular
Rate: 250 beats/minute (atrial);
125 beats/minute (ventricular)
P waves: Two flutter waves to each
QRS complex
PR interval: Not measurable
QRS complex: 0.08 second
Rhythm interpretation: Atrial flutter
with 2:1 AV conduction

Strip 7-100
Rhythm: Regular (basic rhythm);
irregular during pause
Rate: 48 beats/minute (basic
rhythm)
P waves: Sinus (basic rhythm);
absent during pause
PR interval: 0.20 second (basic
rhythm); absent during pause
QRS complex: 0.06 to 0.08 second
(basic rhythm); absent during
pause
Rhythm interpretation: Sinus
bradycardia with sinus arrest

Strip 7-101
Rhythm: Irregular
Rate: 90 beats/minute
P waves: Vary in size, shape, and
direction
PR interval: 0.12 to 0.20 second
QRS complex: 0.06 to 0.08 second
Rhythm interpretation: Wandering
atrial pacemaker

Strip 7-102
Rhythm: Regular (off by one
square)
Rate: 45 to 47 beats/minute
P waves: Sinus
PR interval: 0.16 to 0.20 second
QRS complex: 0.04 to 0.08 second
Rhythm interpretation: Sinus
bradycardia

Strip 7-103
Rhythm: Regular (first and second
rhythms)
Rate: 107 beats/minute (first
rhythm); 214 beats/minute (second
rhythm)
P waves: Sinus (first rhythm);
abnormal, pointed (second
rhythm)
PR interval: 0.16 to 0.18 second (first
rhythm); not measurable (second
rhythm)
QRS complex: 0.08 to 0.10 second
(first and second rhythms)
Rhythm interpretation: Sinus
tachycardia with burst of PAT (8-beat
run initiated by PAC)

Strip 7-104
Rhythm: Irregular
Rate: 100 beats/minute
P waves: Fibrillatory waves
PR interval: Not measurable
QRS complex: 0.08 to 0.10 second
Rhythm interpretation: Atrial
fibrillation

Strip 7-105
Rhythm: Irregular
Rate: 60 beats/minute
P waves: Sinus
PR interval: 0.14 to 0.16 second
QRS complex: 0.06 to 0.08 second
Rhythm interpretation: Sinus
arrhythmia

Strip 7-106
Rhythm: Regular (first rhythm);
irregular (second rhythm)
Rate: 75 beats/minute (first
rhythm); 360 beats/minute atrial
(second rhythm); 140 beats/minute
ventricular (second rhythm)
P waves: Sinus (first rhythm); flutter
waves (second rhythm)
PR interval: 0.12 second (first
rhythm); not measurable (second
rhythm)
QRS complex: 0.06 to 0.08 second
(first and second rhythms)
Rhythm interpretation: Normal sinus
rhythm with PAC (fifth complex)
changing to atrial flutter with
variable AV conduction

Strip 7-107
Rhythm: Regular
Rate: 84 beats/minute
P waves: Sinus
PR interval: 0.12 to 0.14 second
QRS complex: 0.06 to 0.08 second
Rhythm interpretation: Normal sinus
rhythm

Strip 8-1
Rhythm: Regular (basic rhythm);
irregular (PJC)
Rate: 58 beats/minute (basic
rhythm)
P waves: Sinus (basic rhythm);
premature and inverted (PJC)
PR interval: 0.14 to 0.16 second
(basic rhythm); 0.08 second (PJC)
QRS complex: 0.06 second (basic
rhythm and PJC)
Rhythm interpretation: Sinus
bradycardia with one PJC (fifth
complex); a U wave is present.

Strip 8-2
Rhythm: Regular
Rate: 60 beats/minute
P waves: Sinus
PR interval: 0.24 second
QRS complex: 0.06 to 0.08 second
Rhythm interpretation: Normal sinus
rhythm with first-degree AV block;
ST-segment elevation and T-wave
inversion are present.

Strip 8-3
Rhythm: Regular (atrial and
ventricular)
Rate: 96 beats/minute (atrial);
32 beats/minute (ventricular)
P waves: Three sinus P waves before
each QRS complex
PR interval: 0.14 to 0.16 second
(remains consistent)
QRS complex: 0.12 second
Rhythm interpretation: Mobitz II
with 3:1 AV conduction (third P wave
hidden in T waves)

Strip 8-4
Rhythm: Regular (basic rhythm);
irregular (junctional beat)
Rate: 58 beats/minute (basic rhythm)
P waves: Sinus (basic rhythm);
hidden P wave (junctional beat)
PR interval: 0.16 to 0.18 second
(basic rhythm)
QRS complex: 0.08 to 0.10 second
(basic rhythm and junctional beat)
Rhythm interpretation: Sinus
bradycardia with junctional escape
beat (fourth complex) after pause in
basic rhythm; ST-segment depression
is present.

Strip 8-5
Rhythm: Regular (first and second
rhythms)
Rate: 84 beats/minute (first rhythm);
94 beats/minute (second rhythm)
P waves: Sinus (first rhythm);
inverted (second rhythm)
PR interval: 0.12 second (first
rhythm); 0.08 to 0.10 second (second
rhythm)
QRS complex: 0.06 to 0.08 second
(first and second rhythms)
Rhythm interpretation: Normal sinus
rhythm changing to accelerated
junctional rhythm

Strip 8-6
Rhythm: Regular
Rate: 84 beats/minute
P waves: Sinus
PR interval: 0.22 to 0.24 second
QRS complex: 0.08 to 0.10 second
Rhythm interpretation: Normal sinus
rhythm with first-degree AV block

Strip 8-7
Rhythm: Regular
Rate: 65 beats/minute
P waves: Inverted before each QRS
complex
PR interval: 0.08 second
QRS complex: 0.06 to 0.08 second
Rhythm interpretation: Accelerated
junctional rhythm; ST-segment eleva-
tion and T-wave inversion are present.

Strip 8-8
Rhythm: Regular (atrial); irregular
(ventricular)
Rate: 75 beats/minute (atrial);
70 beats/minute (ventricular)
P waves: Sinus
PR interval: Lengthens from 0.28 to
0.32 second
QRS complex: 0.04 to 0.08 second
Rhythm interpretation: Second-degree
AV block, Mobitz I; ST-segment depres-
sion and T-wave inversion are present.

Strip 8-9
Rhythm: Regular
Rate: 47 beats/minute
P waves: Hidden in QRS complex
PR interval: Not measurable
QRS complex: 0.08 second
Rhythm interpretation: Junctional
rhythm; ST-segment depression is
present.

Strip 8-10
Rhythm: Regular (atrial); irregular
(ventricular)
Rate: 75 beats/minute (atrial);
30 beats/minute (ventricular)
P waves: Two sinus P waves before
each QRS complex
PR interval: 0.20 to 0.22 second
QRS complex: 0.08 to 0.10 second
Rhythm interpretation: Second-
degree AV block, Mobitz II (clinical
correlation is suggested to diagnose
Mobitz II when 2:1 conduction is
present with a narrow QRS complex).

Strip 8-11
Rhythm: Regular (atrial and
ventricular)
Rate: 63 beats/minute (atrial);
33 beats/minute (ventricular)
P waves: Sinus (bear no relationship
to the QRS complex; found hidden in
the QRS complex and T waves)
PR interval: Varies greatly
QRS complex: 0.12 second
Rhythm interpretation: Third-degree
AV block; ST-segment depression and
T-wave inversion are present.

Strip 8-12
Rhythm: Regular
Rate: 84 beats/minute
P waves: Hidden in the QRS complex
PR interval: Not measurable
QRS complex: 0.06 to 0.08 second
Rhythm interpretation: Accelerated junctional rhythm; ST-segment depression is present.

Strip 8-13
Rhythm: Regular
Rate: 65 beats/minute
P waves: Sinus
PR interval: 0.44 to 0.48 second
QRS complex: 0.08 to 0.10 second
Rhythm interpretation: Normal sinus rhythm with first-degree AV block; an elevated ST-segment is present.

Strip 8-14
Rhythm: Regular (basic rhythm); irregular (PJC)
Rate: 136 beats/minute (basic rhythm)
P waves: Sinus (basic rhythm); hidden P wave (PJC)
PR interval: 0.12 to 0.14 second
QRS complex: 0.04 to 0.06 second
Rhythm interpretation: Sinus tachycardia with one PJC (thirteenth complex)

Strip 8-15
Rhythm: Regular
Rate: 94 beats/minute
P waves: Sinus
PR interval: 0.26 to 0.28 second
QRS complex: 0.06 second
Rhythm interpretation: Normal sinus rhythm with first-degree AV block; ST-segment depression is present.

Strip 8-16
Rhythm: Regular (basic rhythm); irregular (premature beat)
Rate: 58 beats/minute (basic rhythm)
P waves: Sinus (basic rhythm); inverted (premature beat)
PR interval: 0.16 to 0.18 second (basic rhythm); 0.08 second (PJC)
QRS complex: 0.06 to 0.08 second
Rhythm interpretation: Sinus brady-cardia with one PJC (fourth complex); ST-segment depression is present.

Strip 8-17
Rhythm: Regular (atrial and ventricular)
Rate: 108 beats/minute (atrial); 54 beats/minute (ventricular)
P waves: Two P waves to each QRS complex
PR interval: 0.20 second and constant
QRS complex: 0.08 to 0.10 second
Rhythm interpretation: Second-degree AV block, Mobitz II (clinical correlation is suggested to diagnose Mobitz II when 2:1 conduction is present with a narrow QRS complex). ST-segment elevation and T-wave inversion are present.

Strip 8-18
Rhythm: Regular (atrial); irregular (ventricular)
Rate: 65 beats/minute (atrial); 50 beats/minute (ventricular)
P waves: Sinus
PR interval: Lengthens from 0.20 to 0.48 second
QRS complex: 0.04 second
Rhythm interpretation: Second-degree AV block, Mobitz I

Strip 8-19
Rhythm: Regular
Rate: 125 beats/minute
P waves: Inverted before each QRS complex
PR interval: 0.08 to 0.10 second
QRS complex: 0.06 second
Rhythm interpretation: Junctional tachycardia

Strip 8-20
Rhythm: Regular (atrial and ventricular)
Rate: 100 beats/minute (atrial); 38 beats/minute (ventricular)
P waves: Sinus (bear no relationship to the QRS complex; found hidden in the QRS complex and T waves)
PR interval: Varies greatly
QRS complex: 0.06 to 0.08 second
Rhythm interpretation: Third-degree AV block; ST-segment depression is present.

Strip 8-21
Rhythm: Regular (basic rhythm); irregular (PJC)
Rate: 60 beats/minute (basic rhythm)
P waves: Sinus (basic rhythm); premature and inverted (PJC)
PR interval: 0.12 to 0.14 second (basic rhythm); 0.08 second (PJC)
QRS complex: 0.08 second (basic rhythm and PJC)
Rhythm interpretation: Normal sinus rhythm with one PJC (fourth complex)

Strip 8-22
Rhythm: Regular (basic rhythm) but off by two squares
Rate: 54 to 58 beats/minute
P waves: Sinus (basic rhythm); hidden within QRS complex (junctional beats)
PR interval: 0.16 to 0.18 second (basic rhythm)
QRS complex: 0.08 to 0.10 second (basic rhythm and junctional beats)
Rhythm interpretation: Sinus bradycardia with a pause followed by two junctional escape beats; specific pause (sinus arrest or sinus block) cannot be identified due to the presence of the escape beats.

Strip 8-23
Rhythm: Regular
Rate: 35 beats/minute
P waves: Sinus
PR interval: 0.60 to 0.62 second (remains constant)
QRS complex: 0.06 second
Rhythm interpretation: Sinus bradycardia with first-degree AV block

Strip 8-24
Rhythm: Regular (atrial); irregular (ventricular)
Rate: 68 beats/minute (atrial); 60 beats/minute (ventricular)
P waves: Sinus
PR interval: 0.28 to 0.36 second
QRS complex: 0.08 second
Rhythm interpretation: Second-degree AV block, Mobitz I; a U wave is present.

Strip 8-25
Rhythm: Regular
Rate: 75 beats/minute
P waves: Sinus
PR interval: 0.28 second
QRS complex: 0.08 second
Rhythm interpretation: Sinus rhythm with first-degree AV block

Strip 8-26
Rhythm: Regular (basic rhythm); irregular with premature beats
Rate: 100 beats/minute (basic rhythm)
P waves: Sinus (basic rhythm); pointed P wave (PAC); inverted P wave (PJCs)
PR interval: 0.20 second (basic rhythm); 0.16 second (PAC); 0.06 second (PJCs)
QRS complex: 0.06 to 0.08 second (basic rhythm and premature beats)
Rhythm interpretation: Normal sinus rhythm with one PAC (seventh complex) and paired PJCs (eighth and ninth complexes); ST-segment depression is present.

Strip 8-27
Rhythm: Regular
Rate: 65 beats/minute
P waves: Inverted before each QRS complex
PR interval: 0.08 second
QRS complex: 0.08 second
Rhythm interpretation: Accelerated junctional rhythm; elevated ST segment is present.

Strip 8-28
Rhythm: Regular (basic rhythm); irregular (nonconducted PAC)
Rate: 56 beats/minute (basic rhythm)
P waves: Sinus (basic rhythm); premature, abnormal P wave without a QRS complex
PR interval: 0.24 to 0.26 second (remains constant)
QRS complex: 0.08 second
Rhythm interpretation: Sinus bradycardia with first-degree AV block and nonconducted PAC (follows the fourth QRS complex); ST-segment depression is present.

Strip 8-29
Rhythm: Regular (atrial); irregular (ventricular)
Rate: 72 beats/minute (atrial); 50 beats/minute (ventricular)
P waves: Sinus
PR interval: Lengthens from 0.24 to 0.36 second
QRS complex: 0.08 to 0.10 second
Rhythm interpretation: Mobitz I

Strip 8-30
Rhythm: Regular (atrial and ventricular)
Rate: 79 beats/minute (atrial); 32 beats/minute (ventricular)
P waves: Sinus (bear no relationship to the QRS complex; found hidden in the QRS complex and T waves)
PR interval: Varies greatly
QRS complex: 0.12 second
Rhythm interpretation: Third-degree AV block

Strip 8-31
Rhythm: Atrial and ventricular rhythm regular (both off by two squares)
Rate: 80 beats/minute (atrial); 30 beats/minute (ventricular)
P waves: Three sinus P waves to each QRS complex
PR interval: 0.20 to 0.22 second (remains consistent)
QRS complex: 0.14 to 0.16 second
Rhythm interpretation: Mobitz II with 3:1 AV conduction

Strip 8-32
Rhythm: Regular (atrial and ventricular)
Rate: 75 beats/minute (atrial); 34 beats/minute (ventricular)
P waves: Sinus (bear no relationship to the QRS complex; found hidden in the QRS complex and T waves)
PR interval: Varies greatly
QRS complex: 0.12 to 0.14 second
Rhythm interpretation: Third-degree AV block; ST-segment elevation is present.

Strip 8-33
Rhythm: Regular (basic rhythm); irregular (PAC)
Rate: 100 beats/minute (basic rhythm)
P waves: Inverted before the QRS complex (basic rhythm); upright and pointed (PAC)
PR interval: 0.08 second (basic rhythm); 0.12 second (PAC)
QRS complex: 0.08 second (basic rhythm and PAC)
Rhythm interpretation: Accelerated junctional rhythm with one PAC (sixth complex); ST-segment depression is present.

Strip 8-34
Rhythm: Regular (atrial); irregular (ventricular)
Rate: 75 beats/minute (atrial); 50 beats/minute (ventricular)
P waves: Sinus
PR interval: 0.28 to 0.40 second
QRS complex: 0.08 to 0.10 second
Rhythm interpretation: Second-degree AV block, Mobitz I

Strip 8-35
Rhythm: Regular
Rate: 60 beats/minute
P waves: Sinus
PR interval: 0.24 to 0.26 second
QRS complex: 0.06 to 0.08 second
Rhythm interpretation: Normal sinus rhythm with first-degree AV block

Strip 8-36
Rhythm: Regular
Rate: 41 beats/minute
P waves: Inverted after the QRS complex
PR interval: 0.04 to 0.06 second
QRS complex: 0.06 to 0.08 second
Rhythm interpretation: Junctional rhythm

Strip 8-37
Rhythm: Regular (basic rhythm);
irregular (PJCs)
Rate: 58 beats/minute (basic rhythm)
P waves: Sinus (basic rhythm);
premature and inverted (PJCs)
PR interval: 0.16 second (basic
rhythm); 0.08 to 0.10 second (PJCs)
QRS complex: 0.08 second (basic
rhythm and PJCs)
Rhythm interpretation: Sinus
bradycardia with two PJCs (fourth
and sixth complexes); a U wave is
present.

Strip 8-38
Rhythm: Regular
Rate: 60 beats/minute
P waves: Inverted
PR interval: 0.08 to 0.10 second
QRS complex: 0.06 to 0.08 second
Rhythm interpretation: Junctional
rhythm

Strip 8-39
Rhythm: Regular (atrial and
ventricular)
Rate: 65 beats/minute (atrial);
36 beats/minute (ventricular)
P waves: Sinus
PR interval: Varies (not consistent)
QRS complex: 0.12 to 0.14 second
Rhythm interpretation: Third-degree
AV block

Strip 8-40
Rhythm: Regular (atrial and
ventricular)
Rate: 84 beats/minute (atrial);
30 beats/minute (ventricular)
P waves: Sinus
PR interval: Varies (not consistent)
QRS complex: 0.06 to 0.08 second
Rhythm interpretation: Third-degree
AV block

Strip 8-41
Rhythm: Regular
Rate: 84 beats/minute
P waves: Hidden in QRS complex
PR interval: Not measurable
QRS complex: 0.06 to 0.08 second
Rhythm interpretation: Accelerated
junctional rhythm

Strip 8-42
Rhythm: Regular (atrial and ventricular)
Rate: 125 beats/minute (atrial);
40 beats/minute (ventricular)
P waves: Three sinus P waves before
each QRS complex
PR interval: 0.22 to 0.24 second
(consistent)
QRS complex: 0.12 second
Rhythm interpretation: Mobitz II
second-degree AV block

Strip 8-43
Rhythm: Irregular (first rhythm);
regular (second rhythm)
Rate: 80 beats/minute (first rhythm);
42 beats/minute (second rhythm)
P waves: Fibrillatory waves (first
rhythm); hidden P waves (second
rhythm)
PR interval: Not measurable in either
rhythm
QRS complex: 0.06 to 0.08 second
Rhythm interpretation: Atrial
fibrillation to junctional rhythm;
ST-segment depression is present.

Strip 8-44
Rhythm: Regular (basic rhythm);
irregular (premature beats)
Rate: 60 beats/minute (basic rhythm)
P waves: Sinus (basic rhythm);
premature and abnormal (premature
beats)
PR interval: 0.12 to 0.16 second
(basic rhythm); 0.12 second (PAC);
0.08 second (PJC)
QRS complex: 0.06 to 0.08 second
Rhythm interpretation: Normal
sinus rhythm with one PAC (fourth
complex) and one PJC (fifth
complex); ST-segment depression
and T-wave inversion are present.

Strip 8-45
Rhythm: Regular (atrial and
ventricular)
Rate: 72 beats/minute (atrial);
32 beats/minute (ventricular)
P waves: Sinus (bear no relationship
to the QRS complex; hidden in the
QRS complex and T waves)
PR interval: Varies greatly
QRS complex: 0.12 second
Rhythm interpretation: Third-degree
AV block; ST-segment elevation is
present.

Strip 8-46
Rhythm: Irregular
Rate: 40 beats/minute
P waves: Sinus
PR interval: 0.28 second (remains
constant)
QRS complex: 0.08 to 0.10 second
Rhythm interpretation: Sinus
arrhythmia with bradycardic rate
and first-degree AV block; a U wave is
present.

Strip 8-47
Rhythm: Regular (atrial); irregular
(ventricular)
Rate: 79 beats/minute (atrial);
50 beats/minute (ventricular)
P waves: Sinus
PR interval: Lengthens from 0.24 to
0.40 second
QRS complex: 0.08 to 0.10 second
Rhythm interpretation:
Second-degree AV block, Mobitz I

Strip 8-48
Rhythm: Regular (atrial and
ventricular)
Rate: 108 beats/minute (atrial);
54 beats/minute (ventricular)
P waves: Two sinus P waves before
each QRS complex
PR interval: 0.18 to 0.20 second
(remains constant)
QRS complex: 0.08 second
Rhythm interpretation: Second-
degree AV block, Mobitz II (clinical
correlation is suggested to diagnose
Mobitz II when 2:1 conduction is
present with a narrow QRS complex);
ST-segment elevation and T-wave
inversion are present.

Strip 8-49
Rhythm: Irregular
Rate: 40 beats/minute
P waves: Inverted before each QRS
complex
PR interval: 0.04 to 0.06 second
QRS complex: 0.08 to 0.10 second
Rhythm interpretation: Junctional
rhythm; ST-segment depression is
present.

Strip 8-50
Rhythm: Regular (basic rhythm);
irregular (escape beat)
Rate: 84 beats/minute (basic
rhythm); slows to 75 beats/
minute after escape beat
(temporary rate suppression can
occur after premature or escape
beats; after several cycles rate will
return to basic rate)
P waves: Sinus; P wave hidden with
escape beat
PR interval: 0.14 to 0.16 second
QRS complex: 0.06 to 0.08 second
Rhythm interpretation: Normal
sinus rhythm with junctional escape
beat (fifth complex) after a pause
in the basic rhythm; a U wave is
present.

Strip 8-51
Rhythm: Regular (atrial) but off by
two squares; irregular (ventricular)
Rate: 60 to 65 beats/minute (atrial);
50 beats/minute (ventricular)
P waves: Sinus
PR interval: Lengthens from 0.28 to
0.40 second (not consistent)
QRS complex: 0.08 second
Rhythm interpretation: Mobitz I
second-degree AV block

Strip 8-52
Rhythm: Regular
Rate: 63 beats/minute
P waves: Hidden in the QRS
complex
PR interval: Not measurable
QRS complex: 0.08 second
Rhythm interpretation: Accelerated
junctional rhythm

Strip 8-53
Rhythm: Regular (atrial) but off by
two squares; irregular (ventricular)
Rate: 84 beats/minute (atrial);
40 beats/minute (ventricular)
P waves: Sinus (two or three P waves
before each QRS complex)
PR interval: 0.12 second (consistent)
QRS complex: 0.12 second
Rhythm interpretation: Mobitz II
second-degree AV block with 2:1 and
3:1 AV conduction

Strip 8-54
Rhythm: Regular
Rate: 94 beats/minute
P waves: Inverted before the QRS
complex
PR interval: 0.08 second
QRS complex: 0.06 to 0.08 second
Rhythm interpretation: Accelerated
junctional rhythm

Strip 8-55
Rhythm: Regular (basic rhythm)
Rate: 55 beats/minute (basic rhythm)
P waves: Sinus (basic rhythm); notched
P waves usually indicate left atrial hypertrophy; no P wave seen with fourth
complex; fifth complex has a P wave on
top of the preceding T wave
PR interval: 0.20 second (basic
rhythm)
QRS complex: 0.06 to 0.08 second
Rhythm interpretation: Sinus
bradycardia with a pause followed
by a junctional escape beat (fourth
complex) and a PAC (fifth complex);
abnormal P wave associated with
PAC is observed in preceding T wave.

Strip 8-56
Rhythm: Regular (first and second
rhythms)
Rate: 72 beats/minute (first rhythm);
about 140 beats/minute (second
rhythm)
P waves: Sinus (first rhythm);
inverted (second rhythm)
PR interval: 0.12 second (first rhythm);
0.08 to 0.10 second (second rhythm)
QRS complex: 0.08 second
Rhythm interpretation: Normal
sinus rhythm changing to junctional
tachycardia; ST-segment depression
is present.

Strip 8-57
Rhythm: Regular
Rate: 84 beats/minute
P waves: Sinus
PR interval: 0.30 to 0.32 second
(remains constant)
QRS complex: 0.04 to 0.06 second
Rhythm interpretation: Normal sinus
rhythm with first-degree AV block;
ST-segment elevation is present.

Strip 8-58
Rhythm: Regular (atrial and
ventricular)
Rate: 75 beats/minute (atrial);
30 beats/minute (ventricular)
P waves: Sinus (bear no relationship
to the QRS complex)
PR interval: Varies greatly
QRS complex: 0.12 to 0.14 second
Rhythm interpretation: Third-degree
AV block

Strip 8-59
Rhythm: Regular (atrial and
ventricular)
Rate: 93 beats/minute (atrial);
31 beats/minute (ventricular)
P waves: Three sinus waves to
each QRS complex (one hidden in
T wave)
PR interval: 0.32 to 0.36 second
QRS complex: 0.08 second
Rhythm interpretation: Second-
degree AV block, Mobitz II;
ST-segment depression is present.

Strip 8-60
Rhythm: Regular (basic rhythm);
irregular (premature beats)
Rate: 60 beats/minute (basic
rhythm)
P waves: Sinus (basic rhythm);
premature and abnormal (premature
beats)
PR interval: 0.12 second (basic
rhythm); 0.12 second (PAC); 0.08 to
0.10 second (PJCs)
QRS complex: 0.08 second
Rhythm interpretation: Normal
sinus rhythm with one PAC (third
complex) and paired PJCs (sixth and
seventh complexes)

Strip 8-61
Rhythm: Regular
Rate: 47 beats/minute
P waves: Hidden in the QRS
complex
PR interval: Not measurable
QRS complex: 0.08 second
Rhythm interpretation: Junctional
rhythm

Strip 8-62
Rhythm: Regular (basic rhythm); irregular (nonconducted PAC)
Rate: 79 beats/minute (basic rhythm); slows to 63 beats/minute after a pause (temporary rate suppression is common after a pause in the basic rhythm)
P waves: Sinus (basic rhythm); premature, pointed P wave distorting T wave after the sixth QRS complex
PR interval: 0.24 second (remains constant)
QRS complex: 0.08 second
Rhythm interpretation: Normal sinus rhythm with first-degree AV block; a nonconducted PAC is present after the sixth QRS complex.

Strip 8-63
Rhythm: Regular (atrial); irregular (ventricular)
Rate: 75 beats/minute (atrial); 50 beats/minute (ventricular)
P waves: Sinus
PR interval: Lengthens from 0.24 to 0.32 second
QRS complex: 0.08 second
Rhythm interpretation: Second-degree AV block, Mobitz I

Strip 8-64
Rhythm: Regular (atrial and ventricular)
Rate: 72 beats/minute (atrial); 31 beats/minute (ventricular)
P waves: Sinus (bear no relationship to the QRS complex; hidden in the QRS complex and T waves)
PR interval: Varies greatly
QRS complex: 0.12 second
Rhythm interpretation: Third-degree AV block

Strip 8-65
Rhythm: Regular (atrial and ventricular)
Rate: 90 beats/minute (atrial); 45 beats/minute (ventricular)
P waves: Two sinus waves to each QRS complex
PR interval: 0.26 to 0.28 second (remains constant)
QRS complex: 0.12 second
Rhythm interpretation: Second-degree AV block, Mobitz II; ST-segment elevation is present.

Strip 8-66
Rhythm: Regular
Rate: 79 beats/minute
P waves: Inverted before each QRS complex
PR interval: 0.08 to 0.10 second
QRS complex: 0.06 to 0.08 second
Rhythm interpretation: Accelerated junctional rhythm

Strip 8-67
Rhythm: Regular
Rate: 94 beats/minute
P waves: Sinus
PR interval: 0.24 second
QRS complex: 0.08 second
Rhythm interpretation: Normal sinus rhythm with first-degree AV block

Strip 8-68
Rhythm: Regular (basic rhythm); irregular (premature beats)
Rate: 72 beats/minute (basic rhythm)
P waves: Sinus (basic rhythm); premature and abnormal (premature beats)
PR interval: 0.14 to 0.16 second (basic rhythm); 0.12 second (PACs); 0.10 second (PJC)
QRS complex: 0.06 to 0.08 second
Rhythm interpretation: Normal sinus rhythm with two PACs (third and eighth complexes) and one PJC (fifth complex); a U wave is present.

Strip 8-69
Rhythm: Regular (basic rhythm); irregular (premature beats)
Rate: 52 beats/minute (basic rhythm)
P waves: Hidden (basic rhythm); premature and abnormal (premature beats)
PR interval: Not measurable (basic rhythm); 0.12 to 0.14 second (PACs)
QRS complex: 0.06 to 0.08 second
Rhythm interpretation: Junctional rhythm with two PACs (second and fifth complexes); ST-segment depression is present.

Strip 8-70
Rhythm: Regular (atrial); irregular (ventricular)
Rate: 79 beats/minute (atrial); 70 beats/minute (ventricular)
P waves: Sinus
PR interval: Lengthens from 0.24 to 0.28 second
QRS complex: 0.08 second
Rhythm interpretation: Second-degree AV block, Mobitz I

Strip 8-71
Rhythm: Regular (atrial and ventricular)
Rate: 80 beats/minute (atrial); 40 beats/minute (ventricular)
P waves: Two sinus P waves to each QRS complex
PR interval: 0.24 second (remains constant)
QRS complex: 0.04 to 0.06 second
Rhythm interpretation: Second-degree AV block, Mobitz II (clinical correlation is suggested to diagnose Mobitz II when 2:1 conduction is present with a narrow QRS complex); ST-segment depression is present.

Strip 8-72
Rhythm: Regular (atrial and ventricular)
Rate: 94 beats/minute (atrial); 40 beats/minute (ventricular)
P waves: Sinus (bear no relationship to the QRS complex; hidden in the QRS complex and T waves)
PR interval: Varies greatly
QRS complex: 0.10 second
Rhythm interpretation: Third-degree AV block

Strip 8-73
Rhythm: Regular
Rate: 84 beats/minute
P waves: Hidden in QRS complexes
PR interval: Not measurable
QRS complex: 0.06 second
Rhythm interpretation: Accelerated junctional rhythm; ST-segment depression and T-wave inversion are present.

Strip 8-74
Rhythm: Regular (atrial); irregular (ventricular)
Rate: 54 beats/minute (atrial); 50 beats/minute (ventricular)
P waves: Sinus
PR interval: Lengthens from 0.34 to 0.44 second
QRS complex: 0.08 second
Rhythm interpretation: Second-degree AV block, Mobitz I

Strip 8-75
Rhythm: Regular (basic rhythm); irregular (escape beat)
Rate: 58 beats/minute (basic rhythm)
P waves: Sinus (basic rhythm); hidden P wave (escape beat)
PR interval: 0.16 to 0.18 second
QRS complex: 0.08 to 0.10 second
Rhythm interpretation: Sinus bradycardia with junctional escape beat (fourth complex) after a pause in the basic rhythm

Strip 8-76
Rhythm: Regular
Rate: 47 beats/minute
P waves: Hidden in the QRS complex
PR interval: Not measurable
QRS complex: 0.06 to 0.08 second
Rhythm interpretation: Junctional rhythm; ST-segment depression is present.

Strip 8-77
Rhythm: Regular (atrial and ventricular)
Rate: 94 beats/minute (atrial); 44 beats/minute (ventricular)
P waves: Sinus (bear no relationship to the QRS complex; found hidden in the QRS complex and T waves)
PR interval: Varies greatly
QRS complex: 0.14 to 0.16 second
Rhythm interpretation: Third-degree AV block; ST-segment elevation is present.

Strip 8-78
Rhythm: Regular (basic rhythm); irregular (premature beats)
Rate: 68 beats/minute (basic rhythm)
P waves: Sinus (basic rhythm); premature, abnormal P waves (premature beats)
PR interval: 0.12 to 0.14 second (basic rhythm); 0.14 second (PAC); 0.10 second (PJC)
QRS complex: 0.06 to 0.08 second
Rhythm interpretation: Normal sinus rhythm with one PAC (third complex) and one PJC (seventh complex); a U wave is present.

Strip 8-79
Rhythm: Regular (atrial and ventricular)
Rate: 80 beats/minute (atrial); 40 beats/minute (ventricular)
P waves: Two P waves to each QRS complex
PR interval: 0.12 to 0.14 second (remain constant)
QRS complex: 0.06 to 0.08 second
Rhythm interpretation: Second-degree AV block, Mobitz II (clinical correlation is suggested to diagnose Mobitz II when 2:1 conduction is present with a narrow QRS complex).

Strip 8-80
Rhythm: Regular (basic rhythm); irregular (nonconducted PAC)
Rate: 72 beats/minute (basic rhythm)
P waves: Sinus (basic rhythm); premature, pointed P wave without a QRS complex after the sixth QRS complex
PR interval: 0.22 to 0.24 second (remains constant)
QRS complex: 0.04 to 0.06 second
Rhythm interpretation: Normal sinus rhythm with first-degree AV block and one nonconducted PAC (after the sixth QRS complex); ST-segment depression and T-wave inversion are present.

Strip 8-81
Rhythm: Regular
Rate: 88 beats/minute
P waves: Inverted before each QRS complex
PR interval: 0.08 second
QRS complex: 0.06 to 0.08 second
Rhythm interpretation: Accelerated junctional rhythm

Strip 8-82
Rhythm: regular (atrial); irregular (ventricular)
Rate: 75 beats/minute (atrial); 50 beats/minute (ventricular)
P waves: Sinus P waves present
PR interval: Lengthens from 0.26 to 0.40 second
QRS complex: 0.06 to 0.08 second
Rhythm interpretation: Second-degree AV block, Mobitz I; ST-depression is present.

Strip 8-83
Rhythm: Regular
Rate: 107 beats/minute
P waves: Inverted before each QRS complex
PR interval: 0.08 second
QRS complex: 0.08 to 0.10 second
Rhythm interpretation: Junctional tachycardia

Strip 8-84
Rhythm: Two separate rhythms, both regular
Rate: 79 beats/minute (first rhythm); 84 beats/minute (second rhythm)
P waves: Sinus (first rhythm); inverted (second rhythm)
PR interval: 0.14 to 0.16 second (first rhythm); 0.08 second (second rhythm)
QRS complex: 0.06 to 0.08 second (both rhythms)
Rhythm interpretation: Normal sinus rhythm changing to accelerated junctional rhythm

Strip 8-85
Rhythm: Regular (atrial and ventricular)
Rate: 79 beats/minute (atrial); 31 beats/minute (ventricular)
P waves: Sinus (bear no relationship to the QRS complex; hidden in QRS complexes and T waves)
PR interval: Varies greatly
QRS complex: 0.12 second
Rhythm interpretation: Third-degree AV block

Strip 8-86
Rhythm: Regular
Rate: 60 beats/minute
P waves: Sinus P waves present
PR interval: 0.24 second
QRS complex: 0.08 second
Rhythm interpretation: Normal sinus rhythm with first-degree AV block; ST-segment depression and T-wave inversion are present.

Strip 8-87
Rhythm: Regular (atrial and ventricular)
Rate: 88 beats/minute (atrial); 33 beats/minute (ventricular)
P waves: Sinus (bear no relationship to the QRS complex; found hidden in the QRS complex and T waves)
PR interval: Varies greatly
QRS complex: 0.12 to 0.14 second
Rhythm interpretation: Third-degree AV block

Strip 8-88
Rhythm: Regular (basic rhythm); irregular (premature and escape beats)
Rate: 60 beats/minute (basic rhythm)
P waves: Sinus (basic rhythm); pointed (atrial beat); inverted (junctional beats)
PR interval: 0.12 to 0.14 second (basic rhythm); 0.14 second (atrial beat); 0.08 to 0.10 second (junctional beat)
QRS complex: 0.06 to 0.08 second
Rhythm interpretation: Normal sinus rhythm with one PJC (third complex), one atrial escape beat (fourth complex), and one junctional escape beat (fifth complex)

Strip 8-89
Rhythm: Regular (atrial); irregular (ventricular)
Rate: 65 beats/minute (atrial); 50 beats/minute (ventricular)
P waves: Sinus
PR interval: Lengthens from 0.32 to 0.40 second
QRS complex: 0.08 to 0.10 second
Rhythm interpretation: Second-degree AV block, Mobitz I

Strip 8-90
Rhythm: Regular
Rate: 107 beats/minute
P waves: Inverted before each QRS complex
PR interval: 0.08 to 0.10 second
QRS complex: 0.06 second
Rhythm interpretation: Junctional tachycardia

Strip 8-91
Rhythm: Regular (basic rhythm); irregular (nonconducted PAC)
Rate: 88 beats/minute (basic rhythm)
P waves: Sinus (basic rhythm); premature pointed P wave deforming T wave after the sixth QRS complex; pointed, abnormal P wave with the seventh QRS complex
PR interval: 0.22 to 0.24 second (remains constant)
QRS complex: 0.06 to 0.08 second
Rhythm interpretation: Normal sinus rhythm with first-degree AV block; nonconducted PAC (after the sixth QRS complex); an atrial escape beat (seventh complex) occurs during the pause after the nonconducted PAC (note different P wave when compared with that of underlying rhythm).

Strip 8-92
Rhythm: Regular (atrial); irregular (ventricular)
Rate: 75 beats/minute (atrial); 30 beats/minute (ventricular)
P waves: Sinus (two to three before each QRS complex)
PR interval: 0.16 second (remains constant)
QRS complex: 0.12 second
Rhythm interpretation: Second-degree AV block, Mobitz II with 2:1 and 3:1 AV conduction; ST-segment depression is present.

Strip 8-93
Rhythm: Regular
Rate: 65 beats/minute
P waves: Inverted before each QRS complex
PR interval: 0.08 to 0.10 second
QRS complex: 0.06 second
Rhythm interpretation: Accelerated junctional rhythm; ST-segment elevation is present.

Strip 8-94
Rhythm: Regular (basic rhythm); irregular (PJCs)
Rate: 72 beats/minute (basic rhythm)
P waves: Sinus (basic rhythm); inverted (PJCs)
PR interval: 0.14 second (basic rhythm); 0.08 second (PJCs)
QRS complex: 0.08 second
Rhythm interpretation: Normal sinus rhythm with two PJCs (fourth and sixth complexes)

Strip 8-95
Rhythm: Regular (atrial) but off by two squares; regular (ventricular) off by one square
Rate: 80 beats/minute (atrial); 40 beats/minute (ventricular)
P waves: Two sinus P waves before each QRS complex
PR interval: 0.12 second (consistent)
QRS complex: 0.12 to 0.14 second
Rhythm interpretation: Mobitz II second-degree AV block with 2:1 AV conduction

Strip 8-96
Rhythm: Regular (atrial); irregular (ventricular)
Rate: 75 beats/minute (atrial); 70 beats/minute (ventricular)
P waves: Sinus
PR interval: Lengthens from 0.32 to 0.40 second
QRS complex: 0.04 to 0.06 second
Rhythm interpretation: Second degree AV block, Mobitz I

Strip 8-97
Rhythm: Regular
Rate: 40 beats/minute
P waves: Hidden in the QRS complex
PR interval: Not measurable
QRS complex: 0.10 second
Rhythm interpretation: Junctional rhythm; ST-segment elevation is present.

Strip 8-98
Rhythm: Regular (atrial and ventricular)
Rate: 80 beats/minute (atrial); 40 beats/minute (ventricular)
P waves: Two sinus P waves to each QRS complex
PR interval: 0.22 to 0.24 second (remains constant)
QRS complex: 0.10 second
Rhythm interpretation: Second-degree AV block, Mobitz II (clinical correlation is suggested to diagnose Mobitz II when 2:1 conduction is present with a narrow QRS complex); ST-segment elevation is present.

Strip 8-99
Rhythm: Regular (basic rhythm); irregular (PJC)
Rate: 84 beats/minute (basic rhythm)
P waves: Sinus (basic rhythm); inverted (PJC)
PR interval: 0.12 second (basic rhythm); 0.08 second (PJC)
QRS complex: 0.06 to 0.08 second
Rhythm interpretation: Normal sinus rhythm with one PJC

Strip 8-100
Rhythm: Regular (basic rhythm); irregular after PJC and run of PJT
Rate: 100 beats/minute (basic rhythm); 136 beats/minute (PJT)
P waves: Sinus (basic rhythm); inverted (PJC and PJT)
PR interval: 0.12 to 0.14 second (basic rhythm); 0.08 second (PJC and PJT)
QRS complex: 0.06 to 0.08 second (basic rhythm); 0.08 to 0.10 second (PJC and PJT)
Rhythm interpretation: Normal sinus rhythm with one PJC (fifth complex) and a three-beat run of PJT (eighth, ninth, and tenth complexes)

Strip 8-101
Rhythm: Regular
Rate: 44 beats/minute
P waves: Hidden in the QRS complex
PR interval: Not measurable
QRS complex: 0.08 to 0.10 second
Rhythm interpretation: Junctional rhythm

Strip 8-102
Rhythm: Regular
Rate: 72 beats/minute
P waves: Sinus
PR interval: 0.12 to 0.16 second
QRS complex: 0.06 to 0.08 second
Rhythm interpretation: Normal sinus rhythm

Strip 8-103
Rhythm: Irregular
Rate: 240 beats/minute (atrial); 90 beats/minute (ventricular)
P waves: Flutter waves
PR interval: Not measurable
QRS complex: 0.04 to 0.08 second
Rhythm interpretation: Atrial flutter with variable AV conduction

Strip 8-104
Rhythm: Regular (basic rhythm); irregular with PJC
Rate: 56 beats/minute (basic rhythm)
P waves: Sinus (basic rhythm); inverted P wave (PJC)
PR interval: 0.12 to 0.14 second (basic rhythm); 0.06 second (PJC)
QRS complex: 0.06 to 0.08 second (basic rhythm); 0.10 second (PJC)
Rhythm interpretation: Sinus bradycardia with one PJC (fifth complex)

Strip 8-105
Rhythm: Regular
Rate: 68 beats/minute
P waves: Sinus
PR interval: 0.24 second
QRS complex: 0.08 to 0.10 second
Rhythm interpretation: Normal sinus rhythm with first-degree AV block

Strip 8-106
Rhythm: Irregular
Rate: 90 beats/minute
P waves: Vary in size, shape across strip
PR interval: 0.12 to 0.20 second
QRS complex: 0.04 to 0.08 second
Rhythm interpretation: Wandering atrial pacemaker

Strip 8-107
Rhythm: Regular (basic rhythm); irregular during pause
Rate: 72 beats/minute (basic rhythm before pause); rate slows to 60 beats/minute following pause due to rate suppression.
P waves: Sinus (basic rhythm); absent during pause
PR interval: 0.22 to 0.24 second (basic rhythm); absent during pause
QRS complex: 0.08 to 0.10 second (basic rhythm); absent during pause
Rhythm interpretation: Normal sinus rhythm with first-degree AV block and sinus arrest

Strip 8-108
Rhythm: Regular (atrial and ventricular)
Rate: 82 beats/minute (atrial); 41 beats/minute (ventricular)
P waves: Two sinus P waves to each QRS complex
PR interval: 0.16 to 0.18 second (remains consistent)
QRS complex: 0.12 to 0.14 second
Rhythm interpretation: Mobitz II second-degree AV block

Strip 8-109
Rhythm: Regular
Rate: 115 beats/minute
P waves: Inverted before each QRS complex
PR interval: 0.10 second
QRS complex: 0.06 to 0.08 second
Rhythm interpretation: Junctional tachycardia

Strip 8-110
Rhythm: Regular (basic rhythm)
Rate: 40 beats/minute
P waves: Sinus (basic rhythm); one
premature pointed P wave
PR interval: 0.24 to 0.26 second
QRS complex: 0.08 to 0.10 second
Rhythm interpretation: Sinus brady-
cardia with first-degree AV block and
one nonconducted PAC

Strip 8-111
Rhythm: Irregular
Rate: 80 beats/minute
P waves: Sinus
PR interval: 0.12 to 0.16 second
QRS complex: 0.04 to 0.06 second
Rhythm interpretation: Sinus
arrhythmia

Strip 8-112
Rhythm: Regular (atrial and
ventricular)
Rate: 72 beats/minute (atrial);
35 beats/minute (ventricular)
P waves: Sinus (no relationship to
QRS complex; found hidden in ST
segment, QRS complex)
PR interval: Varies (not consistent)
QRS complex: 0.12 second
Rhythm interpretation: Third-degree
AV block

Strip 8-113
Rhythm: Irregular
Rate: 60 beats/minute
P waves: Fibrillatory waves
PR interval: Not measurable
QRS complex: 0.06 to 0.08 second
Rhythm interpretation: Atrial
fibrillation

Strip 8-114
Rhythm: Regular (off by one
square)
Rate: 48 to 50 beats/minute
P waves: Sinus
PR interval: 0.16 to 0.20 second
QRS complex: 0.06 to 0.08 second
Rhythm interpretation: Sinus
bradycardia

Strip 8-115
Rhythm: Regular
Rate: 167 beats/minute
P waves: TP wave present (P wave
merged with T wave)
PR interval: Not measurable
QRS complex: 0.06 to 0.08 second
Rhythm interpretation: Paroxysmal
atrial tachycardia

Strip 8-116
Rhythm: Regular
Rate: 58 beats/minute
P waves: Hidden within QRS complex
PR interval: Not measurable
QRS complex: 0.08 to 0.10 second
Rhythm interpretation: Junctional
rhythm

Strip 8-117
Rhythm: Regular (atrial); irregular
(ventricular)
Rate: 94 beats/minute (atrial);
60 beats/minute (ventricular)
P waves: Sinus
PR interval: Lengthens from 0.22 to
0.28 second
QRS complex: 0.06 to 0.08 second
Rhythm interpretation: Mobitz I
second-degree AV block

Strip 8-118
Rhythm: Regular
Rate: 107 beats/minute
P waves: Sinus
PR interval: 0.14 to 0.16 second
QRS complex: 0.04 to 0.06 second
Rhythm interpretation: Sinus
tachycardia

Strip 8-119
Rhythm: Regular (basic rhythm);
irregular with premature beat
Rate: 88 beats/minute (basic rhythm)
P waves: Sinus (basic rhythm); small,
pointed P wave with premature beat
PR interval: 0.12 to 0.14 second
(basic rhythm); 0.12 second
(premature beat)
QRS complex: 0.08 second (basic
rhythm and premature beat)
Rhythm interpretation: Normal sinus
rhythm with one PAC

Strip 8-120
Rhythm: Regular
Rate: 65 beats/minute
P waves: Inverted before each QRS
complex
PR interval: 0.08 to 0.10 second
QRS complex: 0.06 to 0.08 second
Rhythm interpretation: Accelerated
junctional rhythm

Strip 9-1
Rhythm: Regular
Rate: 167 beats/minute
P waves: Absent
PR interval: Not measurable
QRS complex: 0.12 to 0.14 second
Rhythm interpretation: Ventricular
tachycardia

Strip 9-2
Rhythm: Regular
Rate: 65 beats/minute
P waves: Sinus; notched P
waves usually indicate left atrial
hypertrophy
PR interval: 0.14 to 0.16 second
QRS complex: 0.12 to 0.14 second
Rhythm interpretation: Normal sinus
rhythm with bundle-branch block;
an elevated ST segment is present.

Strip 9-3
Rhythm: Regular (basic rhythm);
irregular (PVCs)
Rate: 75 beats/minute (basic rhythm)
P waves: Sinus (basic rhythm);
no P waves associated with PVCs;
sinus P waves can be seen after the
PVCs
PR interval: 0.18 to 0.20 second
QRS complex: 0.08 second (basic
rhythm); 0.12 second (PVCs)
Rhythm interpretation: Normal sinus
rhythm with two unifocal PVCs (fifth
and eighth complex)

Strip 9-4
Rhythm: Irregular
Rate: 30 beats/minute
P waves: Absent
PR interval: Not measurable
QRS complex: 0.16 second
Rhythm interpretation:
Idioventricular rhythm

Strip 9-5
Rhythm: 0
Rate: Not measurable
P waves: Chaotic wave deflection of varying height, size, and shape
PR interval: Not measurable
QRS complex: Absent
Rhythm interpretation: Ventricular fibrillation

Strip 9-6
Rhythm: Regular (basic rhythm); irregular (PVCs)
Rate: 100 beats/minute (basic rhythm)
P waves: Sinus (basic rhythm)
PR interval: 0.14 to 0.16 second (basic rhythm)
QRS complex: 0.08 second (basic rhythm); 0.12 second (PVCs)
Rhythm interpretation: Normal sinus rhythm with unifocal PVCs in a bigeminal pattern (second, fourth, sixth, and eighth complexes)

Strip 9-7
Rhythm: First rhythm can't be determined (only one cardiac cycle); second rhythm irregular
Rate: 54 beats/minute (first rhythm); 80 beats/minute (second rhythm)
P waves: Sinus P waves (basic rhythm)
PR interval: 0.16 second (basic rhythm)
QRS complex: 0.08 second (basic rhythm); 0.12 second (ventricular beats)
Rhythm interpretation: Sinus bradycardia changing to accelerated idioventricular rhythm; ST-segment depression is present (basic rhythm).

Strip 9-8
Rhythm: Irregular (first and second rhythms)
Rate: 60 beats/minute (first rhythm); about 200 beats/minute (second rhythm)
P waves: Fibrillation waves (first rhythm); none identified in the second rhythm
PR interval: Not measurable
QRS complex: 0.06 to 0.08 second (first rhythm); 0.12 to 0.14 second (second rhythm)
Rhythm interpretation: Atrial fibrillation with burst of ventricular tachycardia; ST-segment depression with basic rhythm

Strip 9-9
Rhythm: Regular
Rate: 250 beats/minute
P waves: Absent
PR interval: Not measurable
QRS complex: 0.16 to 0.20 second
Rhythm interpretation: Ventricular tachycardia (torsade de pointes)

Strip 9-10
Rhythm: Regular (basic rhythm); irregular (PVCs)
Rate: 79 beats/minute (basic rhythm)
P waves: Sinus (basic rhythm)
PR interval: 0.16 second
QRS complex: 0.06 second (basic rhythm); 0.14 to 0.16 second (PVCs)
Rhythm interpretation: Normal sinus rhythm with paired unifocal PVCs (sixth and seventh complexes)

Strip 9-11
Rhythm: Regular
Rate: 42 beats/minute
P waves: Absent
PR interval: Not measurable
QRS complex: 0.12 to 0.14 second
Rhythm interpretation: Idioventricular rhythm

Strip 9-12
Rhythm: Regular
Rate: 125 beats/minute
P waves: Sinus
PR interval: 0.12 second
QRS complex: 0.12 second
Rhythm interpretation: Sinus tachycardia with bundle-branch block; an elevated ST segment is present.

Strip 9-13
Rhythm: 0
Rate: 0 beats/minute
P waves: None identified
PR interval: Not measurable
QRS complex: None identified
Rhythm interpretation: Ventricular standstill (asystole)

Strip 9-14
Rhythm: Regular
Rate: 214 beats/minute
P waves: None identified
PR interval: Not measurable
QRS complex: 0.16 second
Rhythm interpretation: Ventricular tachycardia

Strip 9-15
Rhythm: Regular (basic rhythm)
Rate: 50 beats/minute (basic rhythm)
P waves: Sinus (basic rhythm)
PR interval: 0.16 to 0.18 second
QRS complex: 0.08 second (basic rhythm); 0.14 second (PVC)
Rhythm interpretation: Sinus bradycardia with one PVC (third complex); ST-segment depression is present.

Strip 9-16
Rhythm: Chaotic
Rate: 0 beats/minute
P waves: Absent; wave deflections are irregular and vary in height, size, and shape
PR interval: Not measurable
QRS complex: Absent
Rhythm interpretation: Ventricular fibrillation

Strip 9-17
Rhythm: Chaotic
Rate: 0 beats/minute
P waves: Wave deflections are chaotic and vary in height, size, and shape
PR interval: Not measurable
QRS complex: Absent
Rhythm interpretation: Ventricular fibrillation is followed by electrical shock and a return to ventricular fibrillation.

Strip 9-18
Rhythm: Regular
Rate: 107 beats/minute
P waves: Sinus
PR interval: 0.16 to 0.18 second
QRS complex: 0.12 second
Rhythm interpretation: Sinus tachycardia with bundle-branch block

Strip 9-19
Rhythm: Irregular
Rate: 300 beats/minute (atrial); 50 beats/minute (ventricular)
P waves: Flutter waves before each QRS complex
PR interval: Not measurable
QRS complex: 0.06 to 0.08 second (basic rhythm); 0.12 second (PVC)
Rhythm interpretation: Atrial flutter with variable AV conduction and one PVC (fifth complex)

Strip 9-20
Rhythm: Regular (atrial)
Rate: 136 beats/minute (atrial);
0 beats/minute (ventricular; no QRS complexes)
P waves: Sinus
PR interval: Not measurable
QRS complex: Absent
Rhythm interpretation: Ventricular standstill

Strip 9-21
Rhythm: Irregular
Rate: 40 beats/minute
P waves: Absent
PR interval: Not measurable
QRS complex: 0.16 second
Rhythm interpretation: Idioventricular rhythm

Strip 9-22
Rhythm: Chaotic
Rate: 0 beats/minute (no QRS complexes)
P waves: None identified
PR interval: Not measurable
QRS complex: Absent
Rhythm interpretation: Ventricular fibrillation

Strip 9-23
Rhythm: Regular
Rate: 88 beats/minute
P waves: Absent
PR interval: Not measurable
QRS complex: 0.12 second
Rhythm interpretation: Accelerated idioventricular rhythm

Strip 9-24
Rhythm: Irregular (basic rhythm)
Rate: 60 beats/minute (basic rhythm)
P waves: Fibrillatory waves
PR interval: Not measurable
QRS complex: 0.06 to 0.08 second (basic rhythm); 0.12 second (PVCs)
Rhythm interpretation: Atrial fibrillation with paired PVCs

Strip 9-25
Rhythm: Regular (basic rhythm)
Rate: 100 beats/minute (first rhythm); 188 beats/minute (second rhythm)
P waves: Sinus (basic rhythm)
PR interval: 0.14 to 0.16 second
QRS complex: 0.08 second (basic rhythm); 0.12 to 0.16 second (ventricular beats)
Rhythm interpretation: Normal sinus rhythm with burst of ventricular tachycardia and paired PVCs

Strip 9-26
Rhythm: Regular (basic rhythm); irregular (PVC)
Rate: 107 beats/minute (basic rhythm)
P waves: Sinus (basic rhythm)
PR interval: 0.18 to 0.20 second
QRS complex: 0.08 to 0.10 second (basic rhythm); 0.16 second (PVC)
Rhythm interpretation: Sinus tachycardia with one PVC (R-on-T pattern); an elevated ST segment is present.

Strip 9-27
Rhythm: Irregular (difficult to determine due to changing polarity of QRS complex)
Rate: 250 beats/minute or greater
P waves: Absent
PR interval: Not measurable
QRS complex: 0.12 second or greater
Rhythm interpretation: Ventricular tachycardia (torsade de pointes)

Strip 9-28
Rhythm: Regular
Rate: 250 beats/minute
P waves: None identified
PR interval: Not measurable
QRS complex: 0.12 to 0.16 second (QRS complexes change in polarity from negative to positive across the strip).
Rhythm interpretation: Ventricular tachycardia (torsades de pointes)

Strip 9-29
Rhythm: Regular
Rate: 84 beats/minute
P waves: None identified
PR interval: Not measurable
QRS complex: 0.14 to 0.16 second
Rhythm interpretation: Accelerated idioventricular rhythm

Strip 9-30
Rhythm: Chaotic
Rate: 0 beats/minute
P waves: Absent; wave deflections are irregular and vary in height, size, and shape.
PR interval: Not measurable
QRS complex: Absent
Rhythm interpretation: Ventricular fibrillation

Strip 9-31
Rhythm: Regular (basic rhythm); irregular (PVCs)
Rate: 115 beats/minute (basic rhythm)
P waves: Sinus (basic rhythm)
PR interval: 0.14 to 0.16 second
QRS complex: 0.04 to 0.06 second (basic rhythm); 0.12 second (PVCs)
Rhythm interpretation: Sinus tachycardia with two unifocal PVCs (fourth and twelfth complexes)

Strip 9-32
Rhythm: Regular (basic rhythm); irregular (PVCs)
Rate: 125 beats/minute (basic rhythm)
P waves: Sinus (basic rhythm)
PR interval: 0.14 to 0.16 second
QRS complex: 0.08 to 0.10 second (basic rhythm); 0.12 second (PVCs)
Rhythm interpretation: Sinus tachycardia with multifocal paired PVCs (eighth and ninth complexes)

Strip 9-33
Rhythm: Regular (basic rhythm)
Rate: 37 beats/minute (basic rhythm)
P waves: Sinus (basic rhythm)
PR interval: 0.14 to 0.16 second
QRS complex: 0.06 to 0.08 second (basic rhythm); 0.12 second (escape beat)
Rhythm interpretation: Sinus bradycardia with one ventricular escape beat (third complex)

Strip 9-34
Rhythm: Regular (first and second rhythms)
Rate: 72 beats/minute (first rhythm); 150 beats/minute (second rhythm)
P waves: Sinus (basic rhythm)
PR interval: 0.18 to 0.20 second
QRS complex: 0.08 second (basic rhythm); 0.12 second (ventricular beats)
Rhythm interpretation: Normal sinus rhythm with a burst of ventricular tachycardia; an inverted T wave is present in basic rhythm.

Strip 9-35
Rhythm: Chaotic
Rate: 0 beats/minute
P waves: Absent; wave deflections vary in height, size, and shape
PR interval: Not measurable
QRS complex: Absent
Rhythm interpretation: Ventricular fibrillation

Strip 9-36
Rhythm: Irregular
Rate: About 30 beats/minute
P waves: Absent
PR interval: Not measurable
QRS complex: 0.12 second
Rhythm interpretation: Idioventricular rhythm; ST-segment elevation is present.

Strip 9-37
Rhythm: Not measurable
Rate: Not measurable (one complex present)
P waves: None identified
PR interval: Not measurable
QRS complex: 0.28 second or wider
Rhythm interpretation: One ventricular complex followed by ventricular standstill

Strip 9-38
Rhythm: Regular
Rate: 84 beats/minute
P waves: None identified
PR interval: Not measurable
QRS complex: 0.14 to 0.16 second
Rhythm interpretation: Accelerated idioventricular rhythm

Strip 9-39
Rhythm: Regular (basic rhythm)
Rate: 115 beats/minute (basic rhythm)
P waves: Inverted before each QRS complex in basic rhythm
PR interval: 0.08 second (basic rhythm)
QRS complex: 0.06 to 0.08 second (basic rhythm); 0.12 second (PVC)
Rhythm interpretation: Junctional tachycardia with one PVC (tenth complex)

Strip 9-40
Rhythm: Regular (atrial)
Rate: 30 beats/minute (atrial); 0 beats/minute (ventricular; no QRS complexes)
P waves: Sinus
PR interval: Not measurable
QRS complex: Absent
Rhythm interpretation: Ventricular standstill

Strip 9-41
Rhythm: Regular (basic rhythm); irregular (PVCs)
Rate: 65 beats/minute (basic rhythm)
P waves: Sinus (basic rhythm)
PR interval: 0.16 second
QRS complex: 0.06 to 0.08 second (basic rhythm); 0.12 second (PVCs)
Rhythm interpretation: Normal sinus rhythm with two unifocal PVCs (third and sixth complexes); ST-segment depression is present.

Strip 9-42
Rhythm: Irregular (first rhythm); regular (second rhythm)
Rate: 100 beats/minute (first rhythm); 167 beats/minute (second rhythm)
P waves: Fibrillation waves (basic rhythm)
PR interval: Not measurable
QRS complex: 0.08 second (basic rhythm); 0.12 second (VT)
Rhythm interpretation: Atrial fibrillation with a burst of ventricular tachycardia

Strip 9-43
Rhythm: Regular (first rhythm); irregular (second rhythm)
Rate: 100 beats/minute (first rhythm); 100 beats/minute (second rhythm)
P waves: Sinus (basic rhythm)
PR interval: 0.12 second
QRS complex: 0.12 to 0.14 second (first rhythm); 0.12 second (second rhythm)
Rhythm interpretation: Normal sinus rhythm with bundle-branch block with transient episode of accelerated idioventricular rhythm

Strip 9-44
Rhythm: First rhythm can't be determined (only one cardiac cycle present); second rhythm regular
Rate: 50 beats/minute (first rhythm); 41 beats/minute (second rhythm)
P waves: Sinus (first rhythm)
PR interval: 0.12 second (first rhythm)
QRS complex: 0.06 to 0.08 second (first rhythm); 0.12 to 0.14 second (second rhythm)
Rhythm interpretation: Sinus bradycardia changing to idioventricular rhythm; a U wave is present.

Strip 9-45
Rhythm: Regular
Rate: 214 beats/minute
P waves: Not identified
PR interval: Not measurable
QRS complex: 0.16 to 0.18 second or wider
Rhythm interpretation: Ventricular tachycardia

Strip 9-46
Rhythm: Regular (basic rhythm); irregular (ventricular beats)
Rate: About 58 beats/minute (basic rhythm)
P waves: Sinus (basic rhythm)
PR interval: 0.20 second
QRS complex: 0.06 second (basic rhythm); 0.16 second (first ventricular beat); 0.12 second (second ventricular beat)
Rhythm interpretation: Sinus bradycardia with one PVC (fourth complex) and one ventricular escape beat (fifth complex); ST-segment depression is present.

Strip 9-47
Rhythm: Regular (basic rhythm)
Rate: 68 beats/minute (basic rhythm)
P waves: Sinus (basic rhythm)
PR interval: 0.12 to 0.14 second
QRS complex: 0.08 to 0.10 second
(basic rhythm); 0.12 to 0.14 second
(PVC)
Rhythm interpretation: Normal sinus
rhythm with one PVC

Strip 9-48
Rhythm: Not measurable
Rate: Not measurable (one complex
present)
P waves: None identified
PR interval: Not measurable
QRS complex: 0.12 second
Rhythm interpretation: One
ventricular complex followed by
ventricular standstill

Strip 9-49
Rhythm: Regular
Rate: 56 beats/minute
P waves: Sinus
PR interval: 0.12 to 0.16 second
QRS complex: 0.12 second
Rhythm interpretation: Sinus
bradycardia with bundle-branch
block; ST-segment depression is
present.

Strip 9-50
Rhythm: Regular
Rate: 188 beats/minute
P waves: Not identified
PR interval: Not measurable
QRS complex: 0.12 second
Rhythm interpretation: Ventricular
tachycardia

Strip 9-51
Rhythm: Regular (atrial); irregular
(ventricular)
Rate: 58 beats/minute (atrial); about
40 beats/minute (ventricular)
P waves: Sinus
PR interval: Lengthens from 0.30 to
0.36 second
QRS complex: 0.08 second (basic
rhythm); 0.12 second (escape beat)
Rhythm interpretation: Second-
degree AV block, Mobitz I with
one ventricular escape beat (third
complex)

Strip 9-52
Rhythm: Regular (first and second
rhythms)
Rate: 72 beats/minute (first rhythm);
72 beats/minute (second rhythm)
P waves: Sinus in first rhythm
PR interval: 0.12 to 0.14 second (first
rhythm)
QRS complex: 0.08 second (first
rhythm); 0.12 to 0.14 second (second
rhythm)
Rhythm interpretation: Normal
sinus rhythm with a transient
episode of accelerated idioventricular
rhythm

Strip 9-53
Rhythm: Slightly irregular (atrial)
Rate: About 40 beats/minute (atrial);
0 beats/minute (ventricular; no QRS
complexes)
P waves: Sinus
PR interval: Not measurable
QRS complex: Absent
Rhythm interpretation: Ventricular
standstill

Strip 9-54
Rhythm: Regular
Rate: 84 beats/minute
P waves: Sinus
PR interval: 0.16 second
QRS complex: 0.12 to 0.14 second
Rhythm interpretation: Normal sinus
rhythm with bundle-branch block; a
depressed ST segment is present.

Strip 9-55
Rhythm: Regular
Rate: 41 beats/minute
P waves: Absent
PR interval: Not measurable
QRS complex: 0.16 second
Rhythm interpretation: Idioventricu-
lar rhythm

Strip 9-56
Rhythm: Regular
Rate: 75 beats/minute
P waves: Sinus
PR interval: 0.12 second
QRS complex: 0.16 to 0.18 second
Rhythm interpretation: Normal sinus
rhythm with bundle-branch block;
T-wave inversion is present

Strip 9-57
Rhythm: Regular (basic rhythm);
irregular (PVCs)
Rate: 72 beats/minute (basic
rhythm)
P waves: Sinus (basic rhythm)
PR interval: 0.12 second
QRS complex: 0.08 second (basic
rhythm); 0.12 to 0.14 second
(PVCs)
Rhythm interpretation: Normal
sinus rhythm with unifocal PVCs
(fourth and eighth complexes) in a
quadrigeminal pattern

Strip 9-58
Rhythm: Regular (atrial); ventricular
not measurable (only one
QRS complex present)
Rate: 29 beats/minute (atrial);
ventricular not measurable (only one
QRS complex present)
P waves: Sinus
PR interval: Not measurable
QRS complex: 0.08 second
Rhythm interpretation: One QRS
complex followed by ventricular
standstill

Strip 9-59
Rhythm: Chaotic
Rate: 0 beats/minute
P waves: Absent; wave deflections
are irregular and chaotic and vary in
size, shape, and height
PR interval: Not measurable
QRS complex: Absent
Rhythm interpretation: Ventricular
fibrillation

Strip 9-60
Rhythm: Not measurable (only one
QRS complex)
Rate: Not measurable (only one QRS
complex)
P waves: None identified
PR interval: Not measurable
QRS complex: 0.12 second or
greater
Rhythm interpretation: One QRS
complex followed by ventricular
standstill

Strip 9-61
Rhythm: Regular (first and second rhythms)
Rate: 100 beats/minute (first rhythm); 100 beats/minute (second rhythm)
P waves: Sinus (first rhythm); none (second rhythm)
PR interval: 0.14 to 0.16 second (first rhythm)
QRS complex: 0.06 to 0.08 second (first rhythm); 0.12 second (second rhythm)
Rhythm interpretation: Normal sinus rhythm changing to accelerated idioventricular rhythm

Strip 9-62
Rhythm: Regular
Rate: 40 beats/minute
P waves: Absent
PR interval: Not measurable
QRS complex: 0.16 second
Rhythm interpretation: Idioventricular rhythm

Strip 9-63
Rhythm: Regular
Rate: 167 beats/minute
P waves: Not identified
PR interval: Not measurable
QRS complex: 0.16 to 0.18 second
Rhythm interpretation: Ventricular tachycardia

Strip 9-64
Rhythm: Regular
Rate: 88 beats/minute
P waves: Sinus
PR interval: 0.22 to 0.24 second
QRS complex: 0.12 second
Rhythm interpretation: Normal sinus rhythm with bundle-branch block and first-degree AV block

Strip 9-65
Rhythm: Irregular
Rate: 80 beats/minute (basic rhythm)
P waves: Fibrillation waves
PR interval: Not measurable
QRS complex: 0.06 to 0.08 second (basic rhythm); 0.12 second (PVCs)
Rhythm interpretation: Atrial fibrillation with paired PVCs

Strip 9-66
Rhythm: Regular (basic rhythm)
Rate: 84 beats/minute (basic rhythm)
P waves: Sinus
PR interval: 0.24 second
QRS complex: 0.08 second
Rhythm interpretation: Normal sinus rhythm with first-degree AV block changing to ventricular standstill

Strip 9-67
Rhythm: Chaotic
Rate: 0 beats/minute
P waves: None identified
PR interval: Not measurable
QRS complex: Absent
Rhythm interpretation: Ventricular fibrillation

Strip 9-68
Rhythm: Regular
Rate: 167 beats/minute
P waves: None identified
PR interval: Not measurable
QRS complex: 0.14 to 0.16 second
Rhythm interpretation: Ventricular tachycardia

Strip 9-69
Rhythm: Regular (first rhythm); slightly irregular (second rhythm)
Rate: 115 beats/minute (first rhythm); about 214 beats/minute (second rhythm)
P waves: Sinus (first rhythm); none identified in the second rhythm
PR interval: 0.12 to 0.14 second (first rhythm)
QRS complex: 0.10 second (first rhythm); 0.12 to 0.16 second (second rhythm)
Rhythm interpretation: Sinus tachycardia with a burst of ventricular tachycardia returning to sinus tachycardia; an inverted T wave is present.

Strip 9-70
Rhythm: Regular
Rate: 40 beats/minute
P waves: Absent
PR interval: Not measurable
QRS complex: 0.16 second
Rhythm interpretation: Idioventricular rhythm

Strip 9-71
Rhythm: Regular
Rate: 100 beats/minute
P waves: Absent
PR interval: Not measurable
QRS complex: 0.12 second
Rhythm interpretation: Accelerated idioventricular rhythm

Strip 9-72
Rhythm: 0 beats/minute (only one QRS complex present)
Rate: 0 beats/minute (only one QRS complex present)
P waves: None identified
PR interval: Not measurable
QRS complex: 0.24 to 0.26 second
Rhythm interpretation: One QRS complex followed by ventricular standstill

Strip 9-73
Rhythm: Regular
Rate: 188 beats/minute
P waves: Not identified
PR interval: Not measurable
QRS complex: 0.16 to 0.20 second or wider
Rhythm interpretation: Ventricular tachycardia followed by electrical shock and return to ventricular tachycardia

Strip 9-74
Rhythm: Regular (basic rhythm); irregular (PVC)
Rate: 100 beats/minute (basic rhythm)
P waves: Sinus (basic rhythm)
PR interval: 0.14 to 0.16 second
QRS complex: 0.08 second (basic rhythm); 0.12 second (PVC)
Rhythm interpretation: Normal sinus rhythm with one PVC (fifth complex)

Strip 9-75
Rhythm: Regular
Rate: 50 beats/minute
P waves: Sinus
PR interval: 0.16 to 0.18 second
QRS complex: 0.12 to 0.14 second
Rhythm interpretation: Sinus bradycardia with bundle-branch block

Strip 9-76
Rhythm: 0 beats/minute
Rate: 0 beats/minute (no QRS complexes)
P waves: Sinus
PR interval: Not measurable
QRS complex: Absent
Rhythm interpretation: Ventricular standstill

Strip 9-77
Rhythm: Regular
Rate: 41 beats/minute
P waves: Absent
PR interval: Not measurable
QRS complex: 0.12 second
Rhythm interpretation: Idioventricular rhythm

Strip 9-78
Rhythm: 0 beats/minute (only one QRS complex)
Rate: 0 beats/minute (only one QRS complex)
P waves: None identified
PR interval: Not measurable
QRS complex: 0.14 second
Rhythm interpretation: One ventricular complex followed by ventricular standstill

Strip 9-79
Rhythm: 0 beats/minute
Rate: 0 beats/minute
P waves: Absent; wave deflections are chaotic and vary in height, size, and shape
PR interval: Not measurable
QRS complex: Absent
Rhythm interpretation: Ventricular fibrillation changing to ventricular standstill

Strip 9-80
Rhythm: Regular (first and second rhythms)
Rate: 94 beats/minute (first rhythm); 75 beats/minute (second rhythm)
P waves: Sinus (first rhythm)
PR interval: 0.16 second
QRS complex: 0.12 second (first rhythm); 0.12 second (second rhythm)
Rhythm interpretation: Normal sinus rhythm with bundle-branch block changing to accelerated idioventricular rhythm and back to normal sinus rhythm with bundle-branch block; T-wave inversion is present.

Strip 9-81
Rhythm: Regular (atrial); ventricular rhythm can't be determined (only one cardiac cycle)
Rate: 94 beats/minute (atrial); 40 beats/minute (ventricular)
P waves: Sinus (bear no relationship to the QRS complex)
PR interval: Varies greatly
QRS complex: 0.14 second
Rhythm interpretation: Third-degree AV block changing to ventricular standstill

Strip 9-82
Rhythm: Regular
Rate: 72 beats/minute
P waves: Sinus
PR interval: 0.16 second
QRS complex: 0.12 second
Rhythm interpretation: Normal sinus rhythm with bundle-branch block

Strip 9-83
Rhythm: Regular (first rhythm); irregular and chaotic (second rhythm)
Rate: 214 beats/minute (first rhythm)
P waves: None identified
PR interval: Not measurable
QRS complex: 0.16 to 0.18 second (first rhythm)
Rhythm interpretation: Ventricular tachycardia changing to ventricular fibrillation

Strip 9-84
Rhythm: Regular
Rate: 32 beats/minute
P waves: Absent
PR interval: Not measurable
QRS complex: 0.20 second
Rhythm interpretation: Idioventricular rhythm

Strip 9-85
Rhythm: Regular (basic rhythm); irregular (PVCs)
Rate: 125 beats/minute (basic rhythm)
P waves: Sinus (basic rhythm)
PR interval: 0.12 second
QRS complex: 0.06 to 0.08 second (basic rhythm); 0.12 second (PVCs)
Rhythm interpretation: Sinus tachycardia with multifocal paired PVCs (eighth and ninth complexes)

Strip 9-86
Rhythm: Regular (atrial)
Rate: 52 beats/minute (atrial); 0 beats/minute (ventricular)
P waves: Sinus
PR interval: Not measurable
QRS complex: Absent
Rhythm interpretation: Ventricular standstill

Strip 9-87
Rhythm: Regular (first rhythm); irregular (second rhythm)
Rate: 68 beats/minute (first rhythm); about 80 beats/minute (second rhythm)
P waves: Sinus (first rhythm)
PR interval: 0.12 to 0.14 second
QRS complex: 0.08 second (first rhythm); 0.12 second (second rhythm)
Rhythm interpretation: Normal sinus rhythm changing to accelerated idioventricular rhythm

Strip 9-88
Rhythm: Regular
Rate: 167 beats/minute
P waves: Not identified
PR interval: Not measurable
QRS complex: 0.16 to 0.20 second
Rhythm interpretation: Ventricular tachycardia (torsades de pointes)

Strip 9-89
Rhythm: Regular (basic rhythm); irregular (PVCs)
Rate: 125 beats/minute (basic rhythm)
P waves: Sinus (basic rhythm)
PR interval: 0.12 second
QRS complex: 0.06 to 0.08 second (basic rhythm); 0.12 second (PVC)
Rhythm interpretation: Sinus tachycardia with paired PVCs (seventh and eighth complexes)

Strip 9-90
Rhythm: Regular (atrial)
Rate: 72 beats/minute (atrial); 0 beats/minute (ventricular)
P waves: Sinus
PR interval: Not measurable
QRS complex: Absent
Rhythm interpretation: Ventricular standstill

Strip 9-91
Rhythm: Regular
Rate: 188 beats/minute
P waves: None identified
PR interval: Not measurable
QRS complex: 0.18 to 0.20 second or wider
Rhythm interpretation: Ventricular tachycardia

Strip 9-92
Rhythm: Chaotic
Rate: 0 beats/minute
P waves: Wave deflections chaotic; vary in size, shape, and direction
PR interval: Not measurable
QRS complex: Absent
Rhythm interpretation: Ventricular fibrillation; 60-cycle (electrical) interference noted on baseline.

Strip 9-93
Rhythm: Regular
Rate: 28 beats/minute
P waves: None
PR interval: Not measurable
QRS complex: 0.20 second or wider
Rhythm interpretation: Idioventricular rhythm

Strip 9-94
Rhythm: Regular
Rate: 79 beats/minute
P waves: Sinus
PR interval: 0.18 to 0.20 second
QRS complex: 0.12 second
Rhythm interpretation: Normal sinus rhythm with bundle-branch block

Strip 9-95
Rhythm: Regular (basic rhythm)
Rate: 68 beats/minute (basic rhythm)
P waves: Sinus (basic rhythm)
PR interval: 0.16 to 0.18 second
QRS complex: 0.06 to 0.08 second (basic rhythm); 0.12 second (PVC)
Rhythm interpretation: Normal sinus rhythm with one interpolated PVC (seventh complex). Interpolated PVCs are sandwiched between two sinus beats and have no compensatory pause. ST-segment depression and T-wave inversion are present.

Strip 9-96
Rhythm: Regular (basic rhythm); irregular (PVCs)
Rate: 72 beats/minute (basic rhythm)
P waves: Sinus (basic rhythm)
PR interval: 0.12 to 0.14 second
QRS complex: 0.08 second (basic rhythm); 0.12 to 0.14 second (PVCs)
Rhythm interpretation: Normal sinus rhythm with PVCs in a trigeminal pattern

Strip 9-97
Rhythm: Irregular
Rate: 80 beats/minute
P waves: Wavy fibrillatory waves
PR interval: Not measurable
QRS complex: 0.14 to 0.16 second
Rhythm interpretation: Atrial fibrillation with bundle-branch block

Strip 9-98
Rhythm: Regular (first rhythm); regular but off by two squares (second rhythm)
Rate: 43 beats/minute (first rhythm); 45 beats/minute (second rhythm)
P waves: Sinus (first rhythm); no associated P waves (second rhythm)
PR interval: 0.14 to 0.16 second (basic rhythm)
QRS complex: 0.10 second (basic rhythm); 0.14 to 0.16 second (second rhythm)
Rhythm interpretation: Sinus bradycardia with three-beat run of idioventricular rhythm

Strip 9-99
Rhythm: Regular (basic rhythm); irregular during pause
Rate: 79 beats/minute (basic rhythm)
P waves: Sinus (basic rhythm); absent during pause
PR interval: 0.20 second
QRS complex: 0.14 to 0.16 second
Rhythm interpretation: Normal sinus rhythm with bundle-branch block and sinus exit block

Strip 9-100
Rhythm: None
Rate: 0 beats/minute
P waves: None identified; wavy baseline
PR interval: Not measurable
QRS complex: Absent
Rhythm interpretation: Ventricular fibrillation changing to ventricular standstill

Strip 9-101
Rhythm: Irregular
Rate: 60 beats/minute
P waves: Sinus
PR interval: 0.16 to 0.20 second
QRS complex: 0.08 second
Rhythm interpretation: Sinus arrhythmia

Strip 9-102
Rhythm: Regular
Rate: 167 beats/minute
P waves: TP waves present
PR interval: Not measurable
QRS complex: 0.08 to 0.10 second
Rhythm interpretation: Paroxysmal atrial tachycardia

Strip 9-103
Rhythm: Regular
Rate: 45 beats/minute
P waves: Hidden within QRS complex
PR interval: Not measurable
QRS complex: 0.06 to 0.08 second
Rhythm interpretation: Junctional rhythm

Strip 9-104
Rhythm: Regular
Rate: 63 beats/minute
P waves: Sinus
PR interval: 0.12 to 0.14 second
QRS complex: 0.14 to 0.16 second
Rhythm interpretation: Normal sinus rhythm with bundle-branch block

Strip 9-105
Rhythm: Regular (atrial); irregular (ventricular)
Rate: 84 beats/minute (atrial); 70 beats/minute (ventricular)
P waves: Sinus
PR interval: Lengthens from 0.20 second to 0.32 second
QRS complex: 0.087 to 0.10 second
Rhythm interpretation: Second-degree AV block, Mobitz I

Strip 9-106
Rhythm: Regular (basic rhythm);
irregular with pause
Rate: 72 beats/minute (basic
rhythm); rate decreases to 65 beats/
minute following pause due to
temporary rate suppression.
P waves: Sinus (basic rhythm);
absent during pause
PR interval: 0.24 second; absent
during pause
QRS complex: 0.06 to 0.08 second;
absent during pause
Rhythm interpretation: Normal sinus
rhythm with first-degree AV block
and sinus arrest

Strip 9-107
Rhythm: Regular (basic rhythm);
irregular with premature beat
Rate: 52 beats/minute (basic rhythm)
P waves: Sinus (basic rhythm); small,
pointed P wave with premature beat
PR interval: 0.14 to 0.16 second (basic
rhythm); 0.12 second (premature beat)
QRS complex: 0.08 to 0.10 second
(basic rhythm); 0.10 second
(premature beat)
Rhythm interpretation: Sinus bradycardia with one PAC

Strip 9-108
Rhythm: Regular (basic rhythm)
Rate: 45 beats/minute (basic rhythm)
P waves: Absent
PR interval: Not measurable
QRS complex: 0.16 to 0.18 second
Rhythm interpretation: Idioventricu-
lar rhythm to ventricular standstill

Strip 9-109
Rhythm: Regular
Rate: 84 beats/minute
P waves: Sinus
PR interval: 0.30 to 0.32 second
QRS complex: 0.08 to 0.10 second
Rhythm interpretation: Normal sinus
rhythm with first-degree AV block

Strip 9-110
Rhythm: Regular (basic rhythm)
Rate: 75 beats/minute (basic rhythm)
P waves: Sinus
PR interval: 0.14 to 0.16 second
QRS complex: 0.06 to 0.08 second (ba-
sic rhythm); 0.12 to 0.14 second (PVC)
Rhythm interpretation: Normal sinus
rhythm with one PVC

Strip 9-111
Rhythm: Regular
Rate: 240 beats/minute (atrial);
60 beats/minute (ventricular)
P waves: Flutter waves
PR interval: Not measurable
QRS complex: 0.08 second
Rhythm interpretation: Atrial flutter
with 4:1 AV conduction

Strip 9-112
Rhythm: Regular
Rate: 115 beats/minute
P waves: Sinus
PR interval: 0.12 to 0.16 second
QRS complex: 0.04 to 0.08 second
Rhythm interpretation: Sinus
tachycardia

Strip 9-113
Rhythm: Not measurable (one
complex)
Rate: Not measurable (one complex)
P waves: Absent
PR interval: Not measurable
QRS complex: 0.20 to 0.24 second
Rhythm interpretation: One ventric-
ular complex to ventricular standstill

Strip 9-114
Rhythm: Regular (basic rhythm) but
off by two squares
Rate: 72 to 75 beats/minute
P waves: Vary in size, shape, direction
PR interval: 0.12 to 0.16 second
QRS complex: 0.04 to 0.08 (basic
rhythm); 0.12 second or greater (pre-
mature beat)
Rhythm interpretation: Wandering
atrial pacemaker with PVC

Strip 9-115
Rhythm: First rhythm probably regular
(only two QRS complexes); second
rhythm regular (off by two squares)
Rate: 75 beats/minute (basic rhythm);
72 to 79 beats/minute (second rhythm)
P waves: Sinus (first rhythm); absent
(second rhythm)
PR interval: 0.18 to 0.20 second (first
rhythm); absent (second rhythm)
QRS complex: 0.06 to 0.08 second
(first rhythm); 0.12 second or greater
(second rhythm)
Rhythm interpretation: Normal sinus
rhythm with episode of accelerated idioventricular rhythm going back to NSR

Strip 9-116
Rhythm: Regular (off by one square)
Rate: 54 to 56 beats/minute
P waves: Sinus
PR interval: 0.14 to 0.16 second
QRS complex: 0.04 second
Rhythm interpretation: Sinus
bradycardia

Strip 9-117
Rhythm: Irregular
Rate: 70 beats/minute
P waves: Fibrillatory waves
PR interval: Not measurable
QRS complex: 0.04 to 0.06 second
Rhythm interpretation: Atrial
fibrillation

Strip 9-118
Rhythm: Regular
Rate: 150 beats/minute
P waves: Absent
PR interval: Not measurable
QRS complex: 0.12 to 0.14 second
Rhythm interpretation: Ventricular
tachycardia

Strip 9-119
Rhythm: Regular
Rate: 100 beats/minute
P waves: Inverted before each QRS
complex
PR interval: 0.08 to 0.10 second
QRS complex: 0.06 to 0.08 second
Rhythm interpretation: Accelerated
junctional rhythm

Strip 9-120
Rhythm: Regular (atrial) but off by
one square; regular (ventricular)
Rate: 88 to 94 beats/minute (atrial);
44 beats/minute (ventricular)
P waves: Sinus
PR interval: Varies greatly (not
consistent)
QRS complex: 0.06 to 0.08 second
Rhythm interpretation: Third-degree
AV block

Strip 9-121
Rhythm: Chaotic and irregular
Rate: 0 beats/minute
P waves: Fibrillatory waves which
are irregular; vary in size, shape,
amplitude
PR interval: Not measurable
QRS complex: Absent
Rhythm interpretation: Ventricular
fibrillation

Strip 9-122
Rhythm: Regular
Rate: 63 beats/minute
P waves: Sinus
PR interval: 0.16 to 0.18 second
QRS complex: 0.08 to 0.10 second
Rhythm interpretation: Normal sinus
rhythm; U wave is present.

Strip 9-123
Rhythm: Regular (basic rhythm)
Rate: 72 beats/minute (basic rhythm)
P waves: Sinus (basic rhythm);
inverted P waves before each
premature beat
PR interval: 0.12 to 0.14 second
(basic rhythm); 0.08 second
(premature beats)
QRS complex: 0.08 second (basic
rhythm and PJCs)
Rhythm interpretation: Normal
sinus rhythm with two premature
junctional contractions

Strip 9-124
Rhythm: Regular (atrial) but off by
two squares; regular (ventricular)
Rate: 65 to 72 beats/minute (atrial);
34 beats/minute (ventricular)
P waves: Sinus (two P waves before
QRS complex)
PR interval: 0.12 to 0.14 second
(consistent)
QRS complex: 0.12 second
Rhythm interpretation:
Second-degree AV block; Mobitz II

Strip 10-1
Analysis: The first four beats are
ventricular paced beats followed
by one intrinsic beat and three
ventricular paced beats.
Interpretation: Ventricular paced
rhythm with one intrinsic beat
(normal pacemaker function)

Strip 10-2
Analysis: The first three beats are
ventricular paced beats followed
by two intrinsic beats, a pacing
spike that occurs too early, an
intrinsic beat, a fusion beat, and two
ventricular paced beats.
Interpretation: Ventricular paced
rhythm with three intrinsic beats, one
fusion beat, and one episode of undersensing (abnormal pacemaker function)

Strip 10-3
Analysis: The first complex is an
intrinsic beat followed by two
ventricular paced beats, an intrinsic
beat, and two ventricular paced
beats.
Interpretation: Ventricular paced
rhythm with two intrinsic beats
(normal pacemaker function)

Strip 10-4
Analysis: The first two complexes are
ventricular paced followed by a pacing spike with failure to capture, a
ventricular paced beat, a pacing spike
with failure to capture, an intrinsic
beat, a ventricular paced beat, a pacing spike with failure to capture, and
an intrinsic beat.
Interpretation: Ventricular paced
rhythm with two intrinsic beats and
three episodes of failure to capture
(abnormal pacemaker function)

Strip 10-5
Analysis: No patient or paced beats
are seen; pacing spikes are present
that fail to capture the ventricles.
Interpretation: Failure to capture
in the presence of ventricular
standstill

Strip 10-6
Analysis: The first five complexes
are intrinsic beats followed by two
ventricular paced beats, two intrinsic
beats, and one ventricular paced
beat.
Interpretation: Ventricular paced
rhythm with seven intrinsic beats
(normal pacemaker function)

Strip 10-7
Analysis: The first complex is an
intrinsic beat followed by a ventricular paced beat that occurs too early,
two ventricular paced beats, a fusion
beat, an intrinsic beat, a pacing spike
that occurs too early, and three
intrinsic beats.
Interpretation: Ventricular paced
rhythm with five intrinsic beats,
one fusion beat, and two episodes
of undersensing (one with capture
and one without capture). This is
abnormal pacemaker function.

Strip 10-8
Analysis: The first five complexes are
ventricular paced followed by a pause
in pacing, a ventricular paced beat
that occurs later than expected, and
a ventricular paced beat.
Interpretation: Ventricular paced
rhythm with one episode of oversensing (pacemaker sensed the small
waveform artifact seen during the
pause). This is abnormal pacemaker
function.

Strip 10-9
Analysis: The first two complexes
are ventricular paced beats followed by a pacing spike that fails
to capture, an intrinsic beat, three
ventricular paced beats, and an
intrinsic beat.
Interpretation: Ventricular paced
rhythm with two intrinsic beats and
one episode of failure to capture
(abnormal pacemaker function)

Strip 10-10
Analysis: All complexes are pacemaker induced.
Interpretation: Ventricular paced
rhythm

Strip 10-11
Analysis: The first three complexes
are ventricular paced beats followed
by an intrinsic beat, a pacing spike
that occurs too early, an intrinsic
beat, a pacing spike with capture
that occurs too early, and three
ventricular paced beats.
Interpretation: Ventricular paced
rhythm with two intrinsic beats and
two episodes of undersensing (one
episode without capture and one
episode with capture). This represents
abnormal pacemaker function.

Strip 10-12
Analysis: The first six complexes are
intrinsic beats followed by two ventricular paced beats and two intrinsic
beats.
Interpretation: Ventricular paced
rhythm with eight intrinsic beats
(normal pacemaker function)

Strip 10-13
Analysis: All complexes are pacemaker induced.
Interpretation: Ventricular paced rhythm (normal pacemaker function)

Strip 10-14
Analysis: The first two complexes are intrinsic beats followed by a fusion beat (note pacing spike at onset of QRS), another fusion beat, and three ventricular paced beats.
Interpretation: Ventricular paced rhythm with two intrinsic beats and two fusion beats (normal pacemaker function)

Strip 10-15
Analysis: The first three complexes are ventricular paced beats; when the pacemaker is turned off the underlying rhythm is ventricular standstill; two ventricular paced beats are seen when the pacemaker is turned back on.
Interpretation: Ventricular paced rhythm with an underlying rhythm of ventricular standstill when the pacemaker is turned off. This strip shows an indication for permanent pacemaker implantation if the underlying rhythm doesn't resolve.

Strip 10-16
Analysis: The first two beats are ventricular paced beats followed by an intrinsic beat, a pacing spike that fails to capture, two ventricular paced beats, two intrinsic beats, and a ventricular paced beat.
Interpretation: Ventricular paced rhythm with three intrinsic beats and one episode of failure to capture (abnormal pacemaker function)

Strip 10-17
Analysis: The first two complexes are ventricular paced beats followed by a fusion beat, two intrinsic beats, a pacing spike that occurs too early, an intrinsic beat, a pacing spike that occurs too early, an intrinsic beat, a pacing spike with capture that occurs too early, and a ventricular paced beat.
Interpretation: Ventricular paced rhythm with four intrinsic beats, one fusion beat, and three episodes of undersensing (two episodes without capture and one episode with capture). This represents abnormal pacemaker function.

Strip 10-18
Analysis: The first two complexes are ventricular paced beats followed by a fusion beat and four intrinsic beats.
Interpretation: Ventricular paced rhythm with one fusion beat and four intrinsic beats (normal pacemaker function)

Strip 10-19
Analysis: The first four complexes are ventricular paced beats followed by an intrinsic beat and three ventricular paced beats.
Interpretation: Ventricular paced rhythm with one intrinsic beat (normal pacemaker function)

Strip 10-20
Analysis: The first complex is a ventricular paced beat followed by two pacing spikes with failure to capture, a ventricular paced beat, a pacing spike with failure to capture, a ventricular paced beat, a pacing spike with failure to capture, two ventricular paced beats, and a pacing spike with failure to capture.
Interpretation: Ventricular paced rhythm with five episodes of failure to capture (abnormal pacemaker function)

Strip 10-21
Analysis: All complexes are pacemaker induced.
Interpretation: Ventricular paced rhythm (normal pacemaker function)

Strip 10-22
Analysis: One ventricular paced beat changing to ventricular tachycardia (torsade de pointes)
Interpretation: Ventricular paced beat changing to torsade de pointes VT

Strip 10-23
Analysis: The first four complexes are ventricular paced beats followed by an intrinsic beat, a pacing spike that occurs too early, a fusion beat, and a ventricular paced beat.
Interpretation: Ventricular paced rhythm with one intrinsic beat, one fusion beat, and one episode of undersensing (abnormal pacemaker function)

Strip 10-24
Analysis: The first complex is a ventricular paced beat followed by a pacing spike with failure to capture, an intrinsic beat, a pacing spike with failure to capture, an intrinsic beat, a ventricular paced beat, a pacing spike with failure to capture, an intrinsic beat, a pacing spike with failure to capture, and an intrinsic beat.
Interpretation: Ventricular paced rhythm with four intrinsic beats, and four episodes of failure to capture (abnormal pacemaker function)

Strip 10-25
Analysis: All complexes are pacemaker induced.
Interpretation: Ventricular paced rhythm (normal pacemaker function)

Strip 10-26
Analysis: The first two beats are ventricular paced beats followed by an intrinsic beat, two ventricular paced beats, a fusion beat, an intrinsic beat, and two ventricular paced beats.
Interpretation: Ventricular paced rhythm with two intrinsic beats, and one fusion beat (normal pacemaker function)

Strip 10-27
Analysis: The first four complexes are ventricular paced beats followed by ventricular standstill (asystole).
Interpretation: Ventricular paced rhythm with failure to fire resulting in ventricular standstill (abnormal pacemaker function)

Strip 10-28
Analysis: The first four complexes are ventricular paced beats followed by two pacing spikes with failure to capture, an intrinsic beat, two pacing spikes with failure to capture, and an intrinsic beat.
Interpretation: Ventricular paced rhythm with two intrinsic beats and four episodes of failure to capture (abnormal pacemaker function)

Strip 10-29
Analysis: The first two complexes are ventricular paced beats followed by three intrinsic beats and three ventricular paced beats.
Interpretation: Ventricular paced rhythm with three intrinsic beats (normal pacemaker function)

Strip 10-30
Analysis: The first complex is a pseudofusion beat (note spike in QRS complex with no change in amplitude or width) followed by two intrinsic beats, three ventricular paced beats, one fusion beat, and one intrinsic beat.
Interpretation: Ventricular paced rhythm with one pseudofusion beat, one fusion beat, and three intrinsic beats (normal pacemaker function)

Strip 10-31
Analysis: The first three complexes are ventricular paced beats followed by two intrinsic beats (paired PVCs) and four ventricular paced beats.
Interpretation: Ventricular paced rhythm with two intrinsic beats (normal pacemaker function)

Strip 10-32
Analysis: The first four complexes are ventricular paced beats followed by one intrinsic beat (PVC), a pacing spike occurring too early, and three ventricular paced beats.
Interpretation: Ventricular paced rhythm with one intrinsic beat and one episode of undersensing malfunction (abnormal pacemaker function)

Strip 10-33
Analysis: The first two complexes are ventricular paced beats followed by two intrinsic beats, a fusion beat, and two ventricular paced beats.
Interpretation: Ventricular paced rhythm with two intrinsic beats and one fusion beat (normal pacemaker function)

Strip 10-34
Analysis: The first four complexes are ventricular paced beats followed by a pacing spike with failure to capture, an intrinsic beat, a pacing spike that occurs too early, and two ventricular paced beats.
Interpretation: Ventricular paced rhythm with one intrinsic beat, one episode of failure to capture, and one episode of undersensing (abnormal pacemaker function)

Strip 10-35
Analysis: The first two complexes are ventricular paced beats followed by an intrinsic beat, a fusion beat, an intrinsic beat, one pacing spike with capture that occurs too early, two ventricular paced beats, and an intrinsic beat.
Interpretation: Ventricular paced rhythm with three intrinsic beats, one fusion beat, and one episode of undersensing (abnormal pacemaker function)

Strip 10-36
Analysis: The first two complexes are ventricular paced beats followed by an intrinsic beat, a pacing spike that occurs too early, three intrinsic beats, and three ventricular paced beats.
Interpretation: Ventricular paced rhythm with four intrinsic beats and one episode of undersensing malfunction (abnormal pacemaker function)

Strip 10-37
Analysis: The first five complexes are ventricular paced beats followed by an intrinsic beat and two ventricular paced beats.
Interpretation: Ventricular paced rhythm with one intrinsic beat (normal pacemaker function)

Strip 10-38
Analysis: The first four complexes are ventricular paced beats followed by a pause in pacing, a ventricular paced beat that occurs later than expected, a ventricular paced beat, and an intrinsic beat.
Interpretation: Ventricular paced rhythm with one intrinsic beat and one episode of oversensing (the pacemaker sensed the large T wave at the start of the pause). This is abnormal pacemaker function.

Strip 10-39
Analysis: The first complex is ventricular paced followed by three intrinsic beats and four ventricular paced beats.
Interpretation: Ventricular paced rhythm with three intrinsic beats (normal pacemaker function)

Strip 10-40
Analysis: The first complex is ventricular paced followed by ventricular standstill (asystole).
Interpretation: Ventricular paced beat with failure to fire resulting in ventricular standstill (abnormal pacemaker function)

Strip 11-1
Rhythm: Regular
Rate: 107 beats/minute
P waves: Sinus
PR interval: 0.12 second
QRS complex: 0.06 to 0.08 second
Rhythm interpretation: Sinus tachycardia

Strip 11-2
Rhythm: Regular
Rate: 58 beats/minute
P waves: Sinus
PR interval: 0.12 to 0.14 second
QRS complex: 0.12 second
Rhythm interpretation: Sinus bradycardia with bundle-branch block; ST-segment depression is present.

Strip 11-3
Rhythm: Regular (atrial); irregular (ventricular)
Rate: 84 beats/minute (atrial); 30 beats/minute (ventricular)
P waves: Sinus (two P waves or four P waves before each QRS complex)
PR interval: 0.24 to 0.28 second (consistent)
QRS complex: 0.08 second
Rhythm interpretation: Mobitz II with 2:1 and 4:1 AV conduction

Strip 11-4
Rhythm: Irregular
Rate: 100 beats/minute
P waves: Fibrillatory waves present; some flutter waves mixed with fib waves
PR interval: Not measurable
QRS complex: 0.04 second
Rhythm interpretation: Atrial fibrillation

Strip 11-5
Rhythm: Regular
Rate: 48 beats/minute
P waves: Hidden in the QRS complex
PR interval: Not measurable
QRS complex: 0.08 second
Rhythm interpretation: Junctional rhythm; ST-segment depression is present.

Strip 11-6
Rhythm: Regular
Rate: 188 beats/minute
P waves: Hidden in preceding T waves
PR interval: Not measurable
QRS complex: 0.10 second
Rhythm interpretation: Paroxysmal atrial tachycardia

Strip 11-7
Analysis: The first four complexes are ventricular paced beats followed by two intrinsic beats, a ventricular paced beat, and two intrinsic beats.
Interpretation: Ventricular paced rhythm with four intrinsic beats (normal pacemaker function)

Strip 11-8
Rhythm: Regular (atrial and ventricular)
Rate: 75 beats/minute (atrial); 26 beats/minute (ventricular)
P waves: Sinus (bear no constant relationship to the QRS complex)
PR interval: Varies
QRS complex: 0.14 to 0.16 second
Rhythm interpretation: Third-degree AV block; ST-segment elevation is present.

Strip 11-9
Rhythm: Regular
Rate: 188 beats/minute
P waves: Not discernible
PR interval: Not discernible
QRS complex: 0.16 to 0.20 second
Rhythm interpretation: Ventricular tachycardia

Strip 11-10
Rhythm: Regular
Rate: 42 beats/minute
P waves: Absent
PR interval: Not measurable
QRS complex: 0.16 second
Rhythm interpretation: Idioventricular rhythm

Strip 11-11
Rhythm: Regular (basic rhythm)
Rate: 56 beats/minute (basic rhythm)
P waves: Sinus (appear notched, which may indicate left atrial hypertrophy)
PR interval: 0.16 second
QRS complex: 0.06 second (basic rhythm); 0.16 second (PVC)
Rhythm interpretation: Sinus bradycardia with one interpolated PVC; ST-segment depression is present.

Strip 11-12
Rhythm: Regular
Rate: 84 beats/minute
P waves: Inverted before each QRS complex
PR interval: 0.10 second
QRS complex: 0.06 to 0.08 second
Rhythm interpretation: Accelerated junctional rhythm

Strip 11-13
Rhythm: Regular
Rate: 232 beats/minute (atrial); 58 beats/minute (ventricular)
P waves: Four flutter waves before each QRS complex
PR interval: Not measurable
QRS complex: 0.06 to 0.08 second
Rhythm interpretation: Atrial flutter with 4:1 AV conduction

Strip 11-14
Rhythm: Regular
Rate: 79 beats/minute
P waves: Sinus
PR interval: 0.16 to 0.18 second
QRS complex: 0.10 second
Rhythm interpretation: Normal sinus rhythm; ST segment elevation is present.

Strip 11-15
Rhythm: Regular
Rate: 88 beats/minute
P waves: Absent
PR interval: Not measurable
QRS complex: 0.14 to 0.16 second
Rhythm interpretation: Accelerated idioventricular rhythm

Strip 11-16
Rhythm: Regular (basic rhythm); irregular with pause
Rate: 75 beats/minute (basic rhythm)
P waves: Sinus (basic rhythm); one premature, abnormal P wave without a QRS complex (after the fifth QRS complex)
PR interval: 0.24 to 0.28 second
QRS complex: 0.06 to 0.08 second
Rhythm interpretation: Normal sinus rhythm with first-degree AV block and one nonconducted PAC (follows the fifth QRS complex)

Strip 11-17
Rhythm: Regular
Rate: 115 beats/minute
P waves: Sinus
PR interval: 0.14 to 0.16 second
QRS complex: 0.06 second
Rhythm interpretation: Sinus tachycardia

Strip 11-18
Rhythm: Regular
Rate: 48 beats/minute
P waves: Sinus
PR interval: 0.12 second
QRS complex: 0.08 to 0.10 second
Rhythm interpretation: Sinus bradycardia; ST-segment elevation is present.

Strip 11-19
Rhythm: Regular (basic rhythm); irregular (premature beats)
Rate: 72 beats/minute (basic rhythm)
P waves: Sinus (basic rhythm); inverted (premature beats)
PR interval: 0.12 to 0.14 second (basic rhythm); 0.08 second (premature beats)
QRS complex: 0.08 second
Rhythm interpretation: Normal sinus rhythm with two premature junctional contractions (fourth and sixth complexes)

Strip 11-20
Rhythm: Regular
Rate: 63 beats/minute
P waves: Vary in size, shape, and position
PR interval: 0.12 to 0.14 second
QRS complex: 0.06 to 0.08 second
Rhythm interpretation: Wandering atrial pacemaker; ST-segment depression is present.

Strip 11-21
Rhythm: Chaotic
Rate: 0 beats/minute (no QRS complexes)
P waves: No P waves; wave deflections are chaotic and irregular and vary in height, size, and shape
PR interval: Not measurable
QRS complex: Absent
Rhythm interpretation: Ventricular fibrillation

Strip 11-22
Rhythm: Regular
Rate: 107 beats/minute
P waves: Inverted before each QRS complex
PR interval: 0.08 second
QRS complex: 0.04 to 0.06 second
Rhythm interpretation: Junctional tachycardia

Strip 11-23
Rhythm: Irregular atrial rhythm
Rate: 40 beats/minute (atrial); 0 beats/minute (ventricular)
P waves: Sinus
PR interval: Not measurable
QRS complex: Absent
Rhythm interpretation: Ventricular standstill

Strip 11-24
Rhythm: Irregular
Rate: 70 beats/minute
P waves: Sinus
PR interval: 0.44 to 0.48 second
QRS complex: 0.08 to 0.10 second
Rhythm interpretation: Sinus arrhythmia with first-degree AV block; ST-segment elevation is present.

Strip 11-25
Rhythm: Regular (basic rhythm)
Rate: 48 beats/minute (basic rhythm)
P waves: Sinus (basic rhythm)
PR interval: 0.36 second
QRS complex: 0.12 to 0.14 second
Rhythm interpretation: Sinus bradycardia with first-degree AV block and sinus arrest

Strip 11-26
Rhythm: Regular (atrial); irregular (ventricular)
Rate: 72 beats/minute (atrial); 40 beats/minute (ventricular)
P waves: Sinus
PR interval: Lengthens from 0.20 to 0.28 second
QRS complex: 0.04 to 0.06 second
Rhythm interpretation: Second-degree AV block, Mobitz I; ST-segment depression is present.

Strip 11-27
Rhythm: Regular
Rate: 72 beats/minute
P waves: Sinus
PR interval: 0.20 second
QRS complex: 0.08 to 0.10 second
Rhythm interpretation: Normal sinus rhythm; ST-segment depression and T-wave inversion are present.

Strip 11-28
Rhythm: Regular (basic rhythm); irregular with pause
Rate: 72 beats/minute (basic rhythm); slows to 63 beats/minute during first cycle after pause; rate suppression can occur for several cycles after an interruption in the basic rhythm.
P waves: Sinus
PR interval: 0.16 to 0.18 second
QRS complex: 0.04 to 0.06 second
Rhythm interpretation: Normal sinus rhythm with sinus arrest

Strip 11-29
Rhythm: Regular (basic rhythm); irregular (premature beat)
Rate: 63 beats/minute (basic rhythm)
P waves: Sinus (basic rhythm); premature and pointed (premature beat)
PR interval: 0.14 to 0.16 second (basic rhythm); 0.12 second (premature beat)
QRS complex: 0.08 second
Rhythm interpretation: Normal sinus rhythm with one PAC (fifth complex)

Strip 11-30
Rhythm: Regular (basic rhythm); irregular (PVCs)
Rate: 72 beats/minute (basic rhythm)
P waves: Sinus
PR interval: 0.12 to 0.14 second
QRS complex: 0.12 second (basic rhythm and PVCs)
Rhythm interpretation: Normal sinus rhythm with bundle-branch block and paired PVCs; a U wave is present.

Strip 11-31
Rhythm: Regular (atrial and ventricular)
Rate: 240 beats/minute (atrial); 60 beats/minute (ventricular)
P waves: Four flutter waves to each QRS complex
PR interval: Not measurable
QRS complex: 0.04 to 0.06 second
Rhythm interpretation: Atrial flutter with 4:1 AV conduction

Strip 11-32
Rhythm: Regular (basic rhythm);
irregular with pause
Rate: 54 beats/minute (basic
rhythm)
P waves: Sinus (basic rhythm); none
(fourth and fifth complexes)
PR interval: 0.18 to 0.20 second
(basic rhythm)
QRS complex: 0.06 to 0.08 second
Rhythm interpretation: Sinus bradycardia with a pause followed by two
junctional escape beats; the specific
pause (sinus arrest or block) can't be
identified due to the presence of the
escape beats.

Strip 11-33
Rhythm: Regular
Rate: 25 beats/minute
P waves: None identified
PR interval: Not measurable
QRS complex: 0.24 second or
greater
Rhythm interpretation:
Idioventricular rhythm

Strip 11-34
Analysis: The first three complexes
are ventricular paced beats
followed by a pacing spike that fails
to capture the ventricle, an intrinsic beat, and two ventricular paced
beats.
Interpretation: Ventricular paced
rhythm with one intrinsic beat and
one episode of failure to capture
(abnormal pacemaker function)

Strip 11-35
Rhythm: Regular
Rate: 84 beats/minute
P waves: Not identified
PR interval: Not measurable
QRS complex: 0.12 to 0.14 second
Rhythm interpretation: Accelerated
idioventricular rhythm

Strip 11-36
Rhythm: Chaotic
Rate: 0 beats/minute
P waves: Absent; wave deflections
are chaotic and irregular and vary in
size, shape, and height
PR interval: Not measurable
QRS complex: Absent
Rhythm interpretation: Ventricular
fibrillation, followed by electrical
shock and return to ventricular
fibrillation

Strip 11-37
Rhythm: Regular
Rate: 52 beats/minute
P waves: Sinus
PR interval: 0.18 to 0.20 second
QRS complex: 0.06 to 0.08 second
Rhythm interpretation: Sinus
bradycardia; a U wave is present.

Strip 11-38
Rhythm: Regular
Rate: 94 beats/minute
P waves: Inverted before each QRS
complex
PR interval: 0.08 to 0.10 second
QRS complex: 0.08 second
Rhythm interpretation: Accelerated
junctional rhythm; baseline artifact
is present.

Strip 11-39
Rhythm: Regular (basic rhythm);
irregular with premature beat
Rate: 72 beats/minute (basic
rhythm)
P waves: Sinus (basic rhythm);
premature abnormal P wave with
premature beat
PR interval: 0.14 to 0.16 second
(basic rhythm); 0.12 second
(premature beat)
QRS complex: 0.04 to 0.08 second
(basic rhythm); 0.08 second
(premature beat)
Rhythm interpretation: Normal sinus
rhythm with one premature atrial
contraction (PAC)

Strip 11-40
Rhythm: Regular (basic rhythm) off
by two squares
Rate: 79 beats/minute (basic
rhythm)
P waves: Sinus (basic rhythm);
premature abnormal P wave without
QRS following fifth QRS complex
PR interval: 0.20 second
QRS complex: 0.08 to 0.10 second
(basic rhythm); 0.08 second
(premature beat)
Rhythm interpretation: Normal sinus
rhythm with nonconducted PAC
followed by a PJC

Strip 11-41
Rhythm: P waves occur regularly
Rate: 88 beats/minute (atrial); 0
(ventricular)
P waves: Sinus
PR interval: Not measurable
QRS complex: Absent
Rhythm interpretation: Ventricular
standstill

Strip 11-42
Rhythm: Regular (basic rhythm);
irregular (premature beats)
Rate: 63 beats/minute (basic
rhythm)
P waves: Sinus (basic rhythm)
PR interval: 0.12 to 0.14 second
QRS complex: 0.08 second (basic
rhythm); 0.12 to 0.16 second (PVC)
Rhythm interpretation: Normal sinus
rhythm with paired multifocal PVCs
(fourth and fifth complexes)

Strip 11-43
Rhythm: Regular (basic rhythm);
irregular (PACs)
Rate: 136 beats/minute (basic
rhythm)
P waves: Sinus (basic rhythm);
premature and pointed (premature
beats)
PR interval: 0.16 to 0.20 second
QRS complex: 0.06 to 0.08 second
Rhythm interpretation: Sinus
tachycardia with two PACs (fourth
and eighth complexes)

Strip 11-44
Rhythm: Regular (basic rhythm); irregular with pause
Rate: 84 beats/minute (basic rhythm); slows after pause but returns to basic rate after four cycles.
P waves: Sinus
PR interval: 0.20 second
QRS complex: 0.08 second
Rhythm interpretation: Normal sinus rhythm with sinus arrest; ST-segment depression and T-wave inversion are present.

Strip 11-45
Analysis: No patient or paced beats are seen; pacing spikes are noted that fail to capture the ventricles.
Interpretation: Failure to capture in the presence of ventricular standstill

Strip 11-46
Analysis: The first two complexes are intrinsic beats followed by a fusion beat, two intrinsic beats, two ventricular paced beats, and a fusion beat.
Interpretation: Ventricular paced rhythm with four intrinsic beats and two fusion beats (normal pacemaker function)

Strip 11-47
Rhythm: Regular
Rate: 42 beats/minute
P waves: Hidden in QRS complex
PR interval: Not measurable
QRS complex: 0.08 to 0.10 second
Rhythm interpretation: Junctional rhythm

Strip 11-48
Rhythm: Regular (atrial); irregular (ventricular)
Rate: 79 beats/minute (atrial); 50 beats/minute (ventricular)
P waves: Sinus
PR interval: Lengthens from 0.20 to 0.32 second
QRS complex: 0.08 to 0.10 second
Rhythm interpretation: Second-degree AV block, Mobitz I

Strip 11-49
Rhythm: Regular (basic rhythm); irregular (premature beat)
Rate: 107 beats/minute
P waves: Inverted before each QRS complex (except the ninth QRS complex, which has a premature, pointed P wave)
PR interval: 0.08 to 0.10 second (basic rhythm); 0.10 second (premature beat)
QRS complex: 0.08 to 0.10 second
Rhythm interpretation: Junctional tachycardia with one PAC (ninth complex)

Strip 11-50
Rhythm: Regular (atrial and ventricular)
Rate: 84 beats/minute (atrial); 28 beats/minute (ventricular)
P waves: Sinus (bear no relationship to the QRS complex)
PR interval: Varies greatly
QRS complex: 0.12 second
Rhythm interpretation: Third-degree AV block; ST-segment depression is present.

Strip 11-51
Rhythm: Irregular
Rate: 70 beats/minute
P waves: Sinus
PR interval: 0.18 to 0.20 second
QRS complex: 0.08 to 0.10 second
Rhythm interpretation: Sinus arrhythmia

Strip 11-52
Rhythm: Regular (basic rhythm); irregular (premature beats)
Rate: 72 beats/minute (basic rhythm)
P waves: Sinus (basic rhythm)
PR interval: 0.16 second
QRS complex: 0.10 second
Rhythm interpretation: Normal sinus rhythm with unifocal PVCs in a trigeminal pattern. ST-segment depression and T-wave inversion are present.

Strip 11-53
Rhythm: Regular
Rate: 93 beats/minute (atrial); 31 beats/minute (ventricular)
P waves: Three sinus P waves to each QRS complex (one hidden in the T wave)
PR interval: 0.36 second (remains constant)
QRS complex: 0.08 second
Rhythm interpretation: Second-degree AV block, Mobitz II

Strip 11-54
Rhythm: Regular (basic rhythm); irregular (PVCs)
Rate: 72 beats/minute (basic rhythm)
P waves: Sinus (basic rhythm)
PR interval: 0.12 to 0.14 second
QRS complex: 0.08 second (basic rhythm); 0.14 to 0.16 second (PVCs)
Rhythm interpretation: Normal sinus rhythm with multifocal PVCs

Strip 11-55
Rhythm: Regular (atrial and ventricular)
Rate: 62 beats/minute (atrial); 31 beats/minute (ventricular)
P waves: Two sinus P waves before each QRS complex
PR interval: 0.44 second (remains constant)
QRS complex: 0.14 to 0.16 second
Rhythm interpretation: Second-degree AV block, Mobitz II

Strip 11-56
Rhythm: Regular
Rate: 65 beats/minute
P waves: Inverted before each QRS complex
PR interval: 0.10 second
QRS complex: 0.04 second
Rhythm interpretation: Accelerated junctional rhythm; ST-segment elevation is present.

Strip 11-57
Rhythm: Regular (basic rhythm);
irregular with pause
Rate: 68 beats/minute (basic rhythm)
P waves: Sinus
PR interval: 0.22 to 0.24 second
QRS complex: 0.08 to 0.10 second
Rhythm interpretation: Normal
sinus rhythm with first-degree AV
block and sinus arrest; ST-segment
elevation is present.

Strip 11-58
Analysis: The first complex is an
intrinsic beat followed by a pacing
spike with failure to capture, an
intrinsic beat, a pacing spike with
failure to capture, two intrinsic
beats, a pacing spike with failure to
capture, an intrinsic beat, a pacing
spike with failure to capture, and an
intrinsic beat.
Interpretation: Strip shows an
intrinsic rhythm (sinus arrhythmia
with first-degree AV block and
two PVCs) with complete failure
to capture (abnormal pacemaker
function); since there were no two
consecutive paced beats or two
consecutive pacing spikes, I used
the interval from the R wave of the
native beat to the pacing spike as my
estimated automatic interval.

Strip 11-59
Rhythm: Regular
Rate: 188 beats/minute
P waves: Not identified
PR interval: Not measurable
QRS complex: 0.06 to 0.08 second
Rhythm interpretation: Paroxysmal
atrial tachycardia

Strip 11-60
Rhythm: Irregular
Rate: 30 beats/minute
P waves: None present
PR interval: Not measurable
QRS complex: 0.16 second
Rhythm interpretation: Idioventricu-
lar rhythm; ST-segment depression
is present.

Strip 11-61
Rhythm: Regular (atrial); irregular
(ventricular)
Rate: 125 beats/minute (atrial);
80 beats/minute (ventricular)
P waves: Sinus
PR interval: Lengthens from 0.12 to
0.24 second
QRS complex: 0.06 to 0.08 second
Rhythm interpretation: Second-
degree AV block, Mobitz I; T-wave
inversion is present.

Strip 11-62
Rhythm: Regular (basic rhythm);
irregular (nonconducted PACs)
Rate: 100 beats/minute (basic
rhythm)
P waves: Sinus; two premature
abnormal P waves without QRS
complex (after the fourth and eighth
complexes)
PR interval: 0.12 second
QRS complex: 0.06 to 0.08 second
Rhythm interpretation: Normal sinus
rhythm with two nonconducted
PACs; T-wave inversion is present.

Strip 11-63
Rhythm: Regular
Rate: 75 beats/minute
P waves: Sinus
PR interval: 0.16 to 0.18 second
QRS complex: 0.12 to 0.14 second
Rhythm interpretation: Normal sinus
rhythm with bundle-branch block;
ST-segment elevation is present.

Strip 11-64
Rhythm: Regular
Rate: 50 beats/minute
P waves: Sinus
PR interval: 0.16 second
QRS complex: 0.06 to 0.08 second
Rhythm interpretation: Sinus
bradycardia; a U wave is present.

Strip 11-65
Analysis: All complexes are
pacemaker induced.
Interpretation: Ventricular paced
rhythm (normal pacemaker
function)

Strip 11-66
Rhythm: Regular
Rate: 78 beats/minute (atrial);
39 beats/minute (ventricular)
P waves: Two sinus P waves to each
QRS complex
PR interval: 0.24 second with a
constant relationship to the QRS
complex
QRS complex: 0.12 to 0.14 second
Rhythm interpretation:
Second-degree AV block, Mobitz II

Strip 11-67
Rhythm: Regular (basic rhythm) but
off by one square
Rate: 52 beats/minute
P waves: No visible P wave (hidden in
QRS complex)
PR interval: Not measurable
QRS complex: 0.06 to 0.08 second
Rhythm interpretation: Junctional
rhythm

Strip 11-68
Analysis: The first four complexes
are ventricular paced followed by a
fusion beat and an intrinsic beat.
Interpretation: Ventricular paced
rhythm with one fusion beat and one
intrinsic beat (normal pacemaker
function)

Strip 11-69
Rhythm: Regular
Rate: 115 beats/minute
P waves: Inverted before each QRS
complex
PR interval: 0.08 to 0.10 second
QRS complex: 0.06 to 0.08 second
Rhythm interpretation: Junctional
tachycardia

Strip 11-70
Rhythm: Regular (basic rhythm);
irregular (PJC)
Rate: 58 beats/minute (basic
rhythm)
P waves: Sinus (basic rhythm);
inverted (PJC)
PR interval: 0.14 to 0.16 second
(basic rhythm); 0.10 second (PJC)
QRS complex: 0.08 second
Rhythm interpretation: Sinus
bradycardia with one PJC

Strip 11-71
Rhythm: Regular (basic rhythm); irregular (nonconducted PAC)
Rate: 63 beats/minute (basic rhythm)
P waves: Sinus (basic rhythm); one premature, abnormal P wave without a QRS complex (after the fourth complex)
PR interval: 0.28 to 0.32 second
QRS complex: 0.12 second
Rhythm interpretation: Normal sinus rhythm with first-degree AV block and bundle-branch block with one nonconducted PAC after the fourth QRS complex; ST-segment elevation and T-wave inversion are present.

Strip 11-72
Rhythm: Regular (basic rhythm); irregular (PVC)
Rate: 50 beats/minute (basic rhythm)
P waves: Sinus (basic rhythm)
PR interval: 0.12 to 0.14 second
QRS complex: 0.08 second (basic rhythm); 0.18 second (PVC)
Rhythm interpretation: Sinus bradycardia with one PVC (after the third QRS complex); ST-segment elevation is present.

Strip 11-73
Analysis: The first two complexes are ventricular paced followed by a fusion beat, a pseudofusion beat (note spike at beginning of R wave), three intrinsic beats, a pacing spike that occurs too early, an intrinsic beat, a pacing spike that occurs too early, an intrinsic beat, and a pacing spike that occurs too early.
Interpretation: Ventricular paced rhythm with one fusion beat, one pseudofusion beat, five intrinsic beats, and three episodes of undersensing (abnormal pacemaker function)

Strip 11-74
Rhythm: Regular
Rate: 50 beats/minute
P waves: None identified
PR interval: Not measurable
QRS complex: 0.04 to 0.06 second
Rhythm interpretation: Junctional rhythm; ST-segment depression and T-wave inversion are present.

Strip 11-75
Rhythm: Irregular atrial rhythm
Rate: 40 beats/minute (atrial); 0 (ventricular)
P waves: Sinus
PR interval: Not measurable
QRS complex: Absent
Rhythm interpretation: Ventricular standstill

Strip 11-76
Rhythm: Irregular
Rate: 60 beats/minute
P waves: Sinus
PR interval: 0.12 to 0.14 second
QRS complex: 0.08 to 0.10 second
Rhythm interpretation: Sinus arrhythmia; ST-segment elevation is present.

Strip 11-77
Rhythm: Regular
Rate: 68 beats/minute
P waves: P waves vary in size, shape, and position
PR interval: 0.14 to 0.16 second
QRS complex: 0.06 to 0.08 second
Rhythm interpretation: Wandering atrial pacemaker; T-wave inversion is present.

Strip 11-78
Rhythm: Regular
Rate: 214 beats/minute
P waves: Hidden
PR interval: Not measurable
QRS complex: 0.06 to 0.08 second
Rhythm interpretation: Paroxysmal atrial tachycardia

Strip 11-79
Rhythm: Regular (first and second rhythms)
Rate: 94 beats/minute (first rhythm); 136 beats/minute (second rhythm)
P waves: Sinus (first rhythm)
PR interval: 0.18 to 0.20 second (first rhythm)
QRS complex: 0.06 to 0.08 second (first rhythm); 0.12 second (second rhythm)
Rhythm interpretation: Normal sinus rhythm changing to ventricular tachycardia

Strip 11-80
Rhythm: Regular (basic rhythm)
Rate: 107 beats/minute (basic rhythm)
P waves: Sinus (basic rhythm)
PR interval: 0.14 to 0.16 second
QRS complex: 0.06 to 0.08 second (basic rhythm); 0.12 second (ventricular beats)
Rhythm interpretation: Sinus tachycardia with a four-beat burst of ventricular tachycardia and paired, unifocal PVCs

Strip 11-81
Rhythm: Irregular
Rate: 260 beats/minute (atrial); 70 beats/minute (ventricular)
P waves: Flutter waves
PR interval: Not measurable
QRS complex: 0.06 to 0.08 second
Rhythm interpretation: Atrial flutter with variable block

Strip 11-82
Rhythm: Regular
Rate: 88 beats/minute
P waves: Sinus
PR interval: 0.12 second
QRS complex: 0.04 to 0.06 second
Rhythm interpretation: Normal sinus rhythm

Strip 11-83
Analysis: The first beat is a pseudofusion beat (note spike inside QRS with complex uncharged) followed by two intrinsic beats, three ventricular paced beats, a fusion beat, and an intrinsic beat.
Interpretation: Ventricular paced rhythm with one pseudofusion beat, one fusion beat, and three intrinsic beats (normal pacemaker function)

Strip 11-84
Rhythm: Regular
Rate: 136 beats/minute
P waves: Sinus
PR interval: 0.12 to 0.14 second
QRS complex: 0.06 to 0.08 second
Rhythm interpretation: Sinus tachycardia

Strip 11-85
Rhythm: Regular
Rate: 54 beats/minute
P waves: Sinus
PR interval: 0.24 to 0.26 second
QRS complex: 0.04 to 0.06 second
Rhythm interpretation: Sinus bradycardia with first-degree AV block

Strip 11-86
Rhythm: Regular (atrial and ventricular)
Rate: 94 beats/minute (atrial); 37 beats/minute (ventricular)
P waves: Sinus (bear no relationship to the QRS complex)
PR interval: Varies
QRS complex: 0.12 to 0.14 second
Rhythm interpretation: Third-degree AV block

Strip 11-87
Rhythm: Regular
Rate: 150 beats/minute
P waves: None identified
PR interval: Not measurable
QRS complex: 0.12 to 0.14 second
Rhythm interpretation: Ventricular tachycardia

Strip 11-88
Rhythm: Regular (basic rhythm); irregular with pause
Rate: 56 beats/minute (basic rhythm)
P waves: Sinus (basic rhythm); absent during pause
PR interval: 0.16 to 0.18 second
QRS complex: 0.08 to 0.10 second
Rhythm interpretation: Sinus bradycardia with sinus arrest; ST-segment depression and T-wave inversion are present.

Strip 11-89
Rhythm: 0 beats/minute
Rate: 0 beats/minute
P waves: Absent
PR interval: Not measurable
QRS complex: Absent
Rhythm interpretation: Ventricular standstill

Strip 11-90
Rhythm: Regular
Rate: 88 beats/minute
P waves: Sinus
PR interval: 0.16 second
QRS complex: 0.06 to 0.08 second
Rhythm interpretation: Normal sinus rhythm; ST-segment depression and T-wave inversion are present.

Strip 11-91
Rhythm: Regular (basic rhythm); irregular (PVC)
Rate: 115 beats/minute (basic rhythm)
P waves: Inverted before each QRS complex
PR interval: 0.08 to 0.10 second
QRS complex: 0.04 to 0.06 second (basic rhythm); 0.12 second (premature beat)
Rhythm interpretation: Junctional tachycardia with one PVC

Strip 11-92
Rhythm: Regular
Rate: 188 beats/minute
P waves: T-P wave (P wave obscured in T wave)
PR interval: Not measurable
QRS complex: 0.08 to 0.10 second
Rhythm interpretation: Paroxysmal atrial tachycardia

Strip 11-93
Rhythm: Chaotic
Rate: 0 beats/minute
P waves: Absent; fibrillatory waves present
PR interval: Not measurable
QRS complex: Absent
Rhythm interpretation: Ventricular fibrillation

Strip 11-94
Rhythm: Regular (basic rhythm); irregular with pause
Rate: 75 beats/minute (basic rhythm)
P waves: Sinus (basic rhythm)
PR interval: 0.24 second
QRS complex: 0.06 to 0.08 second
Rhythm interpretation: Normal sinus rhythm with first-degree AV block and sinus exit block

Strip 11-95
Rhythm: Regular
Rate: 100 beats/minute
P waves: Inverted before each QRS complex
PR interval: 0.08 second
QRS complex: 0.06 to 0.08 second
Rhythm interpretation: Accelerated junctional rhythm

Strip 11-96
Rhythm: Regular (atrial); irregular (ventricular)
Rate: 84 beats/minute (atrial); 70 beats/minute (ventricular)
P waves: Sinus
PR interval: Lengthens from 0.20 to 0.36 second
QRS complex: 0.08 to 0.10 second
Rhythm interpretation: Second-degree AV block, Mobitz I; ST-segment depression is present.

Strip 11-97
Rhythm: Irregular
Rate: 100 beats/minute
P waves: Fibrillatory waves
PR interval: Not measurable
QRS complex: 0.06 to 0.08 second (basic rhythm); 0.12 second (PVC)
Rhythm interpretation: Atrial fibrillation with one PVC

Strip 11-98
Analysis: The first two complexes are ventricular paced beats followed by an intrinsic beat, two ventricular paced beats, a pacing spike with failure to capture, an intrinsic beat, and a ventricular paced beat.
Interpretation: Ventricular paced rhythm with two intrinsic beats and one episode of failure to capture (abnormal pacemaker function)

Strip 11-99
Rhythm: Regular (basic rhythm); irregular (premature beat)
Rate: 125 beats/minute (basic rhythm)
P waves: Sinus
PR interval: 0.12 second
QRS complex: 0.04 to 0.06 second
Rhythm interpretation: Sinus tachycardia with one PAC (twelfth complex)

Strip 11-100
Rhythm: Regular
Rate: 272 beats/minute (atrial);
136 beats/minute (ventricular)
P waves: Two flutter waves to each
QRS complex
PR interval: Not measurable
QRS complex: 0.04 second
Rhythm interpretation: Atrial flutter
with 2:1 AV conduction

Strip 11-101
Rhythm: Irregular
Rate: 60 beats/minute
P waves: Sinus
PR interval: 0.14 to 0.16 second
QRS complex: 0.08 second
Rhythm interpretation: Sinus
arrhythmia

Strip 11-102
Rhythm: Regular
Rate: 48 beats/minute
P waves: Sinus
PR interval: 0.14 to 0.16 second
QRS complex: 0.08 second
Rhythm interpretation: Sinus
bradycardia; a U wave is present.

Strip 11-103
Rhythm: Regular
Rate: 214 beats/minute
P waves: None identified
PR interval: Not measurable
QRS complex: 0.16 second or greater
Rhythm interpretation: Ventricular
tachycardia

Strip 11-104
Rhythm: Irregular
Rate: 60 beats/minute
P waves: Fibrillatory waves
PR interval: Not measurable
QRS complex: 0.06 to 0.08 second
Rhythm interpretation: Atrial
fibrillation

Strip 11-105
Rhythm: Regular (basic rhythm)
Rate: 72 beats/minute (basic rhythm)
P waves: Sinus
PR interval: 0.16 to 0.18 second
QRS complex: 0.06 to 0.08 second
(basic rhythm); 0.12 second (PVC)
Rhythm interpretation: Normal sinus
rhythm with one interpolated PVC;
ST-segment depression is present.

Strip 11-106
Rhythm: Regular (basic rhythm);
irregular (PJC)
Rate: 65 beats/minute (basic rhythm)
P waves: Sinus (basic rhythm);
inverted (PJC)
PR interval: 0.12 to 0.16 second
(basic rhythm); 0.10 second (PJC)
QRS complex: 0.06 to 0.08 second
Rhythm interpretation: Normal sinus
rhythm with one PJC; a U wave is
present.

Strip 11-107
Rhythm: Regular (basic rhythm);
irregular (PVCs)
Rate: 88 beats/minute (basic rhythm)
P waves: Sinus
PR interval: 0.12 to 0.14 second
QRS complex: 0.04 to 0.06 second
Rhythm interpretation: Normal sinus
rhythm with three PVCs

Glossary

Aberrant — Abnormal

Aberrantly conducted supraventricular premature beats — A premature electrical impulse originating in the atria or AV junction may occur so early that the impulse arrives at the bundle of His before the bundle branches have been sufficiently repolarized. Because the right bundle branch is slower to repolarize, the impulse travels down the left bundle branch first, and then stimulates the right bundle branch. Because of this delay in ventricular depolarization the QRS complex will be wide. Premature atrial contractions (PACs) associated with a wide QRS complex are called PACs with aberrant ventricular conduction, indicating that conduction through the ventricles is abnormal. Premature junctional contractions (PJCs) associated with a wide QRS complex are called PJCs with aberrant ventricular conduction. Also known as PACs or PJCs with *aberrancy*.

Absolute refractory period — The period of time during ventricular depolarization and most of repolarization when cardiac cells cannot be stimulated to conduct an electrical impulse. This period begins with the onset of the QRS complex and ends at the peak of the T wave.

Accelerated idioventricular rhythm — An arrhythmia originating in an ectopic site in the ventricles characterized by a regular rhythm, an absence of P waves, and wide QRS complexes at a rate of 50 to 100 beats/minute. The rate is faster than the inherent firing rate of the ventricles, but is slower than ventricular tachycardia. Also known as *AIVR*.

Accelerated junctional rhythm — An arrhythmia originating in the atrioventricular (AV) junction characterized by a regular rhythm; inverted P waves immediately before the QRS,

immediately after the QRS, or hidden within the QRS complex with a short PR interval of 0.10 second or less; a normal duration QRS complex; and a rate between 60 and 100 beats/minute. The rate is faster than the inherent firing rate of the AV junction, but slower than junctional tachycardia.

Accessory conduction pathways — Several abnormal electrical conduction pathways within the heart that allow electrical impulses to bypass the atrioventricular node before entering the ventricles.

Acetylcholine — The chemical neurotransmitter for the parasympathetic nervous system.

Acute myocardial infarction — Necrosis of the myocardium caused by prolonged and complete interruption of blood flow to an area of the myocardial muscle mass.

Agonal rhythm — A rhythm seen in a dying heart, in which the QRS complexes deteriorate into irregular, wide, indistinguishable waveforms just prior to ventricular standstill.

AIVR — *abbr* accelerated idioventricular rhythm

Amplitude — The height or depth of a wave or complex on the ECG measured in millimeters (mm). Also known as *voltage*.

Angina — The term used to describe the pain that results from a reduction in blood supply to the myocardium. The pain is typically described as chest heaviness, pressure, squeezing, or constriction. Associated symptoms include nausea and diaphoresis.

Angioplasty — The insertion of a balloon-tipped catheter into an occluded or narrowed coronary artery to

reopen the artery by inflating the balloon, compressing the atherosclerotic plaque, and dilating the lumen of the artery. Often followed by insertion of a coronary artery stent. Also known as *percutaneous transluminal coronary angioplasty* or *PTCA*.

Anion — An ion with a negative charge.

Antegrade conduction — Conduction of the electrical impulse in a forward direction

Aortic valve — One of two semilunar valves; located between the left ventricle and the aorta.

Apex of the heart — The bottom of the heart formed by the tip of the left ventricle; located to the left of the sternum at approximately the fifth intercostal space, midclavicular line.

Arrhythmia — A general term referring to any cardiac rhythm other than a sinus rhythm. Often used interchangeably with *dysrhythmia*, a more appropriate term, but one used less often.

Artifacts — Distortion of the ECG tracing by activity that is noncardiac in origin, such as patient movement, electrical interference, or muscle tremors. Also known as *interference* or *noise*.

Asystole — Absence of ventricular electrical activity. Tracing will show P waves only or a straight line. Also called *ventricular standstill*.

Atria — The two thin-walled upper chambers of the heart. The right and left atria are separated from the ventricles by the mitral and tricuspid valves.

Atrial fibrillation — An arrhythmia originating in an ectopic site (or numerous sites) in the atria characterized by an atrial rate of 400 beats/minute or more; atrial waveforms appearing as an irregular, wavy baseline; a normal QRS duration; a grossly irregular ventricular rhythm; and a rate that may be fast or slow depending on the number of impulses conducted through the atrioventricular node.

Atrial flutter — An arrhythmia originating in an ectopic site in the atria characterized by an atrial rate between 250 and 400 beats/minute; atrial waveforms appearing in a sawtooth pattern; a normal QRS duration; a regular or irregular ventricular rhythm; and a rate which may be fast or slow depending on the number of impulses conducted through the AV node.

Atrial kick — Blood pushed into the ventricles as a result of atrial contraction to complete filling of the ventricles just before the ventricles contract

Atrioventricular block (AV block) — A delay or failure of conduction of electrical impulses through the AV node.

Atrioventricular junction (AV junction) — Consists of the AV node and the bundle of His.

Atrioventricular node (AV node) — Located in the lower portion of the right atrium near the interatrial septum; only normal pathway for conduction of atrial impulses to the ventricles; primary function is to slow conduction of electrical impulses through the AV node to allow the atria to contract (atrial kick) and complete filling the ventricles.

Atrioventricular valves (AV valves) — The two valves located between the atria and the ventricles. The tricuspid separates the right atrium from the right ventricle, the mitral separates the left atrium from the left ventricle.

Automaticity — Ability of a cell to spontaneously generate an impulse.

Autonomic nervous system — Regulates functions of the body that are involuntary (not under conscious control). Includes the sympathetic and parasympathetic nervous systems, each producing opposite effects when stimulated.

AV — *abbr* atrioventricular

Bachmann's bundle — A branch of the internodal atrial conduction tracts. Conducts the electrical impulses from the sinoatrial node to the left atrium.

Baseline — The straight line between ECG waveforms when no electrical activity is detected.

Base of the heart — Top of the heart located at approximately the level of the second intercostal space.

Beta blockers — A group of drugs that block sympathetic activity. Used to treat tachyarrhythmias, MI, angina, and hypertension.

Bigeminy — An arrhythmia in which every other beat is a premature ectopic beat. The premature beat may be atrial, junctional, or ventricular in origin (i.e., atrial bigeminy, junctional bigeminy, ventricular bigeminy).

Biphasic deflection — A waveform that is part positive and part negative.

Bradycardia — An arrhythmia with a rate of less than 60 beats/minute.

Bundle-branch block — A block of conduction of the electrical impulses through either the right or left bundle branch, resulting in a right or left bundle-branch block.

Bundle branches — A part of the electrical conduction system consisting of the right and left bundle branches that conducts the electrical impulses from the bundle of His to the Purkinje network.

Bundle of His — A part of the electrical conduction system that connects the atrioventricular node to the bundle branches.

Bursts — Three or more consecutive premature ectopic beats (atrial,

junctional, or ventricular). Also known as *salvo* or *run*.

Calcium channel blockers — A group of drugs that block entry of calcium ions into cells, especially those of cardiac and vascular smooth muscle. Used to treat hypertension, angina, and as an antiarrhythmic.

Cardiac cells — Cells of the heart consisting of the myocardial cells responsible for contraction of the heart muscle and the pacemaker cells of the electrical conduction system, which spontaneously generate electrical impulses.

Cardiac cycle — Consists of one heartbeat or one PQRST sequence. Represents atrial contraction and relaxation followed by ventricular contraction and relaxation.

Cardiac tamponade — Compression of the heart due to the effusion of fluid into the pericardial cavity (as occurs in pericarditis) or the accumulation of blood in the pericardium (as occurs in heart rupture or penetrating trauma).

Cardiomyopathy — A disease of the heart muscle. Characterized by chamber dilation, wall thickening, decreased contractility, and conduction disturbances. End result is usually severe dysfunction of the heart muscle, resulting in terminal heart failure.

Cardioversion — An electric shock synchronized to fire during the QRS complex; used to terminate rhythms such as atrial fibrillation or flutter, paroxysmal atrial tachycardia, and ventricular tachycardia to normal sinus rhythm; uses lower joules of electricity. Also known as *synchronized shock*.

Cation — An ion with a positive charge.

Chordae tendineae — Thin strands of fibrous connective tissue that extend from the cusps of the atrioventricular valves to the papillary muscles and prevent the AV valves from bulging back into the atria during ventricular contraction.

Chronic obstructive pulmonary disease — A chronic disease of the lungs characterized by episodes of bronchitis, pneumonia, a chronic productive cough, and dyspnea at rest or with exertion. Also known as *COPD*.

Circulatory system — A closed system consisting of two separate circuits: the systemic circuit and the pulmonary circuit. The systemic circuit consists of the left heart and blood vessels, which carry blood from the left heart to the body and back to the right heart. The pulmonary circuit consists of the right heart and blood vessels, which carry blood to the lungs and back to the left heart.

Collateral circulation — Collateral arteries found throughout the myocardium. They are present at birth, but do not become functionally significant until the myocardium experiences an ischemic insult; collaterals contribute significantly to myocardial perfusion, but blood flow is insufficient to meet the total needs of the myocardium.

Compensatory pause — A pause following a premature beat. A compensatory pause is identified on the ECG by measuring from the R wave before the premature beat to the R wave following the premature beat; if that measurement equals two cardiac cycles (the sum of two R-R intervals), the pause is considered compensatory. A compensatory pause cannot be identified if the underlying rhythm is irregular. Also called *complete pause*.

Conductivity — The ability of a cardiac cell to receive an electrical impulse and conduct that impulse to an adjacent cardiac cell.

Congestive heart failure — An overload of fluid in the lungs and/or body caused by inefficient pumping of the ventricles. Also known as *CHF*.

Contractility — The ability of cardiac cells to cause cardiac muscle contraction in response to an electrical stimulus.

Couplet — Two consecutive premature beats. Also known as *pair*.

Cyanosis — A purplish discoloration of the skin caused by the presence of unoxygenated blood.

Defibrillation — An unsynchronized electrical shock used to terminate ventricular fibrillation and pulseless ventricular tachycardia; uses higher joules of electricity. Also known as *unsynchronized shock*.

Deflection — Refers to the waveforms in the ECG tracing (P wave, QRS complex, T wave, and U wave). A deflection may be positive (upright), negative (inverted), biphasic (having both positive and negative components), or equiphasic (equally positive and negative).

Depolarization — Electrical activation of a cardiac cell due to movement of ions across a cell membrane, causing the inside of the cell to become more positive. Depolarization is an electrical event expected to result in muscle contraction, a mechanical event. Depolarization of the atria produces the P wave. Depolarization of the ventricles produces the QRS complex.

Diaphoresis — Profuse sweating.

Diastole — The period of atrial or ventricular relaxation.

Dying heart — See *agonal rhythm*.

Dyspnea — Shortness of breath.

Dysrhythmia — Any rhythm other than a sinus rhythm. Used interchangeably with *arrhythmia*.

Ectopic — A beat or rhythm originating from a source other than the sinoatrial node.

Electrocardiogram (ECG) — A graphic recording of the electrical activity of the heart generated by the depolarization and repolarization of the atria and ventricles.

Electrocardiograph — A machine used to record the electrocardiogram.

Electrolyte — A substance whose molecules dissociate into charged components when placed in water, producing positively and negatively charged ions.

Endocardium — The innermost layer of the heart, composed of thin, smooth connective tissue.

Enhanced automaticity — An abnormal condition of pacemaker cells in which their firing rate is increased beyond the inherent rate.

Escape beats or rhythms — A term used when the sinus node slows down or fails to initiate an impulse and a secondary pacemaker site assumes pacemaker control of the heart. Escape beats may arise from the atrium (atrial escape beat), the atrioventricular junction (junctional escape beat), or the ventricles (ventricular escape beat). Examples of escape rhythms are junctional escape rhythm and ventricular escape rhythm.

Excitability — The ability of a cardiac cell to respond to an electrical stimulus.

Fascicle — A bundle of muscle or nerve fibers. The left main bundle branch divides into an anterior fascicle and a posterior fascicle, which form the two major divisions of the left bundle branch before it divides into the Purkinje fibers.

First-degree atrioventricular (AV) block — An arrhythmia in which there is a delay in the conduction of the electrical impulses through the AV node. Characterized by sinus P waves with one P wave to each QRS complex; a consistent PR interval that is abnormally prolonged (greater than 0.20 second); and a normal QRS duration.

Heart rate — The number of heartbeats or QRS complexes per minute.

His-Purkinje system — The part of the electrical conduction system consisting of the bundle of His, the bundle branches, and the Purkinje fibers.

Hypertrophy — An increase in the thickness of a heart chamber because of a chronic increase in pressure and/or volume within the chamber. Hypertrophy may occur in both the atria and the ventricles.

Idioventricular rhythm — An arrhythmia arising in an ectopic site in the ventricles characterized by a regular rhythm; an absence of P waves; wide QRS complexes; and a rate between 30 and 40 (sometimes less) beats/minute. This is the inherent rhythm of the ventricles. Also known as *IVR*.

Infarction — Death (necrosis) of tissue caused by an interruption of blood supply to the affected tissue.

Inferior vena cava — One of two large veins that empty venous blood into the right atrium.

Inherent firing rate — The normal rate at which electrical impulses are generated in a pacemaker, whether it is the sinoatrial node or an ectopic pacemaker. Also known as the *intrinsic firing rate*.

Interatrial septum — The wall separating the right and left atria.

Internodal atrial conduction tracts — Part of the electrical conduction system. Consists of three pathways of specialized conducting tissue located in the walls of the right atrium. Conducts impulses from the sinoatrial node to the atrioventricular node.

Interpolated PVC — A premature ventricular contraction (PVC) that falls between two QRS complexes without a pause.

Intraventricular septum — The wall separating the right and left ventricles.

Intrinsic beat — Beats produced by the heart's own electrical conduction system. Also known as *native beat*.

Ion — Electrically charged particle.

Ischemia — Reduced blood flow to tissue caused by narrowing or occlusion of the artery supplying blood to it.

Isoelectric line — See *baseline*.

IVR — *abbr* idioventricular rhythm

J point — The point where the QRS complex and ST segment meet.

Junctional rhythm — An arrhythmia arising in the atrioventricular (AV) junction characterized by a regular rhythm; inverted P waves immediately before the QRS, immediately after the QRS, or hidden within the QRS complex, with a short PR interval of 0.10 second or less; a normal-duration QRS complex; and a rate between 40 and 60 beats/minute. Junctional rhythm is the inherent rhythm of the AV node.

Junctional tachycardia — An arrhythmia arising in the atrioventricular junction characterized by a regular rhythm; inverted P waves immediately before the QRS, immediately after the QRS, or hidden within the QRS complex, with a short PR interval of 0.10 second or less; a normal-duration QRS complex; and a rate greater than 100 beats/minute.

mA — *abbr* milliampere

Mediastinum — Located in the middle of the thoracic cavity. Contains the heart, trachea, esophagus, and great vessels (pulmonary arteries and veins, aorta, and the superior and inferior vena cava).

MI — *abbr* myocardial infarction

Milliampere — Unit of measure of electrical current needed to cause depolarization of the myocardium. A term used most often with pacemakers.

Mitral valve — One of two atrioventricular valves. Located between the left atrium and left ventricle. Similar in structure to the tricuspid valve, but has only two cusps.

Monomorphic — Refers to QRS complexes of the same morphology in the same lead.

Morphology — The shape of a waveform.

Multifocal — Indicates an arrhythmia originating in multiple pacemaker sites.

Multifocal premature ventricular contractions — PVCs originating in multiple pacemaker sites in the ventricles having different QRS morphology in the same lead.

Mural thrombi — Clots in the chambers of the atria caused by ineffective atrial contraction (may occur in atrial fibrillation or flutter)

Myocardium — The middle and thickest layer of the heart composed primarily of cardiac muscle cells and responsible for the heart's ability to contract.

Negative deflection — A waveform that is below baseline.

Noncompensatory pause — A pause following a premature beat. A noncompensatory pause is identified on the ECG by measuring from the R wave before the premature beat to the R wave following the premature beat; if that measurement is less than two cardiac cycles (less than the sum of two R-R intervals), the pause is considered noncompensatory. A noncompensatory pause cannot be identified if the underlying rhythm is irregular. Also known as *incomplete pause*.

Nonconducted premature atrial contraction — A premature abnormal P wave not accompanied by a QRS complex, but followed by a pause.

Normal sinus rhythm — The normal rhythm of the heart originating in the sinoatrial node characterized by a regular rhythm; normal P waves, PR interval, and QRS duration; and a rate between 60 and 100 beats/minute.

Overdrive pacing — Pacing the heart at a rate faster than the tachycardia to terminate the tachyarrhythmia.

PAC — *abbr* premature atrial contraction

Pacemaker — A device that delivers an electric current to the heart to stimulate depolarization.

Papillary muscles — Projections of myocardium arising from the walls of the ventricles connected to fibrous cords called chordae tendineae, which are attached to the valve leaflets. During ventricular contraction the papillary muscles contract and pull on the chordae tendineae, thus preventing inversion of the atrioventricular valve leaflets into the atria.

Parasympathetic nervous system — A part of the autonomic nervous system. Stimulation of this system decreases the heart rate, slows conduction through the atrioventricular node, decreases the force of ventricular contraction, and causes a drop in blood pressure.

Paroxysmal — A term used to describe the sudden onset or cessation of an arrhythmia.

Paroxysmal atrial tachycardia — An arrhythmia originating in the atria characterized by abnormal P waves that are usually hidden in the preceding T waves; a normal QRS duration; and a regular rhythm between 140 and 250 beats/minute.

PAT — *abbr* paroxysmal atrial tachycardia

PJC — *abbr* premature junctional contraction

Polymorphic — Refers to QRS complexes of different morphology in the same lead.

Positive deflection — A waveform that is above baseline.

Premature atrial contraction — An early beat originating in the atria. characterized by a premature, abnormal P wave (usually upright); a PR interval that may be normal or abnormal; and a normal-duration QRS complex followed by a pause. Also known as *PAC*.

Premature junctional contraction — An early beat originating in the atrioventricular junction characterized by a premature inverted P wave occurring immediately before the QRS, immediately after the QRS, or hidden within the QRS complex with a short PR interval of 0.10 second or less and a normal-duration QRS complex followed by a pause. Also known as *PJC*.

Premature ventricular contraction — An early beat originating in the ventricles characterized by a premature, wide QRS complex with no associated P wave and an ST segment and T wave that slope opposite the main QRS deflection followed by a pause. Also known as *PVC*.

PR interval — The period of time from the beginning of atrial depolarization (P wave) to the beginning of ventricular depolarization (QRS complex). The normal PR interval duration is 0.12 to 0.20 second.

Prinzmetal's angina — A type of angina occurring when the coronary arteries experience spasms and constrict.

Proarrhythmic — The effect of certain drugs (especially antiarrhythmics) to induce or worsen ventricular arrhythmias.

PR segment — The portion of the ECG between the end of the P wave and the beginning of the QRS complex.

Pulmonic valve — One of two semilunar valves. Located between the right ventricle and the pulmonary artery.

Pulseless electrical activity — A clinical situation in which an organized cardiac rhythm (excluding pulseless ventricular tachycardia) is observed on the ECG, but no pulse is palpated. Treatment protocols are the same as for ventricular standstill.

Purkinje fibers — A network of fibers that carry electrical impulses directly to ventricular muscle cells.

P wave — The waveform representing depolarization of the right and left atria.

Q wave — The negative deflection of the QRS complex that precedes the R wave.

QRS complex — The waveform that represents depolarization of the ventricles; consists of the Q, R, and S waves. Normal duration is 0.10 second or less.

QT interval — The portion of the ECG between the onset of the QRS complex and the end of the T wave, representing ventricular depolarization and repolarization.

Rate suppression — A decrease in the heart rate for several cycles following a pause in the basic rhythm.

Reciprocal change — A change detected by the ECG in an area of the heart opposite the site of a myocardial infarction.

Relative refractory period — The period of time during ventricular repolarization during which the ventricles can be stimulated to depolarize by an electrical impulse stronger than usual. This period begins at the peak of the T wave and ends with the end of the T wave. Also known as the *vulnerable period of ventricular repolarization*.

Reperfusion rhythms — Rhythms that may occur following reperfusion therapy. Examples of reperfusion rhythms include sinus bradycardia, accelerated idioventricular rhythm, premature ventricular contractions, ventricular tachycardia, and ventricular fibrillation.

Reperfusion therapy — Treatment to reopen an occluded coronary artery using a thrombolytic agent or coronary interventions, such as balloon angioplasty, coronary artery stenting, or atherectomy.

Repolarization — An electrical process by which a depolarized cell returns to its resting state (negative charge) due to the movement of ions across a cell membrane. The repolarization process produces the ST segment, the T wave, and the U wave.

Retrograde — Moving backward or in the opposite direction to that which is considered normal.

R-on-T premature ventricular contraction (PVC) — A PVC that falls on the down slope of the preceding T wave. Stimulation of the ventricle at this time may precipitate repetitive ventricular contractions, resulting in ventricular tachycardia or fibrillation.

R-R interval — The period of time from one R wave to the next consecutive R wave.

R wave — The positive wave in the QRS complex.

SA — *abbr* sinoatrial

Second-degree atrioventricular (AV) block Mobitz I — An arrhythmia in which there is progressive delay in the conduction of electrical impulses through the AV node until an impulse is blocked and not conducted to the ventricles. Characterized by regularly occurring P waves; progressive lengthening of the PR interval until a P wave appears without a QRS, but is followed by a pause; normal QRS duration; and an irregular ventricular rhythm. Also known as *Wenckebach*.

Second-degree atrioventricular block Mobitz II — An arrhythmia in which some electrical impulses are conducted to the ventricles, but most are blocked. Characterized by regularly occurring sinus P waves; consistent PR

intervals with two, three, or more P waves before each QRS complex; a ventricular rhythm that may be regular or irregular depending on the number of impulses conducted to the ventricles; and a QRS complex that may be narrow or wide depending on the site of the conduction disturbance.

Sequential ventricular depolarization — One ventricle depolarizes before the other (instead of simultaneously), resulting in a wide QRS complex.

Sick sinus syndrome — A degenerative disease of the sinus node resulting in bradyarrhythmias alternating with tachyarrhythmias. This syndrome is often accompanied by symptoms such as dizziness, fainting, chest pain, dyspnea, and congestive heart failure. Permanent pacemaker implantation is recommended once the patient becomes symptomatic. Also known as *tachy-brady syndrome*.

Sinus arrest — An arrhythmia caused by a failure of the sinoatrial node to initiate an impulse (a disorder of automaticity). The ECG tracing will show a sudden pause in the sinus rhythm in which one or more beats are missing. The underlying rhythm does not resume on time following the pause.

Sinus arrhythmia — An arrhythmia originating in the sinoatrial (SA) node that occurs when the SA node discharges impulses irregularly. Sinus arrhythmia is a normal phenomenon associated with the phases of respiration. This rhythm is characterized by an irregular rhythm normal P waves, PR interval, and QRS duration, and may be associated with a normal or bradycardic rate.

Sinus bradycardia — An arrhythmia originating in the sinus node characterized by a regular rhythm; normal P waves, PR interval, and QRS duration; and a rate between 40 and 60 beats/minute.

Sinus exit block — An arrhythmia caused by a block in the conduction

of the electrical impulse from the sinoatrial node to the atria (a disorder of conduction). The ECG tracing will show a sudden pause in the sinus rhythm in which one or more beats are missing. The underlying rhythm resumes on time following the pause.

Sinus node — The dominant pacemaker of the heart located in the wall of the right atrium close to the inlet of the superior vena cava.

Sinus tachycardia — An arrhythmia originating in the sinus node characterized by a regular rhythm; normal P waves, PR interval, and QRS duration; and a rate between 100 and 160 beats/minute.

ST segment — The flat line between the QRS complex and the T wave that represents early ventricular repolarization. The ST segment is normally at baseline.

Stokes-Adams attacks — Fainting episodes that occur when the heart rate suddenly slows or stops momentarily; common with second-degree atrioventricular (AV) block, Mobitz II, and third-degree AV block.

Superior vena cava — One of two large veins that empty venous blood into the right atrium.

Supernormal period — The last phase of repolarization during which the cardiac cell can be stimulated to depolarize by a weaker than normal electrical stimulus. This period occurs near the end of the T wave just before the cells have completely repolarized.

Supraventricular — A general term used to describe arrhythmias that originate in sites above the bundle branches (i.e., sinus node, atria, and atrioventricular junction).

S wave — The negative deflection of the QRS complex that follows the R wave.

Sympathetic nervous system — A part of the autonomic nervous system.

Stimulation of this system increases heart rate, speeds conduction through the atrioventricular node, increases the force of ventricular contraction, and causes an increase in blood pressure.

Syncope — Fainting, usually resulting from cardiac or neurologic events.

TCP — *abbr* transcutaneous pacing

TdP — *abbr* torsade de pointes

Third-degree atrioventricular (AV) block — An arrhythmia in which there is no conduction of electrical impulses through the AV node. There is independent beating of the atria and ventricles. The atria are paced by the sinoatrial node at a rate of 60 to 100 beats/minute and the ventricles are paced either by the AV junction at a rate of 40 to 60 beats/minute or by the ventricles at a rate of 30 to 40 beats/minute. This rhythm is characterized by sinus P waves that have no consistent relationship to the QRS complexes (variable PR intervals); P waves found hidden in the QRS complexes, ST segments, and T waves; a regular atrial and ventricular rhythm; a narrow QRS complex if the ventricles are paced by the AV junction; and a wide QRS if paced from a ventricular site. Also known as *complete heart block*.

Torsade de pointes — A form of ventricular tachycardia associated with a prolonged QT interval. The name is derived from a French term meaning "twisting of the points," which describes a QRS complex that changes polarity (from negative to positive and positive to negative) as it twists around the isoelectric line. Also known as *TdP*.

Transcutaneous pacing (TCP) — External cardiac pacing. Consists of two large electrode pads commonly placed in an anterior-posterior position on the patient's chest to conduct electrical impulses through the skin to the heart.

Transvenous pacing — Cardiac pacing through a vein. A lead wire is inserted into a large vein and positioned in the right ventricle. Electrical impulses are conducted from an external power source (pacing generator) through the lead wire to the right ventricle.

Tricuspid valve — One of two atrioventricular valves. Located between the right atrium and the right ventricle. Similar in structure to the mitral valve, but has three cusps.

Trigeminy — An arrhythmia in which every third beat is a premature ectopic beat. The premature beats may be atrial, junctional, or ventricular in origin (i.e., atrial trigeminy, junctional trigeminy, ventricular trigeminy).

T wave — A wave that follows the ST segment. Represents ventricular repolarization.

Unifocal PVCs — Premature ventricular contractions (PVCs) originating in the same site in the ventricle having the same QRS morphology in the same lead.

U wave — A wave that sometimes follows the T wave. Represents late ventricular repolarization.

Vagal maneuvers — Methods used to stimulate vagal (parasympathetic) tone in an attempt to slow the heart rate. Methods include coughing, bearing down (Valsalva maneuver), squatting, breath-holding, carotid sinus pressure, stimulation of the gag reflex, and immersion of the face in ice water.

Valsalva maneuver — Forceful act of expiration with mouth and nose closed producing a "bearing down" action. One of several vagal maneuvers.

Vasovagal reaction — An extreme body response that causes marked bradycardia (due to vagal stimulation) and marked hypotension (due to vasodilation). A vasovagal reaction may result in fainting (vasovagal syncope).

Ventricles — The two thick-walled lower chambers of the heart; they receive blood from the atria and pump it into the pulmonary and systemic circulation. The ventricles are separated from the atria by the mitral and tricuspid valves.

Ventricular fibrillation — An arrhythmia arising from a disorganized, chaotic electrical focus in the ventricles in which the ventricles quiver instead of contracting effectively. The ECG tracing shows an irregular, wavy baseline without QRS complexes.

Ventricular standstill — An arrhythmia in which there is an absence of all ventricular activity. The ECG tracing will show either P waves without QRS complexes or a straight line. Also known as *ventricular asystole*.

Ventricular tachycardia — An arrhythmia arising from an ectopic site in the ventricles. On the ECG the rhythm appears as a series of wide QRS complexes with no associated P waves; a regular or slightly irregular rhythm; and a rate of 140 to 250 beats/minute.

Vulnerable period — The period of time during ventricular repolarization in which the ventricles can be stimulated to depolarize by a strong electrical stimulus. This period corresponds to the down slope of the T wave (relative refractory period). Electrical stimuli occurring during the vulnerable period may lead to ventricular tachycardia or ventricular fibrillation.

Wandering atrial pacemaker — An arrhythmia arising from multiple pacemaker sites in the atria. The ECG tracing will show a normal or slow rate; a regular or irregular rhythm; P waves that vary in size, shape, and direction across the rhythm strip; a PR interval that is usually normal, but may be abnormal because of the different sites of impulse formation; and a normal QRS duration.

Index

i refers to an illustration; t refers to a table.

i refers to an illustration; t refers to a table.

1

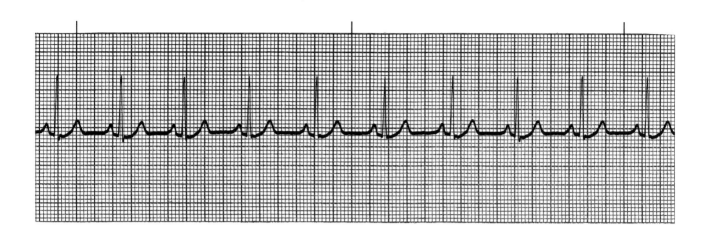

2

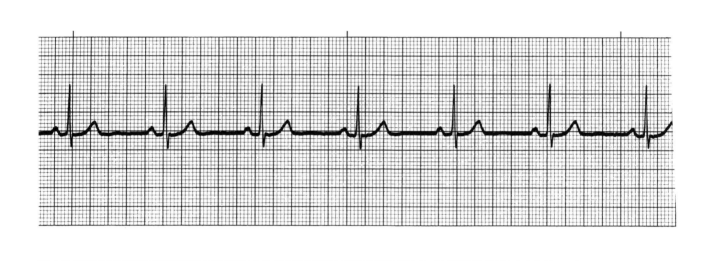

3

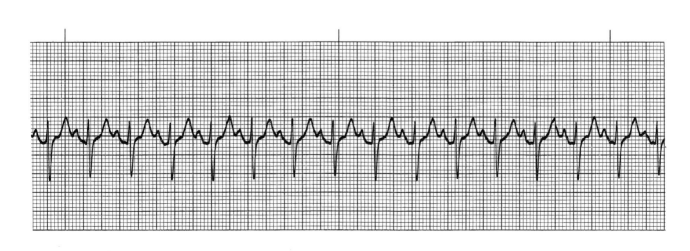

Answer: Normal sinus rhythm

Normal sinus rhythm: Identifying ECG features

Rhythm: Regular

Rate: 60 to 100 beats/minute

P waves: Normal in size, shape, direction; positive in lead II, a positive lead; one P wave precedes each QRS complex

PR interval: Normal (0.12 to 0.20 second)

QRS complex: Normal (0.10 second or less)

2

Answer: Sinus bradycardia

Sinus bradycardia: Identifying ECG features

Rhythm: Regular

Rate: 40 to 60 beats/minute

P waves: Normal in size, shape, direction; positive in lead II, a positive lead; one P wave precedes each QRS complex

PR interval: Normal (0.12 to 0.20 second)

QRS complex: Normal (0.10 second or less)

Answer: Sinus tachycardia

Sinus tachycardia: Identifying ECG features

Rhythm: Regular

Rate: 100 to 160 beats/minute

P waves: Normal in size, shape, direction; positive in lead II, a positive lead; one P wave precedes each QRS complex

PR interval: Normal (0.12 to 0.20 second)

QRS complex: Normal (0.10 second or less)

4

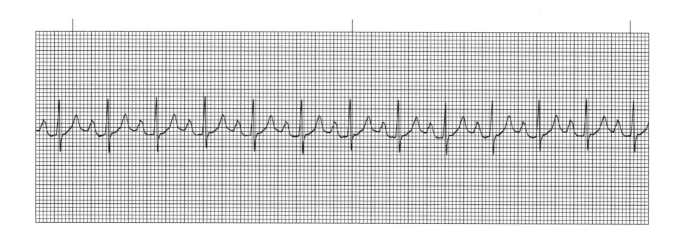

5

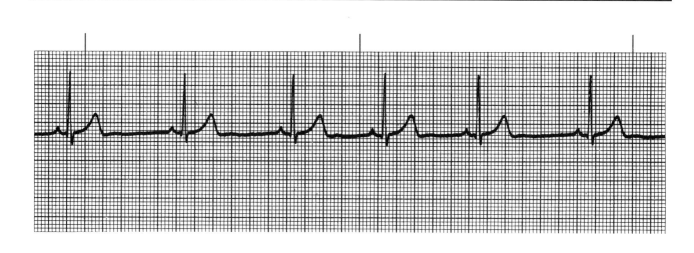

6

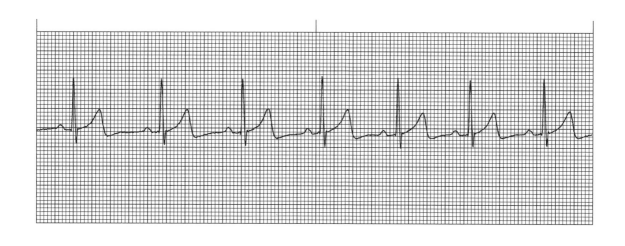

Answer: Sinus tachycardia

Sinus tachycardia: Identifying ECG features

Rhythm: Regular

Rate: 100 to 160 beats/minute

P waves: Normal in size, shape, direction; positive in lead II, a positive lead; one P wave precedes each QRS complex

PR interval: Normal (0.12 to 0.20 second)

QRS complex: Normal (0.10 second)

Answer: Sinus arrhythmia (with bradycardic rate)

Sinus arrhythmia: Identifying ECG features

Rhythm: Irregular

Rate: Normal (60 to 100 beats/minute) or slow (less than 60 beats/minute; often seen with a bradycardic rate)

P waves: Normal in size, shape, direction; positive in lead II, a positive lead; one P wave precedes each QRS complex

PR interval: Normal (0.12 to 0.20 second)

QRS complex: Normal (0.10 second or less)

6

Answer: Sinus arrhythmia

Sinus arrhythmia: Identifying ECG features

Rhythm: Irregular

Rate: Normal (60 to 100 beats/minute) or slow (less than 60 beats/minute; often seen with a bradycardic rate)

P waves: Normal in size, shape, direction; positive in lead II, a positive lead; one P wave precedes each QRS complex

PR interval: Normal (0.12 to 0.20 second)

QRS complex: Normal (0.10 second or less)

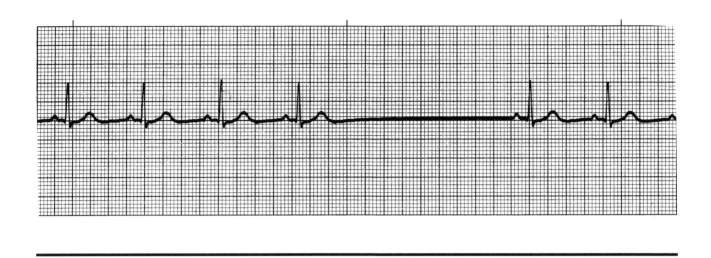

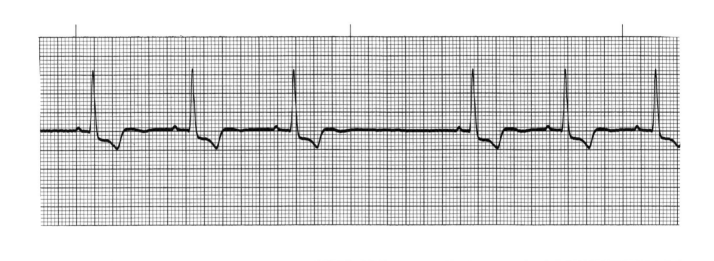

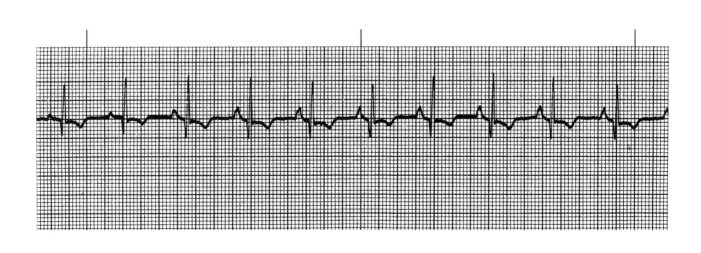

Answer: Normal sinus rhythm with sinus block

Sinus block: Identifying ECG features

Rhythm: Basic rhythm usually regular; sudden pause in basic rhythm (causing irregularity) with one or more missing cardiac cycles; rhythm (R-R regularity) resumes on time following pause; heart rate may slow for several beats following pause (temporary rate suppression), but returns to basic rate after several cycles

Rate: Normal (60 to 100 beats/minute) or slow (less than 60 beats/minute)

P waves: Normal with basic rhythm; absent during pause

PR interval: Normal with basic rhythm; absent during pause

QRS complex: Normal with basic rhythm; absent during pause

Answer: Normal sinus rhythm with sinus arrest

Sinus arrest: Identifying ECG features

Rhythm: Basic rhythm usually regular; sudden pause in basic rhythm (causing irregularity) with one or more missing cardiac cycles; rhythm (R-R regularity) does not resume on time following pause; heart rate may slow for several beats following pause (temporary rate suppression), but returns to basic rate after several cycles

Rate: Normal (60 to 100 beats/minute) or slow (less than 60 beats/minute)

P waves: Normal with basic rhythm; absent during pause

PR interval: Normal with basic rhythm; absent during pause

QRS complex: Normal with basic rhythm; absent during pause

Answer: Wandering atrial pacemaker

Wandering atrial pacemaker: Identifying ECG features

Rhythm: Regular or irregular

Rate: Normal (60 to 100 beats/minute) or slow (less than 60 beats/minute)

P waves: Vary in size, shape, direction across rhythm strip; one P wave precedes each QRS complex

PR interval: Usually normal duration, but may be abnormal depending on changing pacemaker locations

QRS complex: Normal (0.10 second or less)

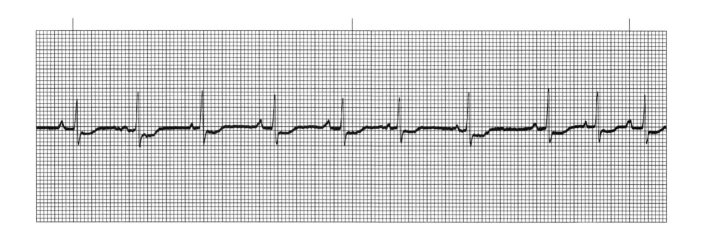

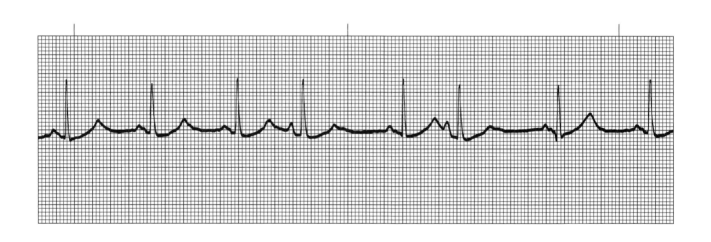

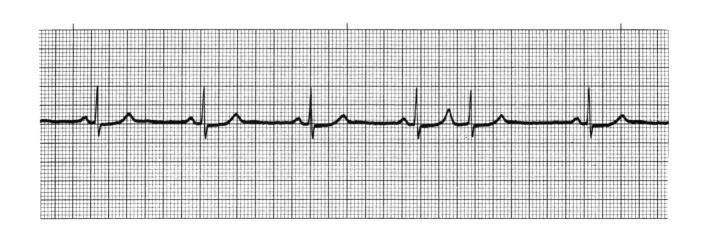

Answer: Wandering atrial pacemaker

Wandering atrial pacemaker: Identifying ECG features

Rhythm: Regular or irregular

Rate: Normal (60 to 100 beats/minute) or slow (less than 60 beats/minute)

P waves: Vary in size, shape, direction across rhythm strip; one P wave precedes each QRS complex

PR interval: Usually normal duration, but may be abnormal depending on changing pacemaker locations

QRS complex: Normal (0.10 second or less)

Answer: Normal sinus rhythm with two PACs

Premature atrial contraction: Identifying ECG features

Rhythm: Underlying rhythm usually regular; irregular with premature beat

Rate: That of underlying rhythm

P waves: P wave associated with PAC is premature, abnormal (commonly appears small, upright, and pointed, but may be inverted or a squiggle); abnormal P wave is often found hidden in preceding T wave, distorting T-wave contour

PR interval: Usually normal but may be abnormal

QRS complex: Premature, normal duration QRS (0.10 second or less); followed by a pause

Answer: Sinus bradycardia with one PAC (abnormal P wave associated with PAC is hidden in preceding T wave, distorting T-wave contour)

Premature atrial contraction: Identifying ECG features

Rhythm: Underlying rhythm usually regular; irregular with premature beat

Rate: That of underlying rhythm

P waves: P wave associated with PAC is premature, abnormal (commonly appears small, upright, and pointed, but may be inverted or a squiggle); abnormal P wave is often found hidden in preceding T wave, distorting T-wave contour

PR interval: Usually normal, but may be abnormal

QRS complex: Premature, normal duration QRS (0.10 second or less); followed by a pause

13

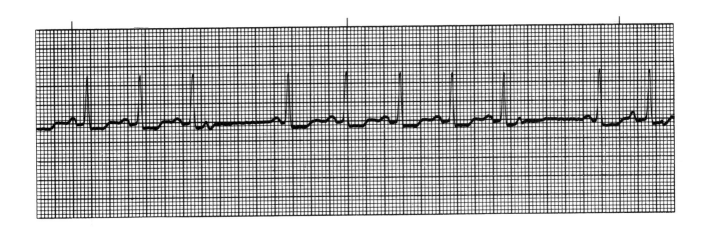

14

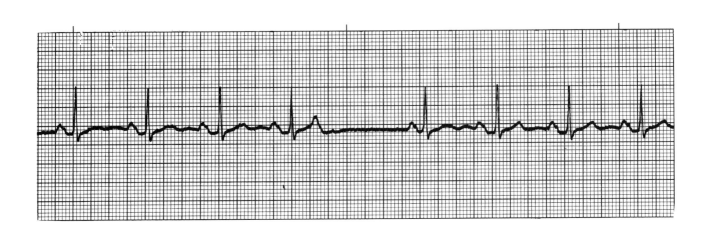

15

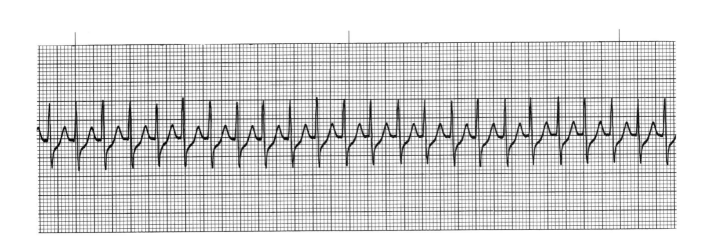

Answer: Sinus tachycardia with two nonconducted PACs

Nonconducted PACs: Identifying ECG features

Rhythm: Underlying rhythm usually regular; irregular with nonconducted PACs

Rate: That of underlying rhythm

P waves: Premature and abnormal; often found hidden in preceding T wave, distorting T-wave contour; a pause follows the nonconducted P wave

PR interval: Absent with nonconducted PAC

QRS complex: Absent with nonconducted PAC

14

Answer: Normal sinus rhythm with one nonconducted PAC (abnormal P wave associated with PAC is hidden in preceding T wave, distorting T-wave contour)

Nonconducted PACs: Identifying ECG features

Rhythm: Underlying rhythm usually regular; irregular with nonconducted PACs

Rate: That of underlying rhythm

P waves: Premature and abnormal; often found hidden in preceding T wave, distorting T-wave contour; a pause follows the nonconducted P wave

PR interval: Absent with nonconducted PAC

QRS complex: Absent with nonconducted PAC

15

Answer: Paroxysmal atrial tachycardia

Paroxysmal atrial tachycardia: Identifying ECG features

Rhythm: Regular

Rate: 140 to 250 beats/minute

P waves: Abnormal (commonly pointed); usually hidden in preceding T wave so that T wave and P wave appear as one wave defection (T-P wave); one P wave to each QRS unless AV block is present

PR interval: Usually not measurable

QRS complex: Normal (0.10 second or less)

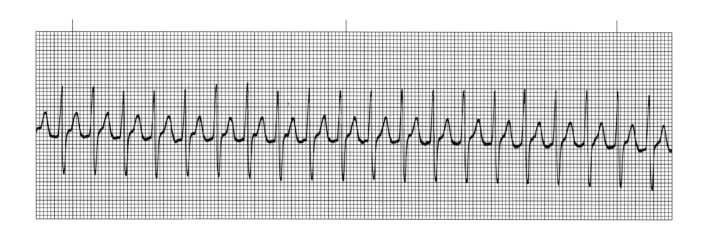

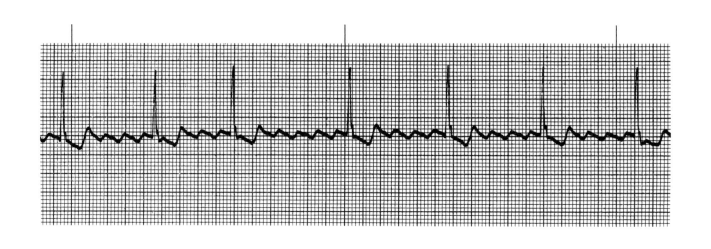

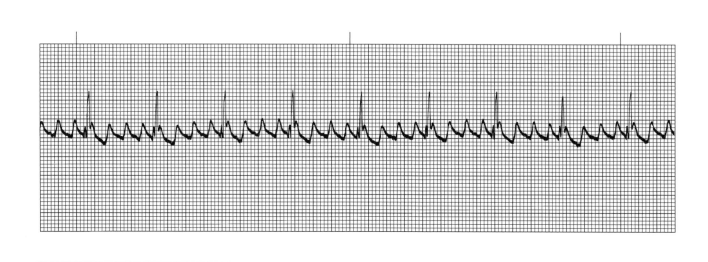

Answer: Paroxysmal atrial tachycardia

Paroxysmal atrial tachycardia: Identifying ECG features

Rhythm: Regular

Rate: 140 to 250 beats/minute

P waves: Abnormal (commonly pointed); usually hidden in preceding T wave so that T wave and P wave appear as one wave defection (T-P wave); one P wave to each QRS unless AV block is present

PR interval: Usually not measurable

QRS complex: Normal (0.10 second or less)

Answer: Atrial flutter with variable AV conduction

Atrial flutter: Identifying ECG features

Rhythm: Regular or irregular (depends on AV conduction ratios)

Rate: Atrial: 250 to 400 beats/minute

   Ventricular: Varies with number of impulses conducted through AV node; will be less than the atrial rate

P waves: Sawtooth wave deflections affecting the entire baseline

PR interval: Not measurable

QRS complex: Normal (0.10 second or less)

Answer: Atrial flutter with 4:1 AV conduction

Atrial flutter: Identifying ECG features

Rhythm: Regular or irregular (depends on AV conduction ratios)

Rate: Atrial: 250 to 400 beats/minute

   Ventricular: Varies with number of impulses conducted through AV node; will be less than the atrial rate

P waves: Sawtooth wave deflections affecting the entire baseline

PR interval: Not measurable

QRS complex: Normal (0.10 second or less)

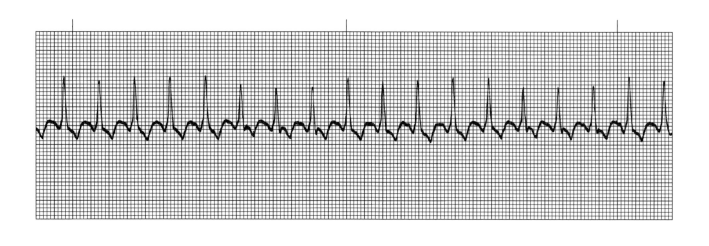

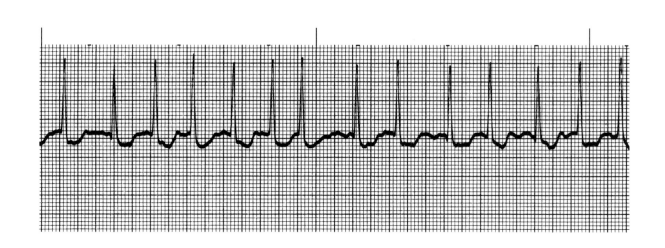

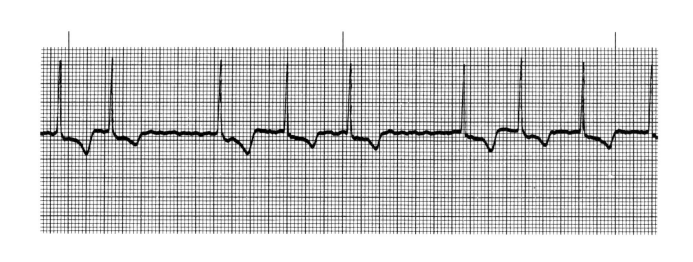

Answer: Atrial flutter with 2:1 AV conduction

Atrial flutter: Identifying ECG features

Rhythm: Regular or irregular (depends on AV conduction ratios)

Rate: Atrial: 250 to 400 beats/minute

  Ventricular: Varies with number of impulses conducted through AV node; will be less than the atrial rate

P waves: Sawtooth wave deflections affecting the entire baseline

PR interval: Not measurable

QRS complex: Normal (0.10 second or less)

Answer: Atrial fibrillation (with uncontrolled ventricular rate)

Atrial fibrillation: Identifying ECG features

Rhythm: Grossly irregular (unless ventricular rate is rapid, in which case the rhythm becomes more regular)

Rate: Atrial: 400 beats/minute or more; not measurable due to wavy baseline

  Ventricular: Varies with number of impulses conducted through AV node to ventricles; ventricular rate is controlled if rate is less than 100 beats/minute; ventricular rate is uncontrolled if rate is greater than 100 beats/minute

P waves: Wavy deflections that affect the entire baseline

PR interval: Not measurable

QRS complex: Normal (0.10 second or less)

Answer: Atrial fibrillation (with controlled ventricular rate)

Atrial fibrillation: Identifying ECG features

Rhythm: Grossly irregular (unless ventricular rate is rapid, in which case the rhythm becomes more regular)

Rate: Atrial: 400 beats/minute or more; not measurable due to wavy baseline

  Ventricular: Varies with number of impulses conducted through AV node to ventricles; ventricular rate is controlled if rate is less than 100 beats/minute; ventricular rate is uncontrolled if rate is greater than 100 beats/minute

P waves: Wavy deflections that affect the entire baseline

PR interval: Not measurable

QRS complex: Normal (0.10 second or less)

22

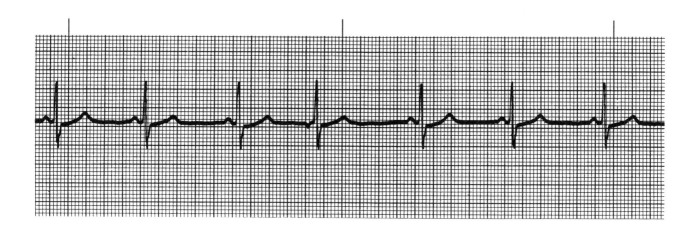

23

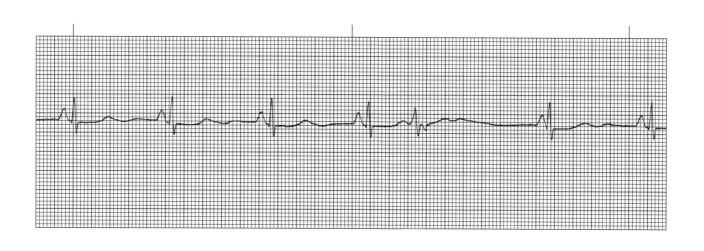

24

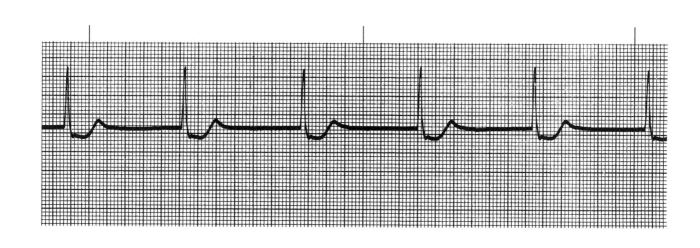

Answer: Normal sinus rhythm with one PJC

Premature junctional contractions: Identifying ECG features

Rhythm: Underlying rhythm usually regular; irregular with PJC

Rate: That of underlying rhythm

P waves: P waves associated with the PJC will be premature, inverted in lead II (a positive lead), and will occur immediately before the QRS, immediately after the QRS, or will be hidden within the QRS complex

PR interval: Short (0.10 second or less)

QRS: Normal (0.10 second or less)

23

Answer: Normal bradycardia with one PJC

Premature junctional contractions: Identifying ECG features

Rhythm: Underlying rhythm usually regular; irregular with PJC

Rate: That of underlying rhythm

P waves: P waves associated with the PJC will be premature, inverted in lead II (a positive lead), and will occur immediately before the QRS, immediately after the QRS, or will be hidden within the QRS complex

PR interval: Short (0.10 second or less)

QRS: Normal (0.10 second or less)

24

Answer: Junctional rhythm

Junctional rhythm: Identifying ECG features

Rhythm: Regular

Rate: 40 to 60 beats/minute

P waves: Inverted in lead II (a positive lead) and will occur immediately before the QRS, immediately after the QRS, or will be hidden within the QRS complex

PR interval: Short (0.10 second or less)

QRS complex: Normal (0.10 second or less)

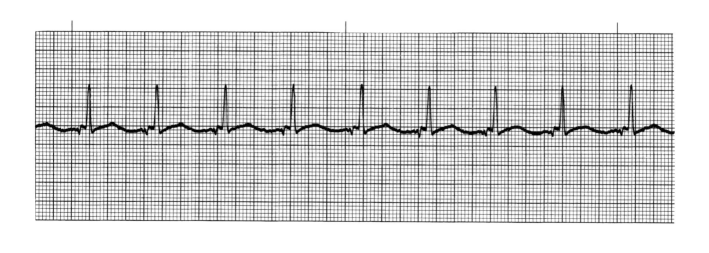

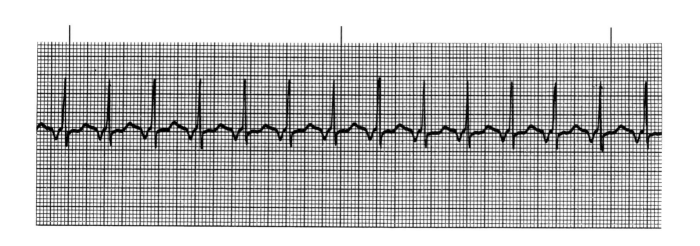

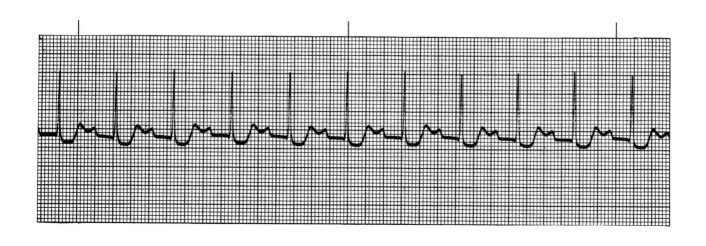

Answer: Accelerated junctional rhythm

Accelerated junctional rhythm: Identifying ECG features

Rhythm: Regular

Rate: 60 to 100 beats/minute

P waves: Inverted in lead II (a positive lead) and will occur immediately before the QRS, immediately after the QRS, or will be hidden within the QRS complex

PR interval: Short (0.10 second or less)

QRS complex: Normal (0.10 second or less)

Answer: Junctional tachycardia

Junctional tachycardia: Identifying ECG features

Rhythm: Regular

Rate: Greater than 100 beats/minute

P waves: Inverted in lead II (a positive lead) and will occur immediately before the QRS, immediately after the QRS, or will be hidden within the QRS complex

PR interval: Short (0.10 second or less)

QRS complex: Normal (0.10 second or less)

Answer: Normal sinus rhythm with first-degree AV block

First-degree AV block: Identifying ECG features

Rhythm: Usually regular

Rate: That of the underlying sinus rhythm

P waves: Sinus; one P wave to each QRS complex

PR interval: Prolonged (greater than 0.20 second); remains consistent

QRS complex: Normal (0.10 second or less)

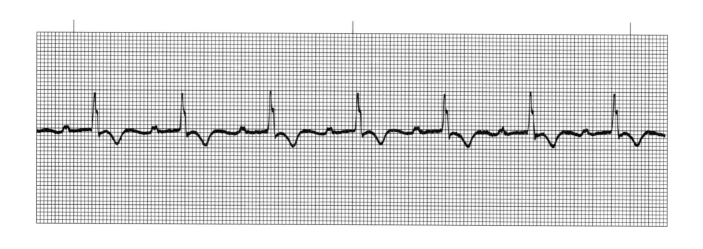

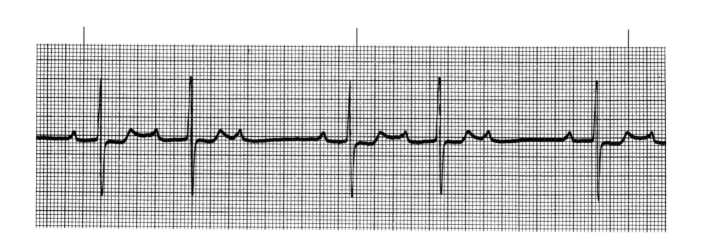

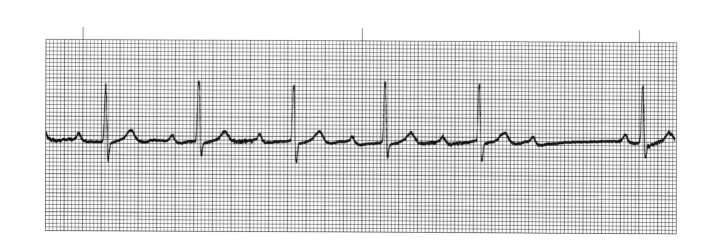

Answer: Normal sinus rhythm with first-degree AV block

First-degree AV block: Identifying ECG features

Rhythm: Usually regular

Rate: That of the underlying sinus rhythm

P waves: Sinus; one P wave to each QRS complex

PR interval: Prolonged (greater than 0.20 second); remains consistent

QRS complex: Normal (0.10 second or less)

Answer: Second-degree AV block, Mobitz I

Mobitz I: Identifying ECG features

Rhythm: Atrial: Regular
　　　　　Ventricular: Irregular

Rate: Atrial: That of underlying rhythm
　　　Ventricular: Depends on number of impulses conducted through AV node; will be less than atrial rate

P waves: Sinus

PR interval: Varies; progressively lengthens until a P wave isn't conducted (P wave appears without QRS complex); a pause follows the dropped QRS complex

QRS complex: Normal (0.10 second or less)

Answer: Second-degree AV block, Mobitz I

Mobitz I: Identifying ECG features

Rhythm: Atrial: Regular
　　　　　Ventricular: Irregular

Rate: Atrial: That of underlying rhythm
　　　Ventricular: Depends on number of impulses conducted through AV node; will be less than atrial rate

P waves: Sinus

PR interval: Varies; progressively lengthens until a P wave isn't conducted (P wave appears without QRS complex); a pause follows the dropped QRS complex

QRS complex: Normal (0.10 second or less)

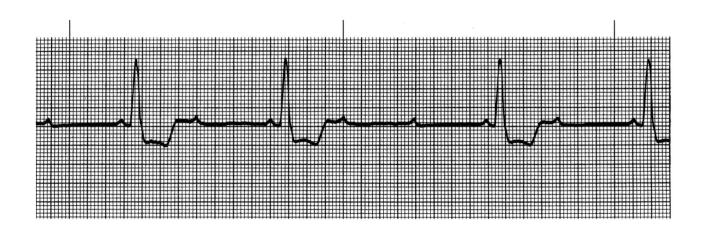

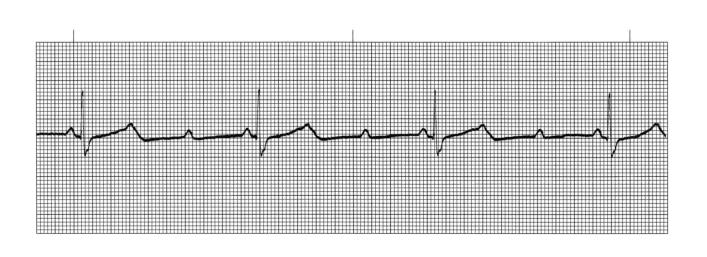

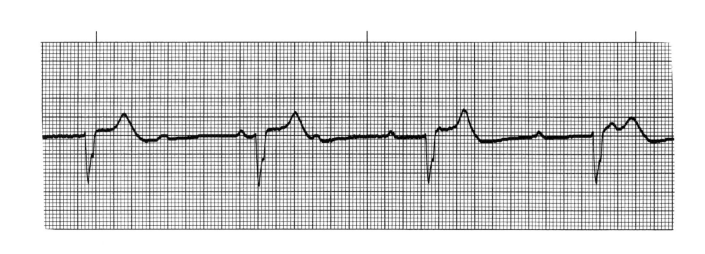

Answer: Second-degree AV block, Mobitz II with 2:1 and 3:1 AV conduction

Mobitz II: Identifying ECG features

Rhythm: Atrial: Regular

  Ventricular: Usually regular; may be irregular if AV conduction ratios vary

Rate: Atrial: That of underlying rhythm

  Ventricular: Depends on number of impulses conducted through AV node; will be less than atrial rate

P waves: Sinus; two or three P waves (sometimes more) before each QRS complex

PR interval: Normal or prolonged; remains consistent

QRS complex: Normal duration if block at bundle of His; wide if block in bundle branches

Answer: Second-degree AV block, Mobitz II with 3:1 AV conduction (one P wave hidden on top of T wave)

Mobitz II: Identifying ECG features

Rhythm: Atrial: Regular

  Ventricular: Usually regular; may be irregular if AV conduction ratios vary

Rate: Atrial: That of underlying rhythm

  Ventricular: Depends on number of impulses conducted through AV node; will be less than atrial rate

P waves: Sinus; two or three P waves (sometimes more) before each QRS complex

PR interval: Normal or prolonged; remains consistent

QRS complex: Normal duration if block at level of bundle of His; wide if block in bundle branches

Answer: Third-degree AV block

Third-degree AV block: Identifying ECG features

Rhythm: Atrial: Regular

  Ventricular: Regular

Rate: Atrial: That of underlying sinus rhythm

  Ventricular: 40 to 60 beats/minute if paced by AV junction; 30 to 40 beats/minute (sometimes less) if paced by the ventricles; rate will be less than the atrial rate

P waves: Sinus P waves with no consistent relationship to the QRS complex; P waves found hidden in QRS complexes, ST segments, and T waves

PR interval: Varies (is not consistent)

QRS complex: Normal duration if block at level of AV node or bundle of His; wide if block in bundle branches

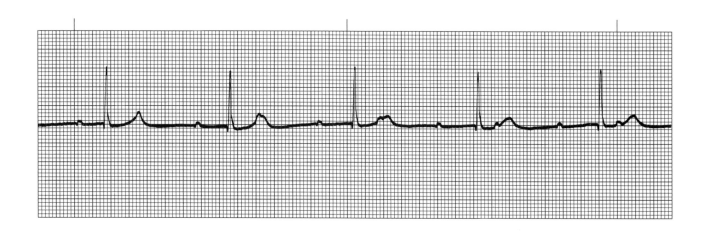

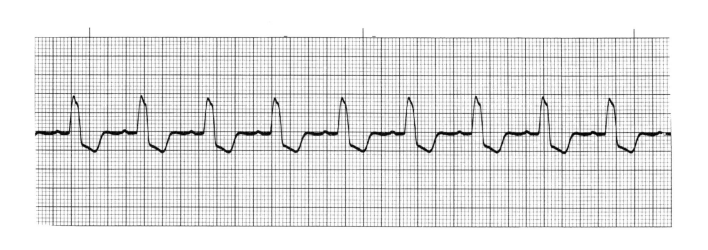

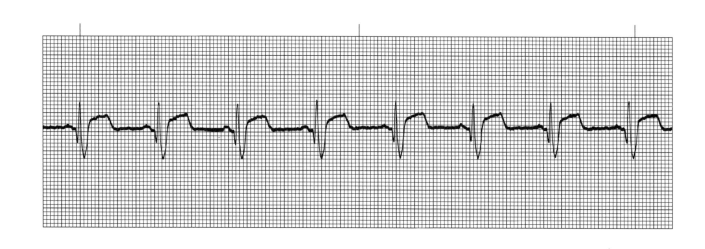

Answer: Third-degree AV block

Third-degree AV block: Identifying ECG features

Rhythm: Atrial: Regular
       Ventricular: Regular

Rate: Atrial: That of underlying sinus rhythm
    Ventricular: 40 to 60 beats/minute if paced by AV junction; 30 to 40 beats/minute (sometimes less) if paced by the ventricles; rate will be less than the atrial rate

P waves: Sinus P waves with no consistent relationship to the QRS complex; P waves found hidden in QRS complexes, ST segments, and T waves

PR interval: Varies (is not consistent)

QRS complex: Normal duration if block at level of AV node or bundle of His; wide if block in bundle branches

Answer: Normal sinus rhythm with bundle-branch block

Bundle-branch block: Identifying ECG features

Rhythm: Usually regular
Rate: That of underlying rhythm (usually sinus)
P waves: Sinus
PR interval: Normal (0.12 to 0.20 second)
QRS complex: Wide (0.12 second or greater)

Answer: Normal sinus rhythm with bundle-branch block

Bundle-branch block: Identifying ECG features

Rhythm: Usually regular
Rate: That of underlying rhythm (usually sinus)
P waves: Sinus
PR interval: Normal (0.12 to 0.20 second)
QRS complex: Wide (0.12 second or greater)

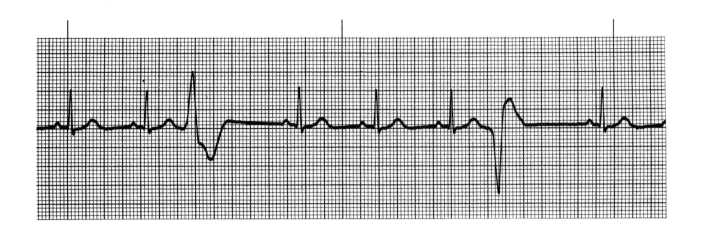

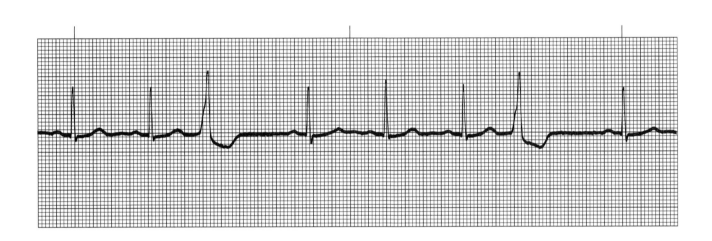

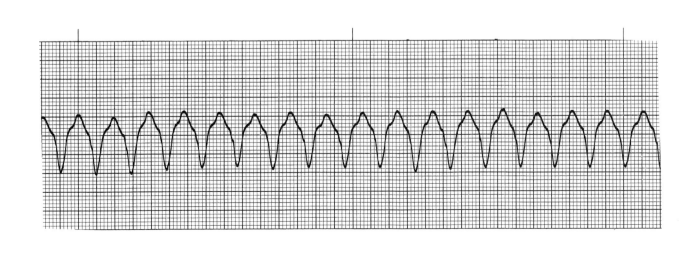

Answer: Normal sinus rhythm with two multifocal PVCs

Premature ventricular contraction: Identifying ECG features

Rhythm: Underlying rhythm usually regular; irregular with PVC

Rate: That of underlying rhythm

P waves: None associated with PVC

PR interval: Not measurable

QRS complex: Premature, wide QRS (0.12 second or greater) with ST segment and T wave sloping opposite the main QRS deflection; followed by a pause

Answer: Normal sinus rhythm with two unifocal PVCs

Premature ventricular contraction: Identifying ECG features

Rhythm: Underlying rhythm usually regular; irregular with PVC

Rate: That of underlying rhythm

P waves: None associated with PVC

PR interval: Not measurable

QRS complex: Premature, wide QRS (0.12 second or greater) with ST segment and T wave sloping opposite the main QRS deflection; followed by a pause

Answer: Ventricular tachycardia

Ventricular tachycardia: Identifying ECG features

Rhythm: Usually regular (may be slightly irregular)

Rate: 140 to 250 beats/minute

P waves: No associated P waves

PR interval: Not measurable

QRS complex: Wide (0.12 second or greater) with ST segments and T waves sloping opposite the main QRS deflection

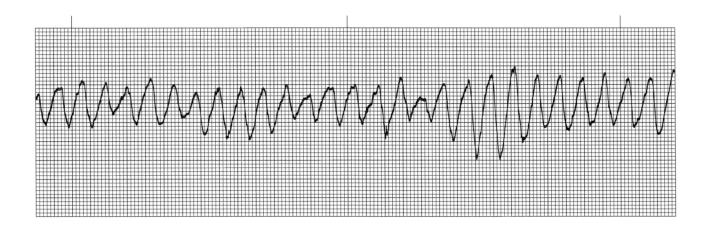

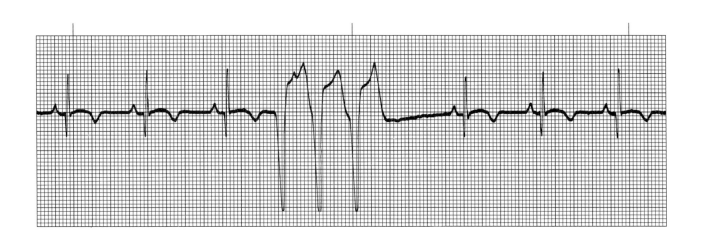

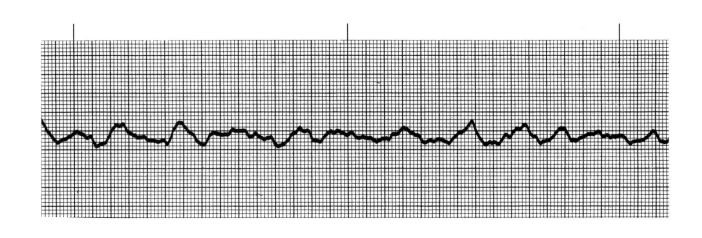

Answer: Ventricular tachycardia (torsade de pointes)

Torsade de pointes: Identifying ECG features

Rhythm: Usually regular (may be slightly irregular)

Rate: 200 beats/minute or more

P waves: None

PR interval: Not measurable

QRS complex: 0.12 second or greater (some much wider than others)

Answer: Normal sinus rhythm with 3-beat run of VT

Ventricular tachycardia: Identifying ECG features

Rhythm: Usually regular (may be slightly irregular)

Rate: 140 to 250 beats/minute

P waves: No associated P waves

PR interval: Not measurable

QRS complex: Wide (0.12 second or greater) with ST segments and T waves sloping opposite the main QRS deflection

Answer: Ventricular fibrillation (coarse deflections present)

Ventricular fibrillation: Identifying ECG features

Rhythm: None (P wave and QRS are absent)

Rate: None (P wave and QRS are absent)

P waves: Wavy, irregular deflection representative of ventricular quivering; deflections may be small (fine ventricular fibrillation) or coarse (coarse ventricular fibrillation)

PR interval: Not measurable

QRS complex: Absent

43

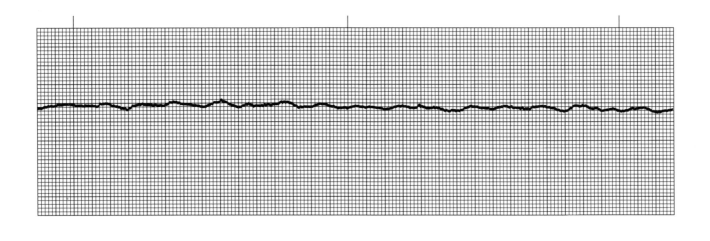

44

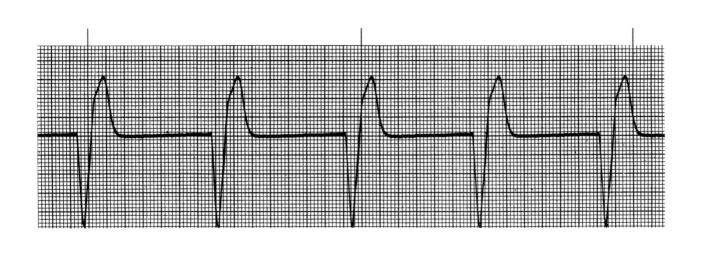

45

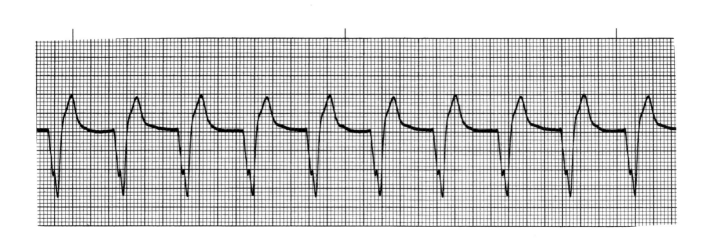

Answer: Ventricular fibrillation (fine deflections present)

Ventricular fibrillation: Identifying ECG features

Rhythm: None (P wave and QRS are absent)

Rate: None (P wave and QRS are absent)

P waves: Wavy, irregular deflections representative of ventricular quivering; deflections may be small (fine ventricular fibrillation) or coarse (coarse ventricular fibrillation)

PR interval: Not measurable

QRS complex: Absent

Answer: Idioventricular rhythm

Idioventricular rhythm: Identifying ECG features

Rhythm: Regular

Rate: 30 to 40 beats/minute (sometimes less)

P waves: Absent

PR interval: Not measurable

QRS complex: Wide (0.12 second or greater)

Answer: Accelerated idioventricular rhythm

Accelerated idioventricular rhythm: Identifying ECG features

Rhythm: Regular

Rate: 50 to 100 beats/minute

P waves: Absent

PR interval: Not measurable

QRS complex: Wide (0.12 second or greater)

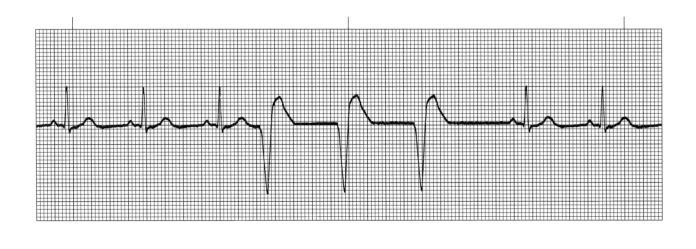

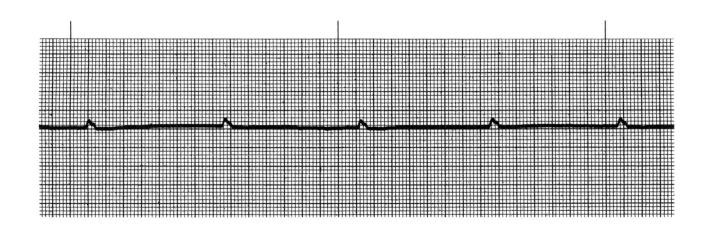

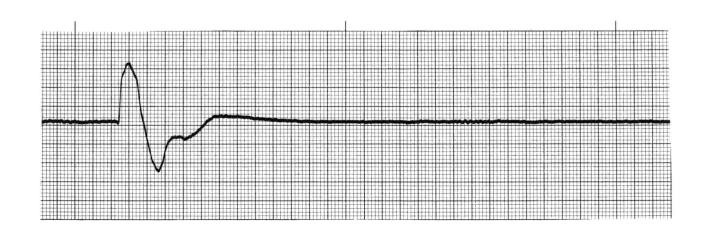

Answer: Normal sinus rhythm with 3-beat run AIVR

Accelerated idioventricular rhythm: Identifying ECG features

Rhythm: Regular
Rate: 50 to 100 beats/minute
P wave: Absent
PR interval: Not measurable
QRS complex: Wide (0.12 second or greater)

Answer: Ventricular standstill (asystole)

Ventricular standstill: Identifying ECG features

Rhythm: Atrial: If waves present, will have atrial rhythm
   Ventricular: None; no QRS complexes are present
Rate: Atrial: If P waves present, will have atrial rate
  Ventricular: None; no QRS complexes are present
P waves: Tracing will show only P waves or a straight line
PR interval: Not measurable
QRS complex: Absent

Answer: Ventricular standstill (asystole)

Ventricular standstill: Identifying ECG features

Rhythm: Atrial: If P waves present, will have atrial rhythm
   Ventricular: None; no QRS complexes are present
Rate: Atrial: If P waves present, will have atrial rate
  Ventricular: None; no QRS complexes are present
P waves: Tracing will show only P waves or a straight line
PR interval: Not measurable
QRS complex: Absent